Maxillary Sinus: A Comprehensive Guide

AF873795

Goran Latif Omer • Stefano Di Girolamo
Editors

Maxillary Sinus: A Comprehensive Guide

Anatomy, Pathologies, and Therapeutic Approaches

Springer

Editors
Goran Latif Omer
Department of Clinical Sciences
College of Medicine
University of Sulaimani
Sulaymaniyah, KRI, Iraq

Stefano Di Girolamo
Department of Otorhinolaryngology
University of Rome Tor Vergata
Roma, Italy

ISBN 978-3-031-83470-7   ISBN 978-3-031-83468-4 (eBook)
https://doi.org/10.1007/978-3-031-83468-4

© The Editor(s) (if applicable) and The Author(s), under exclusive license to Springer Nature Switzerland AG 2025

This work is subject to copyright. All rights are solely and exclusively licensed by the Publisher, whether the whole or part of the material is concerned, specifically the rights of translation, reprinting, reuse of illustrations, recitation, broadcasting, reproduction on microfilms or in any other physical way, and transmission or information storage and retrieval, electronic adaptation, computer software, or by similar or dissimilar methodology now known or hereafter developed.
The use of general descriptive names, registered names, trademarks, service marks, etc. in this publication does not imply, even in the absence of a specific statement, that such names are exempt from the relevant protective laws and regulations and therefore free for general use.
The publisher, the authors and the editors are safe to assume that the advice and information in this book are believed to be true and accurate at the date of publication. Neither the publisher nor the authors or the editors give a warranty, expressed or implied, with respect to the material contained herein or for any errors or omissions that may have been made. The publisher remains neutral with regard to jurisdictional claims in published maps and institutional affiliations.

This Springer imprint is published by the registered company Springer Nature Switzerland AG
The registered company address is: Gewerbestrasse 11, 6330 Cham, Switzerland

If disposing of this product, please recycle the paper.

In dedication to my wife, Dr. Sawen, my children, Yani, Dani, and Bani, and my mother and father who gave me strength and the will to always do better. I want to thank them for their perseverance, support, and love.

This book is also dedicated to Prof. Stefano Di Girolamo, Dr. Nzar Sayda Fatah, Dr. Yousif Chalabi, and Dr. Süreyya Şeneldir for their trust in my abilities and whose words of encouragement and push of tenacity ring in my ears.

Preface

The maxillary sinus, being the largest of the paranasal sinuses, is a complex hollow space with many pathologies affecting it. Since the development of functional endoscopic sinus surgery, surgeons all over the world continue to discover new and efficient techniques to tackle pathologies in this intricate space. However, due to the many different approaches and ideals, the literature lacks a single resource where most ideas are gathered and summarized, so that newer generations have a better and more efficient understanding of what the sinus is, its pathologies, and a comprehensive guide toward managing them.

The authors of this book have tried to dig deep into the sea of knowledge the literature has about the maxillary sinus and to equip this book with the necessary information regarding most, if not all, of the sinus's sophistication, from the basic scientific knowledge regarding its anatomy and physiology to the more compound and innovative procedures that are done for the rarest of pathologies. To all of these authors, I want to present my deepest gratitude and appreciation, together we made this idea a reality. Finally, I would like to thank my students, Sahand and Aland, and my work coordinator, Hawnaz Anwar (RN), for their help, keeping up with my work, and always making sure we are on schedule.

Sulaymaniyah, Iraq　　　　Goran Latif Omer

Competing Interest There was no competing interest to declare.

Ethics Approval This was not a primary study. Also, only one patient is identifiable from the figures, from whom consent was obtained and a participation form was signed.

Contents

Editors and Contributors

About the Editors

Goran Latif Omer is an otorhinolaryngologist and skull base surgeon affiliated with the University of Sulaimani in Iraq and the University of Rome Tor Vergata in Italy. He has received double board certification in his field, as well as additional fellowships in anterior skull base surgery, lateral skull base surgery, and rhinoplasty. Additionally, Dr. Goran holds a PhD degree in Rhinology and Skull Base Surgery.

He has directed many research projects throughout his career, thus making many contributions to the medical community at large, and his inventive spirit has led to the development of new techniques in functional endoscopic sinus surgery, 360° skull base surgery, middle ear surgery, and rhinoplasty, thus participating in the advancement of standards of care in these areas.

Stefano Di Girolamo is a highly accomplished professional in the field of Otorhinolaryngology and Audiology. He graduated with top honors from the University of Rome "La Sapienza" in 1991 and earned his specialization in Otorhinolaryngology from the University of Siena in 1995. Additionally, he obtained a diploma in Audiology from the University of Rome "La Sapienza" in 2001. Prof. Stefano Di Girolamo has held various prestigious academic positions, including Associate Professor and later promoted to Full Professor at the University of Rome "Tor Vergata." He currently serves as the Head of the Otorhinolaryngology Unit at the University Hospital "Policlinico Universitario Tor Vergata." With an exceptional commitment to education, Prof. Stefano Di Girolamo also serves as the Director of the Specialization School in Otorhinolaryngology and Cervico-Facial Surgery at the same university. His expertise and dedication have made a significant impact on the medical community, both through his academic contributions and his leadership in clinical practice.

Contributors

Dastan Tahir Abdallah, BDS, MSc, FKHCMS Royal Hospital, Sulaymaniyah, KRI, Iraq

Aland Salih Abdullah Department of Clinical Sciences, College of Medicine, University of Sulaimani, Sulaymaniyah, KRI, Iraq

Fouad Ahmed Abdullah, MBChB, DLO (ORL) Royal Hospital, Sulaymaniyah, KRI, Iraq

Ahmed Qadir Ahmed, MBChB, MSc Royal Hospital, Sulaymaniyah, KRI, Iraq

Aran Aso Ahmed, MD Royal Hospital, Sulaymaniyah, KRI, Iraq

Aso Khasraw Ahmed, MBChB, CABMS (ORL HNS) Royal Hospital, Sulaymaniyah, KRI, Iraq

Avar Fuad Ahmed, MD Royal Hospital, Sulaymaniyah, KRI, Iraq

Raz Haider Ahmed, MBChB, HD Hiwa Hospital, Sulaymaniyah, KRI, Iraq

Talar Sabir Ahmed, MBChB, HD Royal Hospital, Sulaymaniyah, KRI, Iraq

Arianna Alagna, MD Department of Otorhinolaryngology, University of Rome Tor Vergata, Rome, Italy

Sahand Soran Ali, MD Department of Clinical Sciences, College of Medicine, University of Sulaimani, Sulaymaniyah, KRI, Iraq

Sazgar Shahab Ali, MD Royal Hospital, Sulaymaniyah, KRI, Iraq

Davide Balletta, MD Department of Otorhinolaryngology, University of Rome Tor Vergata, Rome, Italy

Laura Borghesi, MD Department of Otorhinolaryngology, University of Rome Tor Vergata, Rome, Italy

Saman W. Boskani, HDD, AAAM, FIBMS Royal Hospital, Sulaymaniyah, KRI, Iraq

Andrea Bravetti, MD Department of Otorhinolaryngology, University of Rome Tor Vergata, Rome, Italy

Stefano Di Girolamo, MD, ORL HNS, PhD Department of Otorhinolaryngology, University of Rome Tor Vergata, Rome, Italy

Massimi Erika, MD Department of Otorhinolaryngology, University of Rome Tor Vergata, Rome, Italy

Beatrice Francavilla, MD Department of Otorhinolaryngology, University of Rome Tor Vergata, Rome, Italy

Pier Giorgio Giacomini, MD, ORL HNS, PhD Department of Otorhinolaryngology, University of Rome Tor Vergata, Rome, Italy

Andrea Gravina, MD Department of Otorhinolaryngology, University of Rome Tor Vergata, Rome, Italy

Mohammed Gubari, DCM, BPH, HDCM, MSc, PhD Department of Clinical Sciences, College of Medicine, University of Sulaimani, Sulaymaniyah, KRI, Iraq

Amanj Hamaamin Hamaamin, MBChB, CABMS (ORL HNS) Royal Hospital, Sulaymaniyah, KRI, Iraq

Hawre Abdulsattar Hasan, MBChB, FICMS Royal Hospital, Sulaymaniyah, KRI, Iraq

Zhwan Sabah Hassan, MBChB, FICMS Royal Hospital, Sulaymaniyah, KRI, Iraq

Othman Hussein, MBChB, DLO (ORL) Royal Hospital, Sulaymaniyah, KRI, Iraq

Fabbri Ilenia, MD Department of Otorhinolaryngology, University of Rome Tor Vergata, Rome, Italy

Rekawt Hama Rashid Kareem, MBChB, DLO, FEB ORL HNS, PhD Royal Hospital, Sulaymaniyah, KRI, Iraq

Amir Murad Khudadad, MBChB, FICMS Department of Clinical Sciences, College of Medicine, University of Sulaimani, Sulaymaniyah, KRI, Iraq

Silvani Lorenzo, MD Department of Otorhinolaryngology, University of Rome Tor Vergata, Rome, Italy

Maria Grazia Maglie, MD Department of Otorhinolaryngology, University of Rome Tor Vergata, Rome, Italy

Kawa Abdullah Mahmood, MBChB, FIBMS Department of Clinical Sciences, College of Medicine, University of Sulaimani, Sulaymaniyah, KRI, Iraq

Giulia Marzocchella, MD Department of Otorhinolaryngology, University of Rome Tor Vergata, Rome, Italy

Sara Maurantonio, MD Department of Otorhinolaryngology, University of Rome Tor Vergata, Rome, Italy

Riccardo Maurizi, MD Department of Otorhinolaryngology, University of Rome Tor Vergata, Rome, Italy

Ahmed Maki Merza, FIBMS, FIAOMS, FIBCSOMS Royal Hospital, Sulaymaniyah, KRI, Iraq

Attar Abdul Kareem Nadir, MBChB, HD Royal Hospital, Sulaymaniyah, KRI, Iraq

Kosar Hama Noori, MBChB, DLO (ORL) Royal Hospital, Sulaymaniyah, KRI, Iraq

Goran Latif Omer, MBChB, FIBMS, FEB ORL HNS, PhD Department of Clinical Sciences, College of Medicine, University of Sulaimani, Sulaymaniyah, KRI, Iraq

Hemn Hussein Othman, MBChB, FIBMS (ORL HNS) Royal Hospital, Sulaymaniyah, KRI, Iraq

Francesco Maria Passali, MD, ORL HNS, PhD Department of Otorhinolaryngology, University of Rome Tor Vergata, Rome, Italy

Marco Perla, MD Department of Otorhinolaryngology, University of Rome Tor Vergata, Rome, Italy

Vyan Hiwa Mohammed Rouf, MD Royal Hospital, Sulaymaniyah, KRI, Iraq

Karwan Shahin, MBChB, FICMS (ORL HNS) Royal Hospital, Sulaymaniyah, KRI, Iraq

Mahabad Abdalaziz Salih, MBChB, CABMS Department of Clinical Sciences, College of Medicine, University of Sulaimani, Sulaymaniyah, KRI, Iraq

Mithra Sara, MBBS, MS (ORL HNS) KM Cherian Institute of Medical Sciences, Chengannur, Kerala, India

Vivek Sasindran, MBBS, MS, FACS (ORL HNS) KM Cherian Institute of Medical Sciences, Chengannur, Kerala, India

Gianluca Scialla, MD Department of Otorhinolaryngology, University of Rome Tor Vergata, Rome, Italy

Fiorela Shemsiu Department of Otorhinolaryngology, University of Rome Tor Vergata, Rome, Italy

Brian Sommerlad Great Ormond Street Hospital, London, UK

Stefania Tilotta, MD Department of Otorhinolaryngology, University of Rome Tor Vergata, Rome, Italy

Gianluca Velletrani, MD Department of Otorhinolaryngology, University of Rome Tor Vergata, Rome, Italy

Sveva Viola, MD Department of Otorhinolaryngology, University of Rome Tor Vergata, Rome, Italy

Anatomy

1

Goran Latif Omer, Beatrice Francavilla, Massimi Erika, Gianluca Velletrani, Riccardo Maurizi, Hemn Hussein Othman, Sahand Soran Ali, Stefano Di Girolamo, and Aland Salih Abdullah

Anatomy of the Maxillary Sinus

The maxillary sinus, also known as the "antrum of Highmore", is the largest of the paranasal sinuses, typically holding a volume of approximately 15 cm^3 and featuring a pyramidal shape (Hollinshead 1982). Located within the maxillary bone, its inferior boundary is situated just above the maxillary teeth, extending superiorly to below the orbit (Tiwana et al. 2006). The nasal wall of the maxillary sinus contains a large, irregular aperture that communicates with the nasal cavity (Anastasi 2020). The maxillary sinus communicates with the nasal cavity via the maxillary ostium, situated in the semilunar hiatus of the lateral nasal wall, which facilitates the drainage of mucous and lymphatic fluids (Chiapasco 2020; Prasanna and Mamatha 2010).

The average dimensions of the maxillary sinus are approximately 33 mm in height, 23 mm in width, and 34 mm in anterior–posterior length. Notably, the floor of the sinus may contain alveolar processes, and the roof forms part of the orbital floor, traversed by the infraorbital nerves and vessels. The presence of "Underwood's septa," or maxillary sinus septa, may occasionally divide the sinus into asymmetrical compartments. This can be seen in Fig. 1.1 (Nelke et al. 2023).

G. L. Omer (✉) · S. S. Ali · A. S. Abdullah
Department of Clinical Sciences, College of Medicine, University of Sulaimani, Sulaymaniyah, KRI, Iraq

B. Francavilla · M. Erika · G. Velletrani · R. Maurizi · S. Di Girolamo
Department of Otorhinolaryngology, University of Rome Tor Vergata, Rome, Italy

H. H. Othman
Royal Hospital, Sulaymaniyah, KRI, Iraq

© The Author(s), under exclusive license to Springer Nature Switzerland AG 2025
G. L. Omer, S. Di Girolamo (eds.), *Maxillary Sinus: A Comprehensive Guide*, https://doi.org/10.1007/978-3-031-83468-4_1

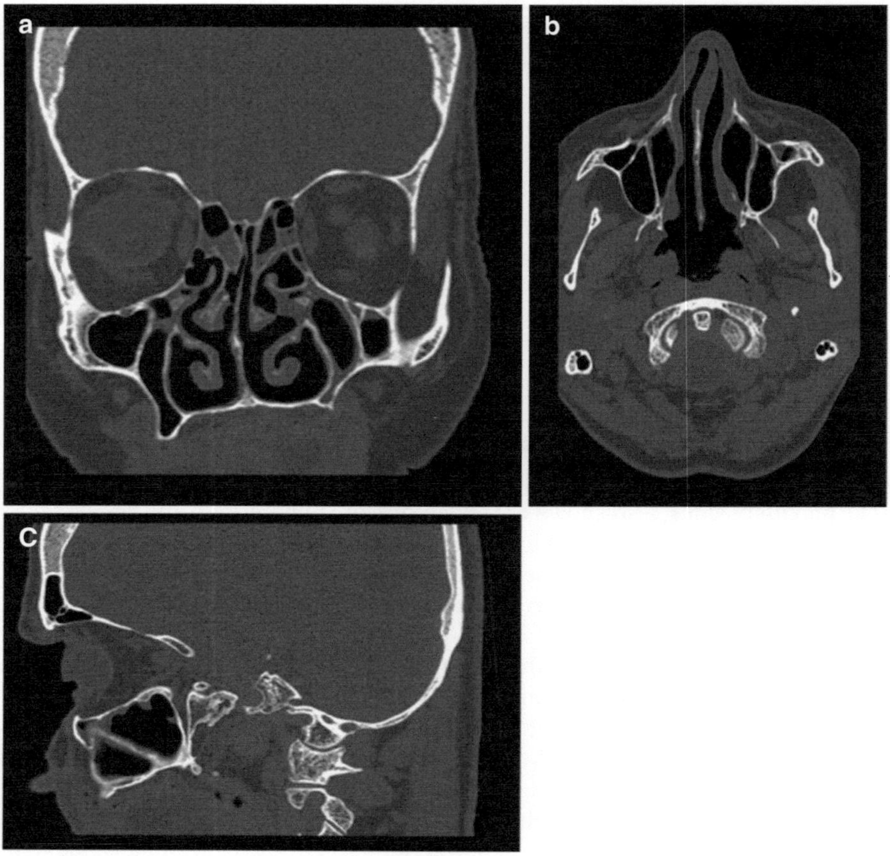

Fig. 1.1 Bilateral, thin, complete, and vertical bony septa traversing the maxillary sinus cavities (**a**) coronal view, (**b**) axial view, (**c**) sagittal view)

Embryology and Normal Development

The maxillary sinus is the first of the paranasal sinuses to develop during foetal life. Its development begins around the tenth week of gestation, and at birth, it initially presents as a rudimentary, aerated, or fluid-filled slit oriented along the anteroposterior axis (Whyte and Boeddinghaus 2019). It is common for the maxillary sinus to exhibit partial or complete opacification in the first few years of life, which is considered a normal developmental phenomenon (Scuderi et al. 1993).

The growth of the maxillary sinus is closely tied to the overall growth of the facial bones, occurring in distinct phases. The first phase of growth happens during the first 3 years of life, during which the sinus extends laterally to reach the infraorbital canal. The second phase, occurring between ages 6 and 12, involves a further lateral extension to the zygomatic recess of the maxilla and inferior extension to the level of the hard palate by around 9 years of age. The third phase of sinus expansion is marked by pneumatization of the maxillary alveolus, which accompanies the eruption of the permanent molar and premolar teeth, resulting in the sinus floor descending 4–5 mm below the floor of the nasal cavity (Whyte and Boeddinghaus 2019).

The level of sinus development is influenced by several factors, including the pressure exerted by the eyeball on the orbital wall, the pull of facial muscles on the lower jaw, and the onset of permanent dentition (Chanavaz 1990; Lang 1989; Lorkiewicz-Muszyńska et al. 2015). The height of the maxillary sinus continues to increase up to the age of 18 years, whereas the width and anteroposterior length typically reach adult proportions by the age of 12 (Whyte and Boeddinghaus 2019). Asymmetry in sinus size and shape is common, with unilateral agenesis occurring in about 7% of adults and bilateral agenesis in 2% (Scuderi et al. 1993). Interestingly, despite the inferior expansion of the maxillary sinus that can occur following the loss of a posterior maxillary tooth, particularly the first molar, studies generally indicate that sinus volume is not significantly affected by dentition status and may even decrease with advancing age (Lovasova et al. 2018). This suggests that other factors, such as age-related changes in bone density and structure, play a more substantial role in the overall volume of the maxillary sinus over time.

Blood Supply

The vascular supply to the maxillary sinus is primarily derived from branches of the maxillary artery, specifically the posterior superior alveolar artery (PSAA), the infraorbital artery, and the posterior lateral nasal artery (Bell et al. 2011; Flanagan 2005; Kqiku et al. 2013), as shown in Fig. 1.2. The posterior superior alveolar artery

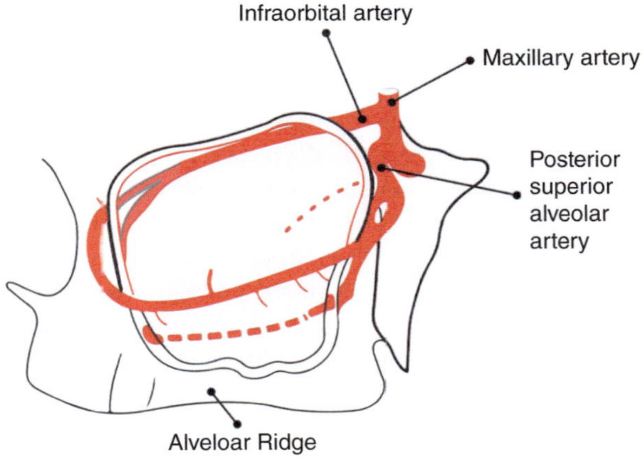

Fig. 1.2 Arterial supply of the maxillary sinus

(PSAA) branches from the maxillary artery as it enters the pterygopalatine fossa. This artery descends along the maxillary tuberosity, providing numerous branches that enter the alveolar process to supply the lining of the antrum, the posterior teeth, and the maxillary gingiva. It can also course along the medial wall of the sinus. Clinically, the PSAA is significant because it can be encountered during procedures involving the maxillary second or third molar, potentially leading to bleeding complications (Flanagan 2005; Iwanaga et al. 2019).

The infraorbital artery is another branch of the maxillary artery. It travels along the infraorbital groove and canal, under the orbit, and exits through the infraorbital foramen on the facial surface of the maxilla. This artery is accompanied by the infraorbital nerve. It supplies the anterior part of the maxillary sinus, as well as the infraorbital region, including the lower eyelid, side of the nose, and upper lip. The infraorbital artery anastomoses with the PSAA along the anterolateral wall of the sinus, forming an extraosseous anastomosis that supplies the mucous membrane of the nasal chambers and sinus lining (Flanagan 2005; Iwanaga et al. 2019).

The posterior lateral nasal artery branches from the sphenopalatine artery, and the latter is a branch of the maxillary artery. The posterior lateral nasal artery enters the nasal cavity through the sphenopalatine foramen and courses along the medial wall of the maxillary sinus. As it continues anteriorly, it branches extensively to supply the posterior and medial walls of the sinus. This artery is crucial in providing blood to the nasal cavity and sinuses, including the conchae and meatuses, and it often anastomoses with branches of the facial and ethmoidal arteries, forming a robust vascular network (Flanagan 2005; Iwanaga et al. 2019).

Innervation

The maxillary sinus receives its sensory innervation primarily from branches of the maxillary nerve (V2), a division of the trigeminal nerve (cranial nerve V). The main contributors to this innervation are the infraorbital nerve and the anterior, middle, and posterior superior alveolar branches (Fig. 1.3) (Bell et al. 2011; Chanavaz 1990; Rodella et al. 2012).

The posterior superior alveolar nerve provides the majority of sensory innervation to the maxillary sinus, particularly to the posterior region, including the mucosa and the roots of the molar and premolar teeth. This nerve typically has two to three branches that spread throughout these areas (Iganawa). The anterior superior alveolar nerve, a branch of the infraorbital nerve, innervates the anterior portion of the maxillary sinus. It runs beneath the Schneiderian membrane and also contributes to the innervation of the superior dental plexus, affecting the upper anterior teeth. The middle superior alveolar nerve provides secondary innervation to the sinus mucosa, primarily in the central region of the sinus.

Additional innervation includes the greater palatine nerve, which supplies the area around the maxillary ostium, and the anterior ethmoidal nerve (a branch of the ophthalmic nerve V1), which innervates the infundibulum. Parasympathetic

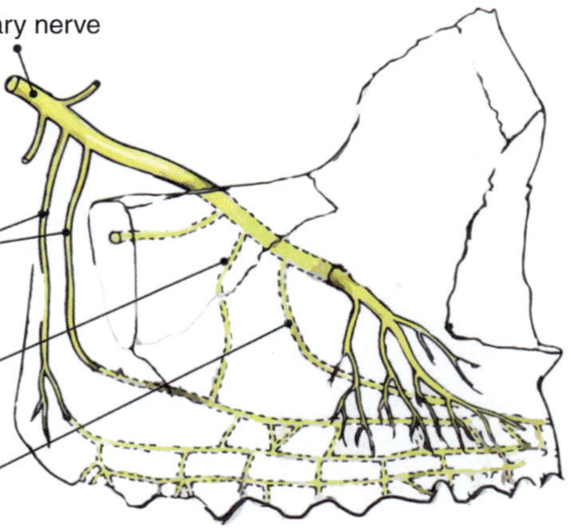

Fig. 1.3 Nervous supply of the maxillary sinus

secretomotor fibres, originating from the nervus intermedius of the facial nerve, synapse in the pterygopalatine ganglion. These fibres then travel alongside the sensory branches of the trigeminal nerve to reach the sinus mucosa, playing a role in glandular secretion within the sinus (Iganawa).

Relation of Maxillary Sinus with Surrounding Structures and Border

Maxillary sinuses are paired air-filled cavities with a pyramidal shape located in the mid-face region, surrounded by the orbit superiorly and medially by the nasal cavity, with its lateral limit being the zygoma. Posterior to the maxillary sinus is the infratemporal fossa, and its posteromedial limit is the pterygopalatine fossa (Whyte and Boeddinghaus 2019).

It is essential to know the areas and structures that bind the maxillary sinus due to the critical structures that are present in these areas and the multiple surgical approaches (open and endoscopic) that use the maxillary sinus and its surrounding areas and structures as a corridor to treat various pathologies of the nose, sinus, skull base, and orbit. The maxillary sinus is closely related to multiple vital structures: the pterygopalatine fossa, the orbit, the lateral wall of the nose, and the lacrimal apparatus.

Pterygopalatine Fossa

It is a narrow space (Fig. 1.4a) with an inverted pyramidal shape between the posterior surface of the maxilla, the pterygoid plates of the sphenoid bone, and the

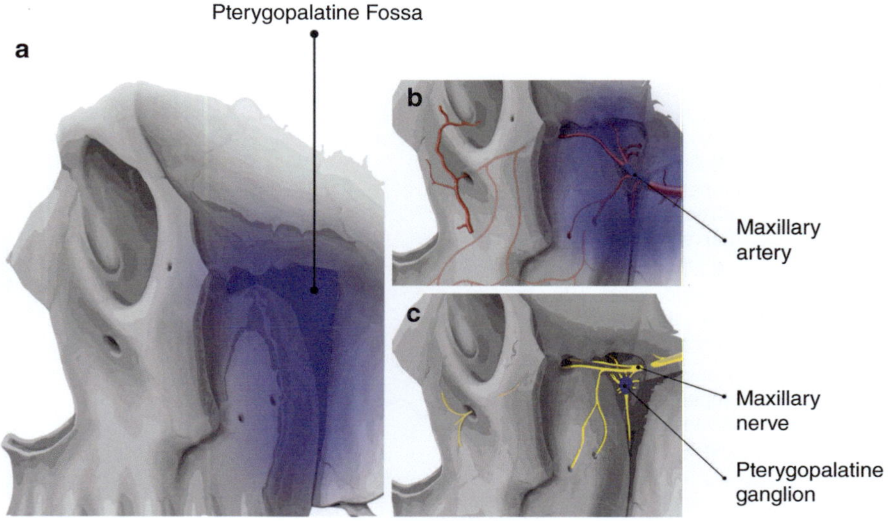

Fig. 1.4 The Pterygopalatine fossa (**a**) with its arterial supply (**b**) and nerve supply (**c**)

palatine bone. According to a radiological study using HRCT done by H.S. Kim et al., it was found that on axial view, PPF, in its most inferior part, has a slightly oval shape rostrally that is 10 mm. Its width is about 10 mm, and it has a height of 4 mm. In the coronal plane, it has a quadrangular shape (Kim et al. 1996).

The pterygopalatine fossa's clinical relevance lies in the neural and vascular structures that are present in the fossa, including the terminal part of the maxillary artery (Fig. 1.4b), the maxillary division of the trigeminal nerve (V2), and the pterygopalatine ganglion (Fig. 1.4c), along with their locations and close relationships with the nasal cavity, orbit, middle cranial fossa, oral cavity, and infratemporal fossa. This close relationship makes it a crossroads for the transmission of neoplastic and inflammatory conditions to and from these surrounding structures. Generally, the vascular contents lie anteriorly and the neural contents posteriorly; also, the neural structures in the PPF play a crucial role in the pathophysiology of cranial nerve neuralgias and pain conditions (Fortes et al. 2008; Piagkou et al. 2011).

Boundaries of the PPF

Anteriorly is the posterior surface of maxillary bone; medially is the vertical plate of palatine bone; and posteriorly is the sphenoid bone at the origin of pterygoid plates. The medial and lateral pterygoid plates fuse with the pyramidal process of the palatine bone and form the floor and posteroinferior border of the PPF (Daniels et al. 1998).

PPF Communications

In its posterior part, PPF communicates with three openings, from lateral to medial; they are the foramen rotundum, the pterygoid canal, and the palatovaginal canal.

- *Foramen rotundum:* It connects the middle cranial fossa to the posterior part of the PPF and transmits the maxillary division of the trigeminal nerve (V2) and emissary veins. It lies superolateral to the pterygoid canal, is closely related to the lateral wall of the sphenoid sinus, and could, hence, be affected by its pathology.
- *The pterygoid canal:* It connects the foramen lacerum to the PPF between the sphenoid sinus and pterygoid process and transmits the Vidian nerve, which is formed by the connection of the deep and greater petrosal nerves and carries parasympathetic nerve supply to the pterygopalatine ganglion, and the Vidian artery, which in 30% of the cases is a branch of the internal carotid artery. The relation of the Vidian canal to the sphenoid sinus floor changes according to the sinus pneumatization, and the anterior genu of the internal carotid artery is superior and medial to the pterygoid canal.
- *Palatovaginal canal:* It connects the nasopharynx to the PPF and is between the vaginal process of the pterygoid bone and the sphenoid process of the palatine bone. It contains small arteries and nerves that supply the nasopharynx (Daniels et al. 1998; Kim et al. 1996; Vescan et al. 2007).

Other Communications from the PPF (von Arx 2017; Scanavine et al. 2009; Turvey and Golden 2012)

1. *Pterygopalatine canal*: this is the lowermost communication of PPF to the oral cavity, which is divided into the greater and lesser palatine canals shortly after entering the hard palate. The greater palatine canal is located at the junction of the horizontal and vertical parts of the palatine bone at the level of the second to third molar tooth. It transmits the greater palatine artery and nerve. The lesser palatine canal, which lies in the pyramidal process of the palatine bone, transmits the lesser palatine artery and nerve.
2. *The sphenopalatine foramen*: lies in the medial wall of the PPF between the orbital and sphenoidal processes of the Palatine bone united with the floor of the sphenoid and communicates the PPF to the nasal cavity mainly through one foramen, but multiple foramina are also reported. Its location in the nasal cavity is either in the superior or middle meatus, and the direction of the bony crest of the middle turbinate helps localise it. The foramen transmits the sphenopalatine artery, vein, and nasal branches of V2, and the sphenopalatine artery divides into the lateral nasal artery and posterior septal artery.

3. *Inferior Orbital Fissure (IOF)*: It connects the PPF to the floor of the orbit and is formed by the zygomatic bone laterally, the greater wing of the sphenoid posterolaterally, the palatine bone and body of the sphenoid medially, and the maxillary bone anteriorly, form its anterior part a small canal running through the orbital floor to exit on the facial surface of the maxilla it transmits:
   (a) *The infraorbital nerve*, which is a terminal branch of the V2, gives off small dental branches (anterior, superior, and middle alveolar nerves) before exiting facially on the anterior surface of the maxilla.
   (b) *The infraorbital artery and ophthalmic vein*, which drain into the pterygoid plexus.
4. *Pterygomaxillary fissure*: This connects the PPF fossa laterally to the infratemporal fossa and transmits the maxillary artery to become the third part of the artery in the PPF.

PPF Contents

Maxillary Division of Trigeminal Nerve V2

It is a purely sensory branch which supplies sensation to the structure of the midface and perimaxilla (side of the nose, lower eyelid, upper lip, maxillary sinus, soft palate, maxillary teeth, the roof of the mouth and palatine tonsils). It runs beneath the dura below the level where the medial and lateral walls of cavernous sinus join at the lower level of V1, passes through the foramen rotundum to enter the PPF and gives the following branches in it:

1. *Ganglionic branches*: which carry post-ganglionic parasympathetic branches to the pterygopalatine ganglion (PPG) and pass to join the zygomatic branch of V2 and supply the lacrimal glands through its connection to the lacrimal nerve.
2. *Zygomatic nerve*: This enters the orbit through the inferior orbital fissure, passes through the lateral orbital wall and divides into zygomaticotemporal and zygomatico-facial branches. The zygomaticotemporal branch passes from the inferolateral angle of orbit into a bony canal in the zygomatic bone to enter the temporal fossa and supply the skin above the zygomatic arch. The zygomatico-facial branch goes out to the face through a foramen in the zygomatic bone to supply the skin of the cheek.
3. *Posterosuperior Alveolar nerve*: This comes off the V2 before it enters the infraorbital canal as 1–3 branches. It passes on the posterior wall of the maxillary bone before it enters the maxillary sinus, and with the middle alveolar nerve from the dental plexus, it supplies part of the gum and cheek.
4. *Infraorbital nerve (ION)*: After passing through the upper part of PPF, it enters the infraorbital groove and canal, runs downward and medially through the roof of the maxilla, and comes out to the face through the infraorbital foramen. In the infraorbital canal, it branches into:

(a) *The middle superior alveolar nerve* emerges from ION in the infraorbital groove. It goes into the lateral wall of the maxillary sinus, which is connected to the superior dental plexus and posterior alveolar nerve.
(b) *The anterior superior alveolar nerve*, which emerges from the ION just before its exit to the face, passes through the anterior wall of the maxillary sinus, forms the superior dental plexus with the middle superior alveolar nerve to supply the canine and incisors and supplies the anterior area of the lateral wall and floor of the nasal cavity.

On the face, the ION, which is the terminal branch of V2, emerges through the infraorbital foramen 1 cm below the orbital rim and is divided into:

(a) *Inferior palpebral branches* ascend to the orbicularis oculi muscle to supply the skin and conjunctiva of the lower eyelid.
(b) *Nasal branches:* External and internal, which supply the lateral wall of the nose.
(c) *Superior labial branches*: multiple branches descend to the levator labii superior muscle to supply the skin of the anterior part of the cheek, lip, and oral mucosa.

5. *Palatine Nerve*: also conveys taste impulses from the palate via the Vidian nerve and PPG to the nervus intermedius. It is divided into:
   (a) *Greater Palatine Nerve*: descends through the greater palatine foramen located at the inferior tip of the PPF and runs forward in a groove on the inferior surface of the hard palate; also, it anastomoses with the Nasopalatine nerve, which is a branch of the sphenopalatine nerve.
   (b) *Lesser palatine nerve*: passes through the lesser palatine foramen and supplies the soft palate (palatine tonsils and uvula), anastomoses with branches of the glossopharyngeal nerve to form a plexus around the palatine tonsils.
6. *Nasal branches*: They enter the nose through the sphenopalatine foramen and include the following:
   (a) *The lateral posterosuperior nasal nerve*, usually six in number, innervates the mucosa of the posterior part of the superior and middle turbinate.
   (b) *Medial posterosuperior nasal nerves*: 2–3 in number, cross the nasal root to supply the mucosa of the posterior part of the roof and the nasal septum.
   (c) *Nasopalatine nerve*: reaches the septum through the sphenopalatine foramen below the sphenoid sinus opening, runs between the periosteum and mucosa of the septum, exits the nasal cavity through the incisive foramen, communicates with the greater palatine nerve, supplies the nasal septum and mucosa of the anterior part of the hard palate and runs along the nasal floor.
7. *Pharyngeal nerve*: emerges from the posterior part of PPG and enters the palate vaginal canal with the pharyngeal branch of the maxillary artery to supply the nasopharynx and auditory tube (Joo et al. 2013; Ziyal et al. 2004).

Pterygopalatine Ganglion (PPG)

It is a mass of nervous tissue located in the PPF in front of the Vidian canal opening, with the foramen rotundum superior and lateral to it. It acts as a transfer station between the superior salivary nucleus and the mucous glands of the eye, nose, and palate.

Connections of the Pterygopalatine Fossa

Greater Superficial Petrosal Nerve (GSPN)

GSPN carries preganglionic parasympathetic fibres from the superior salivary nucleus of the pons carried through the facial nerve and pass through the geniculate ganglion without synapsing to join the deep petrosal nerve to form the Vidian nerve. Its post-ganglionic fibres pass to the zygomatic branch of V2 and reach the lacrimal gland through the lacrimal branch of the ophthalmic nerve. Sympathetic neurons of the intermediate horns of the spinal cord give rise to preganglionic fibres, which pass to the superior cervical ganglion, and its post-ganglionic fibres pass with the internal carotid artery and give rise to the deep petrosal nerve. The deep petrosal nerve passes through the PPG ganglion without synapsing after joining the GSPN to form the Vidian nerve in the foramen lacerum. The maxillary division of the trigeminal nerve is purely sensory, comes out from the foramen rotundum and gives branches to PPG. The cell bodies in the ganglion are parasympathetic only, and only the GSPN synapse in the ganglion, but there is a mixture of sympathetic, parasympathetic, and sensory fibres in all post-ganglionic fibres that come out from the PPG. Several small branches enter the orbital periosteum and supply the muscle and periosteum of the orbit to the posterior part of the ethmoid and sphenoid sinuses. The greater palatine and lesser palatine nerves come out from the inferior part of PPG. The greater palatine nerve supplies the oral surface of the hard palate and gives posterior branches to the nose to supply the nasal floor and inferior turbinate; on the other hand, the lesser palatine nerve carries sensation and taste from GSPN to the soft palate uvula and tonsils. There are several posterosuperior nasal branches which pass through the sphenopalatine foramen and supply the roof and lateral wall of the nose; the largest one is the Nasopalatine branch, which supplies the Vomer, passes through the hard palate to supply the incisors and joins the greater palatine nerve on the anterior part of the hard palate (Khonsary et al. 2013; Sinnatamby 2013; Piagkou et al. 2011).

Maxillary Artery

The last part of MA enters the PPF after passing through the pterygomaxillary fissure in the superior medial and anterior direction. After giving off the buccal branch, which is sometimes absent and not consistent, it gives several branches in the PPF, which have different branching patterns. These branches are at the level of the upper third of the posterior and posterolateral wall of the maxillary sinus, which is mentioned below (Allen et al. 1973; Choi and Park 2003; Tanoue et al. 2013):

1. Posterosuperior alveolar artery (PSAA) is the first branch of the third segment. It originates from the lateral side of MA, branches on the posterior wall of the maxilla and enters the posterosuperior alveolar foramen with the Posterosuperior

alveolar nerve. It gives off branches to the buccal mucosa and buccinator muscle and supplies the posterior and lateral walls of the maxillary sinus, maxillary molar and premolar teeth. Finally, it can anastomose with the descending palatine artery.

2. The inferior orbital artery branches from the last segment of MA on its anterior side, either from a common branch with PSAA or separately. It passes on the posterior surface of the maxillary sinus to enter the inferior orbital fissure, which is anterosuperior to the PPF and then enters the infraorbital groove and canal to exit the orbit from the orbital foramen with the infraorbital nerve. It gives branches to the orbital muscles and lacrimal sac, and after its exit from the foramen, it supplies the lateral wall of the nose, upper lip, and anterior maxilla.
3. The pharyngeal artery, which is a small branch of MA, comes out from its posterior surface and courses through the palatovaginal canal to supply the upper part of the eustachian tube and nasopharynx.
4. Descending palatine artery: which branches from the inferior surface of the MA 24.8 ± 2.8 mm from the most inferior border of the pterygomaxillary joint and is divided into the greater palatine artery (GPA) and lesser palatine artery (LPA), which passes through their respective foramen with similar named nerves and supply the hard palate, soft palate, and palatine tonsils. The GPA anastomoses with branches of the sphenopalatine artery after passing through the incisive canal to the nasal cavity.
5. Vidian artery: which branches from the MA posteriorly to the Vidian canal and supplies the nasopharynx, pharyngeal recess, and part of the tympanic cavity; it may join the ascending pharyngeal artery, accessory meningeal, and branches of the petrous carotid artery (CA).
6. Artery of the foramen rotundum: courses along the maxillary nerve to the foramen rotundum posterosuperiorly after branching from the MA, and it may anastomose with branches of the cavernous CA.
7. The sphenopalatine artery, which is the terminal branch of the maxillary artery, enters the nasal cavity through the Sphenopalatine foramen at the level of the superior meatus, either in single or multiple foramina. It is divided into the lateral nasal artery, which supplies the lateral wall of the nose, and the posterior septal branch, which gives multiple branches to the septum. The sphenopalatine artery branches anastomose with the anterior ethmoid, superior labial, and greater palatine artery. Morton and Khan classified SPA and DPA morphologically as they branch from the MA into Y, intermediate, and M types.

Infratemporal Fossa (ITF)

It is a space in the lateral skull base and includes the area between the posterior border of the maxilla, the greater wing of the sphenoid, and the ascending ramus of the mandible. Its medial border is the lateral pterygoid plate with tensor veli palatini posterior to it and superiorly, the pharyngeal constrictor, anterior to the lateral pterygoid plate is pterygomaxillary fissure where ITF communicates with PPF, its anterior border is the posterior wall of maxilla laterally bounded by ramus of mandible and posteriorly is styloid process and tympanic part of temporal bone. Its roof is formed by the greater wing of the sphenoid superomedially, with F. ovale and F. spinosum connecting it to the middle cranial fossa. Its superolateral part has no roof and continues with infratemporal fossa. It has no definite floor and continues with the upper part of the neck and parapharyngeal space. Due to its proximity to various nearby structures and regions like the orbit-nasopharynx, maxilla, and middle cranial fossa, ITF is a potential area for tumour invasion in the surrounding area. Also, due to its content, which includes the mandibular branch of the trigeminal nerve, part of the maxillary artery, pterygoid muscles and pterygoid venous plexus, it has the potential for various nerve entrapments and neuropathic conditions by nerve compression from the muscles and arteries present in the fossa. Additionally, the management of haemorrhage from the maxillary artery during various head, neck, and neurosurgical procedures may mandate access to the fossa (von Arx 2017; Chaurasia 2013; Gerges et al. 2020; Sinnatamby 2013).

Contents of the Infratemporal Fossa

(Allen et al. 1973; von Arx 2017; Khonsary et al. 2013; Sinnatamby 2013; Tanoue et al. 2013; Ziyal et al. 2004)

1. Maxillary artery: The maxillary and superficial temporal arteries are the terminal branches of the external carotid artery (ECA) which arise from the ECA below the superior border of the external auditory meatus at the level of mandibular neck and pass between the ECA and the sphenomandibular ligament with internal maxillary vein to the infratemporal fossa, either deep or superficial to the bellies of lateral pterygoid muscle and ends in the pterygopalatine fossa after giving off several branches with supply the deep components of the face, maxilla, mandible, nose, and dura.

   The maxillary artery is divided into three parts, with two of them having a course in the ITF:

   (a) ***Mandibular part***: After giving off from its origin, it immediately gives off two small branches: anterior tympanic and deep auricular arteries, which supply the external auditory canal and tympanic membrane. It passes deep to the auriculotemporal nerve and then goes horizontally. Apart from these two arteries, it gives off three other branches:

   - *Middle meningeal artery:* which branches off from the maxillary artery in an ascending direction at 114 mm from the origin of the maxillary artery. It is the largest and most constant branch of the maxillary artery with a diameter of 0.9–1.5 mm. It also passes through the foramen spinosum to supply the Dura mater. It is divided into four branches: anterior division, posterior division, petrosal branch, and petrosquamous branch. Its anterior division supplies the orbital region and dura of the anterior cranial fossa, the posterior division supplies the dura of the temporoparietal region, the petrous branch supplies the facial nerve and the petrosquamous part, after branching from the petrous part, supplies the dura of the posterior fossa.

- *Accessory meningeal arteries are* sometimes present and branch either from the maxillary artery or the MMA, or from both, and run superomedially through the foramen ovale to supply the Dura, Eustachian tube and pharynx.
- *Inferior alveolar nerve*: which originates from the first part of the maxillary artery at 15.6 mm from the origin of MA and gives a branch to the omohyoid muscle, then it goes inferiorly in a straight course with the inferior alveolar nerve and vein through the mandibular canal in the interior part of the mandible to supply the gums and teeth. After exiting from the mental foramen, it anastomoses with branches of the facial artery and reaches the midline to link to its contralateral branch.

(b) ***Pterygoid part***:

It runs upward and medially in the infratemporal fossa and courses either superficially or deep into the lateral pterygoid muscle. It has the following branches, which mainly supply the muscles of mastication and buccinators:

- Deep temporal artery: It has two branches which supply the temporalis muscle: the anterior and posterior deep temporal arteries; the anterior branch arises from the distal part of MA and ascends along the anterior surface of the temporalis muscle, while the posterior deep temporal artery, which is the main supply of the temporalis muscle, passes deep into it and creates a notch on the anterior surface of the squamous part of the temporal bone.
- Pterygoid arteries: Supply the pterygoid muscles.
- Masseteric artery: after originating from the second segment of MA, it enters the mandibular notch and supplies the masseter muscle.
- Buccal artery: it is a branch of the second segment of MA; it courses between the medial pterygoid and temporal muscles, supplies the buccinators, and could join the facial artery.

2. Lateral Pterygoid Muscle: It arises in two heads: the upper head arises from the crest of the greater wing of the sphenoid, and the lower head, which is larger, arises from the lateral surface of the lateral pterygoid plate, and they both insert as a single tendon to the neck of the mandible and posterolateral articular surface of the temporomandibular joint. It is supplied by the anterior division of V1, and its action is to help open the mouth and side-to-side movement of the mouth.
3. Medial pterygoid muscle: Has a quadrilateral shape with a small superficial and large deep head; the superficial head originates from maxillary tuberosity, and the deep head from the medial surface of the lateral pterygoid plate; they both insert to the medial surface of the angle of the mandible when the ramus of the mandible joins it, supplied by a branch from the main trunk of V1. Its action is to elevate the mandible and help its protrusion, as well as aid in the side-to-side movement.

4. Pterygoid venous plexus: composed of an extensive network of small vessels that spread between the muscles of the ITF and around its nerves, it receives blood from all the structures surrounding the ITF and communicates with the brain and cavernous sinus through various emissary veins in F. ovale, F. spinosum, and F. lacerum.
5. Mandibular Division of Trigeminal Nerve V1: It is the largest division of the trigeminal nerve and is composed of large sensory and smaller motor parts; the sensory division comes out of the foramen ovale from the lateral part of the trigeminal ganglion to enter the infratemporal fossa. Medial to the lateral pterygoid muscle is the motor branch and unites with the sensory part just outside the f. ovale. Its branches are as follows:
   (a) *Undivided trunk*: about 7.7 mm from F. ovale to the bifurcation, after the sensory and motor branches unite near the otic ganglion, they give rise to:
      - *Meningeal branch*: which ascends in the F. spinosum with the meningeal artery and supplies the middle fossa dura.
      - *Medial pterygoid nerve*: arises from the medial aspect of the main trunk below the f. ovale, close to the otic ganglion, and descends to supply sensation, motor, and proprioceptive fibres to MPM.
      - *Tensor veli palatine*: comes out of the medial aspect of the main trunk and passes through the otic ganglion to innervate the tensor veli palatine.
      - *Tensor tympani nerve*: passes through the otic ganglion, pierces the cartilage of the external auditory canal, and enters the tensor tympani muscle.

   (b) Anterior division: Its branches are:
      - Buccal nerve: it passes between the two heads of the lateral pterygoid, deep to the masseter muscle, to course on its anterior border and unite with the buccal branch of the facial nerve; it supplies sensory innervation to the buccal mucosa, corner of the mouse and buccinators muscle sensation.
      - Lateral pterygoid nerve: this branch could arise from the buccal branch and go deep into the muscle. Because of its inconsistent landmark, the LPM could receive innervations from other nerves, like the buccal and deep temporal nerves.
      - Masseter Nerve: It passes laterally on the pterygoid muscle in front of the temporomandibular joint and runs deep to the deep surface of the masseter to supply it by two branches.
      - The deep temporal nerve arises in the anterior and posterior divisions and passes above the LPM to enter the infratemporal fossa to supply the anterior and posterior parts of the temporal muscle. It has an anterior branch that arises from the buccal nerve and a posterior branch that arises in common with the masseter nerve.

   (c) Posterior division: is the larger division and mainly has sensory branches.
      - Auriculotemporal nerve: It arises as two branches encircle the MMA and run backwards. Medial to the LPM, it passes between the neck of the mandible and the sphenomandibular ligament, gives a branch to the

parotid gland, then goes upward between the TMJ and EAC and divides into superficial temporal branches.

- Lingual nerve: Branches about 13.5 mm from the F. ovale. It runs down between tensor veli palatini and LPM, with its inferior border joined by the chorda tympani branch of the facial nerve, which contains taste fibres from the Geniculate Ganglion and Pre ganglionic parasympathetic fibres. From this point, the lingual nerve contains fibres for general sensation, taste fibres and preganglionic parasympathetic fibres for submandibular ganglion, and then, it passes between the ramus of the mandible and MPM. After passing the superior constrictor and entering the gingiva, it passes onto the side of the tongue and ends in a terminal branch under the lingual mucosa.
- Inferior alveolar nerve: It arises from the posterolateral surface of the main mandibular trunk and descends deep to the LPM between the ramus of the mandible and the sphenomandibular ligament to enter the mandibular foramen. It gives three sensory and one motor branches. The sensory nerves are incisive, mental, and nerve to lower premolars and molars; they form the inferior dental plexus. The mental nerve is a large branch that leaves the inferior border of the mandible to supply the skin of the chin, lower lip, and mucosa with the adjacent gum.

6. Otic Ganglion (René 2006; Turvey and Golden 2012 It is the relay station for parasympathetic secretomotor fibres to the parotid gland, anatomically located in the infratemporal fossa below the F. ovale, it lies medial to the undivided trunk of V3, but its function is related to the glossopharyngeal nerve. The preganglionic parasympathetic fibres from the inferior salivary nucleus reach the otic ganglion as the lesser superficial petrosal nerve after passing into the tympanic cavity and joining the tympanic plexus. The post-ganglionic fibres from the ganglion join the auriculotemporal nerve to reach the parotid gland. The sympathetic roots do not synapse in the ganglion and carry post-ganglionic fibres from the superior salivary nucleus via a plexus of nerves running with MMA to supply blood vessels in the parotid gland.

The Orbit

It is a bony cavity located in the mid-facial region. It has a pyramidal shape, the apex lies proximally, and its base, which is rectangular, opens on the facial skeleton. Its walls contain foramina and fissures, and several ligaments and muscles attach to it. It is lined by orbital fascia, which continues at the apex as dura matter and contains ocular muscles and orbital fat in addition. Several important neurovascular structures surround the organs of vision. Its height is 35 mm, its width is 40 mm, and it is widest inside the orbital rim, which has a volume of 30 mL. Its length from the medial orbital rim to the orbital apex is 45 mm, which is 1 cm shorter on the lateral side, which means that it rotated laterally to facilitate vision. It is surrounded medially by the nasal cavity and ethmoid sinuses, superiorly related to the anterior cranial fossa and frontal lobe of the brain; inferior to it is the maxillary sinus, posterolaterally related to middle cranial fossa and infratemporal fossa. There are various foramens and fissures that connect the orbit to the surrounding structure, which could lead to the transmission of disease to and from the orbit.

Walls of Orbit

1. Medial wall:
   Extends from the anterior lacrimal crest to the orbital apex and contains the lacrimal sac in the lacrimal fossa between the anterior and posterior lacrimal crest. The medial wall is composed mainly of a thin paper-like bone called lamina papyracea, which overlays the ethmoid sinuses and a small contribution from the body of the sphenoid posteriorly. This wall unites superiorly with the frontal bone at the frontoethmoidal suture, which contains anterior and posterior ethmoidal foramina, which transmit corresponding arteries and nerves. It is inferiorly connected to the orbital process of the maxilla at the maxillo-ethmoidal suture.
2. The Floor of Orbit
   The floor corresponds to the maxillary roof and is composed of the orbital process of the maxilla, mainly zygoma anterolaterally, and contribution from palatine bone posteriorly. It goes gradually upward to merge with the medial wall at the maxillo-ethmoidal suture. In its posterolateral part, it is separated from the lateral wall by an inferior orbital fissure, which is composed of the greater wing of the sphenoid and zygoma laterally and the orbital process of the maxilla medially. The infraorbital branch of the maxillary artery, inferior ophthalmic vein and autonomic branch of PPG pass through the infraorbital fissure in the company of the infraorbital nerve branch of V2 crossing the PPF, and exit 1 cm below the lower orbital rim, the infraorbital nerve, medial to the infraorbital wall, the orbital floor is thin and fractured easily.
3. Lateral Wall
   It is composed of the greater wing of the sphenoid and zygoma, separated from the floor by the inferior orbital fissure and from the roof by the superior orbital fissure. It has an attachment to the frontal bone through the sphenofrontal suture and to the zygomatic bone through the sphenozygomatic suture. Zygomaticofacial and zygomaticotemporal pass through their corresponding foramina in the lateral wall. The lateral tubercle is 3–4 mm behind the lateral orbital rim and gives rise to several important ligaments and tendons of the orbit.
4. The Roof of the Orbit
   It is mainly composed of frontal bone with a small contribution posteriorly by the lesser wing of the sphenoid. It is the floor of the anterior cranial fossa with variable pneumatization from the frontal sinus in its anteromedial part. At the anteromedial part of the rim, there is a fossa that contains the trochlea and superior orbital foramen. At the junction of the medial third and lateral two-thirds of the superior orbital rim, there is the supraorbital neurovascular bundle. The paired roof goes down medially towards the cribriform plate.

5. The Orbital Apex
   It consists of the optic canal, supraorbital fissure, and inferior orbital fissure, which are all connected and related to each other at the back of the orbit and contain multiple important neurovascular structures. The optic canal is in the lesser wing of the sphenoid in the most posterior and medial part of the orbit and passes medially and upward. It is less than 1 cm in length and 5 mm in diameter, bounded medially by an indentation on the sphenoid sinus and sometimes by the posterior ethmoidal cells when there is an Onodi cell extended posteriorly. The roof is composed of the lesser wing of the sphenoid, and the wall is composed of the greater wing. It connects the orbit to the middle cranial fossa, and the optic nerve and ophthalmic artery pass through it.

Structures of the Orbit

1. Orbital fascia (periorbita): The orbit is lined by a fibrous membrane, which is a continuation of dura matter inside the orbit from its periosteum. Orbital septum forms from its condensation at the margins and is firmly attached to it. The periorbita gives processes to bridge the lacrimal groove and form a pulley for the tendon of the superior oblique muscle.
2. Orbital fat: Structures of the orbit are surrounded by orbital fat, which is divided into the posterior or intramuscular part. It is dense and contributes to the maintenance of globe projection. The extramuscular fat is dispersed anteriorly, which is the fat that is reduced during blepharoplasty.
3. Orbital Ligaments:
   (a) Tenon's capsule: Forms a fibrous, thin membrane around the eyeball beneath the intermuscular orbital fat that extends from the optic nerve to the sclera corneal junction. It is pierced by tendons of various extraocular muscles, ciliary vessels, and nerves at the optic nerve entrance and is continuous with the fascia or orbital muscles.
   (b) Lockwood ligament: It is formed by the union of the inferior rectus sheath margin and inferior oblique muscles with the medial and lateral check ligaments to suspend the globe and prevent its anterior and posterior displacement.
   (c) Superior check ligament (Whitnall's ligament): A fascial sling medially attached to the trochlea and laterally to Whitnall's tubercle and lateral wall of the orbit that holds the tendon of the superior oblique muscle and has attachments to the superior rectus, conjunctiva, and tenons' capsule.
   (d) Medial check ligament: It is the expansion of the medial rectus muscle, which extends from the orbital septum to the posterior lacrimal crest.
   (e) Lateral check ligament: It is the expansion of the lateral rectus muscle, which attaches to the zygomatic bone with a contribution from the bulbous sheath.
   (f) Inferior check ligament: The inferior rectus and inferior oblique, which cover the inferior orbital fissure, serve as inferior check ligaments.

Muscles of the Orbit

A tight fibrous ring known as the annulus of Zinn, which encloses the optic canal and middle part of the superior orbital fissure, is the origin of four recti orbital muscles;

1. Medial rectus: It's closely related to the medial orbital wall and prone to entrapment in medial orbital wall fractures; its action is to move the globe medially in the horizontal plane.
2. Lateral rectus: Separated from the lateral orbital wall by fat, the lacrimal gland and lacrimal artery lie superior to it and posteriorly separated from the optic nerve by the ciliary ganglion; its action is to move the globe laterally in the horizontal plane.
3. Inferior rectus: It lies close to the floor posteriorly and has fat between it and the floor anteriorly; it is liable to herniation into the maxillary antrum in an orbital floor fracture; its action is to move the globe downward and inward.
4. Levator palpebrae superiors: Originate from the lesser wing of the sphenoid superomedial to the origin of the superior rectus muscle, and both are related to each other; the superior rectus travels inferiorly to insert to the globe and the levator palpebrae after becoming an aponeurosis divided into superior (voluntary) and inferior (involuntary) lamellae. The superior lamellae are inserted into the anterior surface of the superior tarsus and the skin of the upper eyelid. Inferior lamellae insert into the upper margin of the superior tarsus and conjuctival fornix. All the recti muscles are inserted into the sclera posterior to the limbus.
5. Superior oblique muscle: Arises from the annulus of the zin and body of the sphenoid superomedial to the optic canal. It crosses above the frontoethmoidal suture to reach the trochlea, then beneath the superior rectus to reach the globe in a broad fashion and extends to its posterolateral aspect; its action is to move the globe down and outward.
6. Inferior oblique muscle: It arises from the orbital surface of the maxilla lateral to the lacrimal groove, courses laterally and posteriorly below the inferior rectus, and inserts into the inferolateral aspect of the globe; its action is to move the globe up and outward.

Ophthalmic Division of Trigeminal Nerve V1

Originates from the trigeminal ganglion, goes upward and travels in the lateral wall of the cavernous sinus to reach the superior orbital fissure. It is the smallest division of the trigeminal nerve and has three branches:

1. *The frontal nerve* is the largest division of V1. After passing on the lateral wall of the cavernous sinus, it enters the lateral part of SOF, runs forward between the levator palpebral muscle and periorbita, travels outside of the annular tendon and divides into:
   (a) *Supratrochlear nerve*: which goes above the trochlea of the superior oblique muscle with the superior trochlear artery and exits between the trochlea and supraorbital foramen. It is located medially to the supraorbital nerve, sup-

plying the conjunctiva and skin of the upper eyelid and the skin of the forehead near the midline.

(b) *Supraorbital nerve*: it exits the supraorbital notch after passing between the levator palpebrae muscle and the orbital roof; it supplies the upper eyelid and mucous membrane of the frontal sinus and ascends on the forehead to supply part of the skin of the scalp.

2. *Nasociliary nerve*: arises from the medial part of V1 and courses medial to it; then, it reaches the medial part of the orbit after crossing between two divisions of the oculomotor nerve and above the optic nerve to give rise to the anterior and posterior ethmoidal and infratrochlear nerves.
3. *The lacrimal nerve*, which is the smallest branch of V1, originates from its lateral part. After passing on the lateral side of SOF, it enters the orbit and courses on the superior margin of the lateral rectus. It is joined by the zygomatic branch of V2, which carries post-ganglionic parasympathetic secretomotor fibres to reach the lacrimal gland via the lacrimal nerve and also provides sensation to the area around the gland (Joo et al. 2013; Ziyal et al. 2004).

Ciliary Ganglion

It is a small aggregate of neural cells that is located below the optic nerve and on the medial side of the lateral rectus. It receives parasympathetic, sympathetic, and sensory roots. The parasympathetic fibres form the nucleus of the oculomotor nerve in the midbrain synapse in the ganglion and give rise to the short ciliary nerve, which supplies the ciliary muscle and pupil sphincter. The sympathetic fibres move along with the internal ophthalmic artery and do not synapse in the ganglion. The sensory root from the Nasociliary nerve supplies sensation to the cornea and globe via short ciliary nerves (Joo et al. 2013; Sinnatamby 2013; Ziyal et al. 2004).

Motor Nerve

The extraocular muscles are supplied by the oculomotor nerve except the lateral rectus, which is supplied by the abducens nerve, and the superior oblique, which is supplied by the trochlear nerve. The oculomotor nerve divides in the cavernous sinus into superior and inferior divisions; the superior divisions supply the levator and superior rectus, while the inferior divisions supply the medial rectus, inferior rectus, and inferior oblique. The trochlear nerve enters the orbit outside of the annulus; it is superior to the oculomotor in the lateral wall of the cavernous sinus. It crosses from lateral to medial to enter the lateral border of the superior oblique. The abducens nerve enters the orbit within the cone, travels along the medial surface of the lateral rectus, and pierces it.

Blood Supply

The main arterial supply of the orbit is through the ophthalmic artery (OA), which branches from the ICA right when it comes off the cavernous sinus and enters the optic canal below the optic nerve; the central retinal artery enters the optic nerve 1 cm behind the globe; other branches of the OA are multiple ciliary arteries to supply the ciliary body and the iris. The lacrimal artery supplies the lacrimal gland and the anterior and posterior ethmoid arteries, which enter their respective foramen to the ethmoid sinus. Other branches of the OA, like the supraorbital, supratrochlear, and palpebral arteries supply the upper eyelid. The lower eyelid and the orbital fat receive blood supply from the inferior orbital artery, a terminal branch of the maxillary artery.

Venous Drainage

Drainage of the orbit is via superior and inferior orbital veins; the superior orbital vein, which is the larger one, forms superomedially from the union of the supraorbital, supratrochlear, and angular vein and passes to the superior orbital fissure. The inferior orbital vein forms as a plexus within the inferomedial orbital fat travels posteriorly to drain into the superior orbital vein and communicates with the pterygoid plexus via the inferior orbital fissure. The inferior orbital vein receives from muscular and collateral veins.

Orbital Septum

The periorbita from the lid margin to the tarsal plate becomes the orbital septum; its main function is confinement of infection and prevention of its spread from the eyelid to the orbital compartment.

Tarsal Plate

Thick fibrous condensation of the orbital septum at the lid margin (1 cm behind the upper lid margin and 0.5 cm behind the lower lid margin), which receives attachment of the levator aponeurosis in the upper lid, gives rigidity to the lid, and there is the Meibomian gland behind it.

Eyelid Layers

From outward to inward, the eyelid is covered by a loose layer of skin that becomes oedematous easily during infection and trauma. Underneath the skin is the palpebral part of the orbicularis oculi muscle, which is continuous with the parietal fascia. Beneath them are the orbital septum and tarsal plates, followed by the conjunctiva. Beneath the lower tarsus and deep surface of the levator aponeurosis is a layer of smooth muscle known as Müller's muscle, which is supplied by the lacrimal nerve carrying sympathetic supply from the supracervical ganglion and causes reflex closure of the eyelid.

Medial Canthal Ligament

This is the mainly tendinous attachment of the orbicularis oculi muscle to the anterior and posterior lacrimal crests; between them is the lacrimal sac, which receives canaliculi from the lacrimal gland. The main contribution is from the anterior attachment to the anterior lacrimal crest on the frontal process of the maxilla; a minor contribution is from the posterior attachment to the posterior lacrimal crest, also known as Horner's muscle.

Lateral Canthal Ligament

At the lateral side of the eye, both upper and lower eyelids attach firmly to a tubercle on the lateral wall of the orbit, which also receives levator aponeurosis and the lateral check ligament of the lateral rectus, and they extend until the orbital septum, but the fusion of upper and lower orbicularis oculi occurs superficial to the septum at the lateral palpebral raphe and continues with the temporoparietal fascia.

Lateral Wall of Nose

The maxillary sinus is bounded medially by the lateral wall of the nose, which is formed anterosuperiorly by the nasal bone, lacrimal bone and frontal process of maxilla, inferiorly by inferior turbinate, which is a separate bone that articulates with the maxilla anteriorly and palatine process of maxilla posteriorly and has inferior meatus beneath it which receive the nasolacrimal duct opening. The medial pterygoid plate forms the posteroinferior part of the lateral nasal wall posteriorly till the choanae. At its middle and superior part, ethmoid bone forms the majority of the lateral nasal wall; a thin paper-like bony structure known as lamina papyracea separates the orbit from the nasal cavity and ethmoid sinuses. *Agger nasi* is the most anterior ethmoid cell and forms a projection on the lateral nasal wall. Also, the ethmoid labyrinth gives off two bony projections, which are covered by connective tissue and mucosa; they are the middle and superior turbinates in the nasal cavity. Beneath them lies their corresponding meatus. In the middle meatus, there is the ethmoidal bulla, which is a large anterior ethmoid cell attached to the lamina papyracea laterally. Its pneumatization may reach the skull base. Just beneath the bulla is the basal lamella, which is a thin bone through which the entire length of the middle turbinate attaches to the lateral wall of the nose and separates the anterior and posterior groups of ethmoid cells. The uncinate process (UP), which is a thin movable part of the ethmoid labyrinth, attaches to the frontal process of the maxilla superiorly and the ethmoid process of inferior turbinate inferiorly. Between the ethmoidal bulla and posterior part of UP is a two-dimensional space known as infundibulum; lateral to it lies the hiatus semilunaris that receives the drainage of the maxillary, anterior ethmoid and frontal sinus, while the superior meatus receives drainage from posterior ethmoidal cells (Chastain and Sindwani 2006).

Lacrimal Apparatus

The structures that create and drain tears are known as lacrimal apparatus and include the lacrimal gland and its ducts, lacrimal puncta and canaliculi, and nasolacrimal duct. The lacrimal secretion apparatus consists of the main lacrimal gland with its multiple secreting ducts in the upper conjunctival fornix, multiple accessory glands in the conjunctiva fornix and palpebral conjunctiva. There are two parts of the conjunctiva: the palpebral, which lines the eyelid, and the bulbar, which covers the. Ell. The potential space between them is called the conjunctival sac. By eye blinking, the tear moves laterally and is propelled deep into the eyelid and medially to enter the lacrimal canaliculi through up the upper and lower punctae. Both the lower and upper canaliculi have a vertical part, which is 2 mm, and a horizontal part, which is about 8 mm; the upper and lower canaliculi unite to form the common canaliculi and drain to the lateral part of the lacrimal sac. The lacrimal sac is located between the two limbs of the medial canthal ligament in a fossa just outside the orbit, which is formed by the frontal process of the maxilla anteriorly and lacrimal bone posteriorly. It is about 12 mm long and 5 mm wide and extends 3–5 mm above the medial canthal ligament. Intranasally, it is 6–8 mm above the middle turbinate insertion. The lower part of the lacrimal sac connects to the membranous nasolacrimal duct, which travels in the bony nasolacrimal canal downward, laterally and posteriorly for about 18 mm, to open in the inferior meatus 4–6 mm posterior to the head of the inferior turbinate and 15 mm above the nasal floor, with the mucosal valve of Hasner present at this opening (Chastain and Sindwani 2006).

References

Allen WF, Kier EL, Rothman SLG (1973) The maxillary artery: normal arteriographic anatomy. Am J Roentgenol 118:517–527. https://doi.org/10.2214/ajr.118.3.517

Anastasi G (2020) Trattato di anatomia umana sistematica e funzionale. 5ª ed. Milano: Edi-Ermes. ISBN: 978-88-7051-706-4

Bell GW, Joshi BB, Macleod RI (2011) Maxillary sinus disease: diagnosis and treatment. Br Dent J 210:113–118. https://doi.org/10.1038/sj.bdj.2011.47

Chanavaz M (1990) Maxillary sinus: anatomy, physiology, surgery, and bone grafting related to implantology—eleven years of surgical experience (1979–1990). J Oral Implantol 16(3):199–209

Chastain JB, Sindwani R (2006) Anatomy of the orbit, lacrimal apparatus, and lateral nasal wall. Otolaryngol Clin N Am 39:855–864. https://doi.org/10.1016/j.otc.2006.07.003

Chaurasia BD (2013) BD Chaurasia's Human Anatomy: Regional and Applied Dissection and Clinical (Vol. 1–4). CBS Publishers & Distributors

Chiapasco M (2020) Manuale illustrato di chirurgia orale. 4ª ed. Milano: Edra. ISBN: 978-88-214-5314-4

Choi J, Park H-S (2003) The clinical anatomy of the maxillary artery in the pterygopalatine fossa. J Oral Maxillofac Surg 61:72–78. https://doi.org/10.1053/joms.2003.50012

Daniels DL, Mark LP, Ulmer JL et al (1998) Osseous anatomy of the pterygopalatine fossa. AJNR Am J Neuroradiol 19(8):1423–1432

Flanagan D (2005) Arterial supply of maxillary sinus and potential for bleeding complication during lateral approach sinus elevation. Implant Dent 14:336–339. https://doi.org/10.1097/01.id.0000188437.66363.7c

Fortes FSG, Sennes LU, Carrau RL et al (2008) Endoscopic anatomy of the pterygopalatine fossa and the transpterygoid approach: development of a surgical instruction model. Laryngoscope 118:44–49. https://doi.org/10.1097/mlg.0b013e318155a492

Gerges MM, Godil SS, Younus I et al (2020) Endoscopic transorbital approach to the infratemporal fossa and parapharyngeal space: a cadaveric study. J Neurosurg 133:1948–1959. https://doi.org/10.3171/2019.7.jns191743

Hollinshead WH (1982) Anatomy for surgeons, vol 1, 3rd edn. Lippincott Williams and Wilkins, Philadelphia—References—Scientific Research Publishing. https://www.scirp.org/reference/referencespapers?referenceid=2321196

Iwanaga J, Wilson C, Lachkar S, Tomaszewski KA, Walocha JA, Tubbs RS (2019) Clinical anatomy of the maxillary sinus: application to sinus floor augmentation. Anat Cell Biol 52(1):17–24. https://doi.org/10.5115/acb.2019.52.1.17

Joo W, Yoshioka F, Funaki T et al (2013) Microsurgical anatomy of the trigeminal nerve. Clin Anat 27:61–88. https://doi.org/10.1002/ca.22330

Khonsary SA, Ma Q, Villablanca P et al (2013) Clinical functional anatomy of the pterygopalatine ganglion, cephalgia and related dysautonomias: a review. Surg Neurol Int 4:422. https://doi.org/10.4103/2152-7806.121628

Kim DI, Kim HS, Chung IH (1996) High-resolution CT of the pterygopalatine fossa and its communications. Neuroradiology 38:S120–S126. https://doi.org/10.1007/bf02278138

Kqiku L, Biblekaj R, Weiglein AH et al (2013) Arterial blood architecture of the maxillary sinus in dentate specimens. Croat Med J 54:180–184. https://doi.org/10.3325/cmj.2013.54.180

Lang J (1989) Clinical anatomy of the nose, nasal cavity, and paranasal sinuses. Thieme Medical Publishers, New York

Lorkiewicz-Muszyńska D, Kociemba W, Rewekant A et al (2015) Development of the maxillary sinus from birth to age 18. Postnatal growth pattern. Int J Pediatr Otorhinolaryngol 79:1393–1400. https://doi.org/10.1016/j.ijporl.2015.05.032

Lovasova K, Kachlik D, Rozpravkova M, Matusevska M, Ferkova J, Kluchova D (2018) Three-dimensional CAD/CAM imaging of the maxillary sinus in ageing process. Ann Anat 218:69–82. https://doi.org/10.1016/j.aanat.2018.01.008

Nelke K, Diakowska D, Morawska-Kochman M et al (2023) The CBCT retrospective study on underwood septa and their related factors in maxillary sinuses—a proposal of classification. J Pers Med 13:1258. https://doi.org/10.3390/jpm13081258

Piagkou M, Demesticha T, Troupis T et al (2011) The pterygopalatine ganglion and its role in various pain syndromes: from anatomy to clinical practice. Pain Pract 12:399–412. https://doi.org/10.1111/j.1533-2500.2011.00507.x

Prasanna LC, Mamatha H (2010) The location of maxillary sinus ostium and its clinical application. Indian J Otolaryngol Head Neck Surg 62:335–337. https://doi.org/10.1007/s12070-010-0047-z

René C (2006) Update on orbital anatomy. Eye 20:1119–1129. https://doi.org/10.1038/sj.eye.6702376

Rodella LF, Buffoli B, Labanca M, Rezzani R (2012) A review of the mandibular and maxillary nerve supplies and their clinical relevance. Arch Oral Biol 57:323–334. https://doi.org/10.1016/j.archoralbio.2011.09.007

Scanavine AB, Navarro JA, Megale SR, Anselmo-Lima WT (2009) Anatomical study of the sphenopalatine foramen. Braz J Otorhinolaryngol 75:37–41. https://doi.org/10.1016/s1808-8694(15)30829-5

Scuderi AJ, Harnsberger HR, Boyer RS (1993) Pneumatization of the paranasal sinuses: normal features of importance to the accurate interpretation of CT scans and MR images. Am J Roentgenol 160:1101–1104. https://doi.org/10.2214/ajr.160.5.8470585

Sinnatamby CS (2013) Last's anatomy: regional and applied, 12th ed. Ann R Coll Surg Engl 95:230. https://doi.org/10.1308/rcsann.2013.95.3.230a

Tanoue S, Kiyosue H, Mori H et al (2013) Maxillary artery: functional and imaging anatomy for safe and effective transcatheter treatment. Radiographics 33:e209–e224. https://doi.org/10.1148/rg.337125173

Tiwana PS, Kushner GM, Haug RH (2006) Maxillary sinus augmentation. Dent Clin N Am 50:409–424. https://doi.org/10.1016/j.cden.2006.03.004

Turvey TA, Golden BA (2012) Orbital anatomy for the surgeon. Oral Maxillofac Surg Clin North Am 24(4):525–536

Vescan AD, Snyderman CH, Carrau RL et al (2007) Vidian canal: analysis and relationship to the internal carotid artery. Laryngoscope 117:1338–1342. https://doi.org/10.1097/mlg.0b013e31806146cd

von Arx T, Lozanoff S (2017). Clinical oral anatomy: A comprehensive review for dental practitioners and researchers. Springer International Publishing. https://doi.org/10.1007/978-3-319-41993-0

Whyte A, Boeddinghaus R (2019) The maxillary sinus: physiology, development and imaging anatomy. Dentomaxillofac Radiol 48:20190205. https://doi.org/10.1259/dmfr.20190205

Ziyal IM, Sekhar LN, Özgen T et al (2004) The trigeminal nerve and ganglion: an anatomical, histological, and radiological study addressing the transtrigeminal approach. Surg Neurol 61:564–573. https://doi.org/10.1016/j.surneu.2003.07.009

2 Maxillary Sinus Physiology

Goran Latif Omer, Gianluca Velletrani, Beatrice Francavilla, Rekawt Hama Rashid Kareem, Talar Sabir Ahmed, Sahand Soran Ali, Aland Salih Abdullah, and Stefano Di Girolamo

Functions of the Maxillary Sinus

The maxillary sinus, like the other paranasal sinuses, has numerous roles and functions within the head and neck region. Some of these are as follows:

- As an air-filled cavity, it works to lower the weight of the skull (Wilk 1999). This weight reduction is necessary as it reduces the workload on the neck muscles required to move the region. Additionally, a lighter skull is easier to balance and move on the neck (Amorosa and Latini 2016).
- It plays a role in humidifying and increasing the temperature of inspired air as well as enhancing voice resonance (Wilk 1999). However, due to the minimal exchange of air between the nose and the paranasal sinuses, air humidification and warming are not considered the primary functions of the sinus (Björn et al. 1967).
- It contributes to heat conservation from the nasal fossae.

G. L. Omer (✉) · S. S. Ali · A. S. Abdullah
Department of Clinical Sciences, College of Medicine, University of Sulaimani, Sulaymaniyah, KRI, Iraq

G. Velletrani · B. Francavilla · S. Di Girolamo
Department of Otorhinolaryngology, University of Rome Tor Vergata, Rome, Italy

R. H. R. Kareem · T. S. Ahmed
Royal Hospital, Sulaymaniyah, KRI, Iraq

© The Author(s), under exclusive license to Springer Nature Switzerland AG 2025

G. L. Omer, S. Di Girolamo (eds.), *Maxillary Sinus: A Comprehensive Guide*,
https://doi.org/10.1007/978-3-031-83468-4_2

- It participates in both the formation and storage of nasal mucus (Wilk 1999). Compared to the total mucus available in the nasal cavity, the amount contributed by the maxillary sinus is relatively small.
- The sinus also acts as a cushion, dampening and absorbing a portion of impact forces to help prevent concussions (Amorosa and Latini 2016; Wilk 1999).
- Interestingly, the maxillary sinus has been hypothesised to have an immunological role. It produces nitric oxide (NO), which has antimicrobial properties, and provides a sterile secretion that dilutes mucus and includes protective factors such as lysozyme and immunoglobulin A (IgA) (Amorosa and Latini 2016; Lundberg 2008).

Histology of the Maxillary Sinus

There is no periosteum in the inner lining of the maxillary sinus, leaving the respiratory epithelium, which is a form of pseudostratified columnar epithelium that is ciliated and forms mucus (Fig. 2.1), as the sole layer in the sinus lining (Iwanaga et al. 2019). Since the cilia help with clearance, their number increases as you approach the ostium of the maxillary sinus. This type of epithelium is shared by the majority of the respiratory system, from the nasal cavity to the bronchi. However, starting from the bronchioles and continuing further down the respiratory tract, the epithelium changes to simple columnar epithelium and cuboidal epithelium, with the alveoli being lined by a thin squamous epithelium (Kia'i and Bajaj 2023).

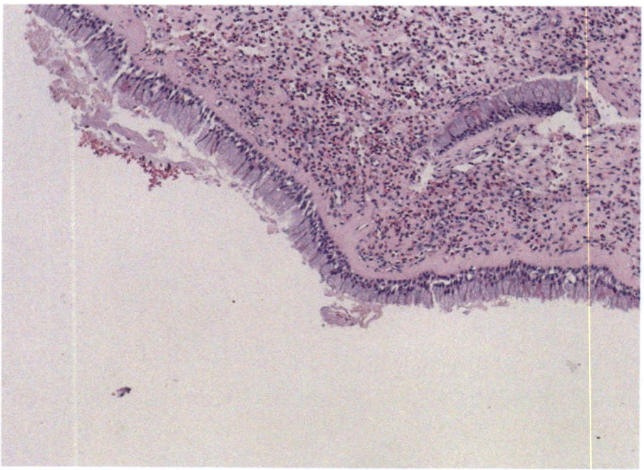

Fig. 2.1 Respiratory epithelium is a type of ciliated pseudostratified columnar epithelium that is made of a single cell layer along the basement membrane. Although only a single layer, due to the nonplanar alignment of the nuclei, the epithelium appears as multiple layers

Mucociliary Clearance

Mucociliary clearance is the process by which the respiratory epithelium transports and expels particles and pathogens out of the airway (Schnoor et al. 2022). It acts as a physical barrier and is considered an essential part of innate immunity. The cilia transport both debris and mucus in a spiral fashion toward the sinus ostium. Goblet cells produce a mucociliary blanket composed mostly of water and a small amount of mucin and inorganic salts (Wilk 1999). To move this mucociliary blanket, the cilia beat at a rate of 1000 times/min (Watzek et al. 1997). The speed of transport varies among individuals, ranging from 5 to 20 mm/min (Ballenger and Ballenger 1952).

The flow of mucociliary transport can be either a smooth flow at a rate of 0.84 cm/min, a jerky flow at 0.3 cm/min, or a mucostasis flow at less than 0.3 cm/min (Wilk 1999). This mucociliary transport is particularly crucial in the maxillary sinus due to the sinus ostium's superior location along the sinus's medial wall, making sinus drainage largely dependent on this mucociliary escalator (Fig. 2.2) (Standring 2015).

The mucus is swept away from the primary ostium superiorly through the infundibulum of the ethmoid. It is then swept from the posterior uncinate process, through the middle meatus, into the ethmoidal bulla, and finally propelled through the middle meatus into the nasopharynx for swallowing (Duncavage and Becker 2011). Under normal physiological conditions, the cilia can clear the sinuses in 10–30 min (Stammberger 1986). Although very durable, many substances can damage the cilia, either reversibly or irreversibly. Interestingly, unlike the tracheobronchial tree, mucociliary clearance of the nasal mucosa increases when irritated. Factors that impact this physiological process include inflammatory mediators and local factors.

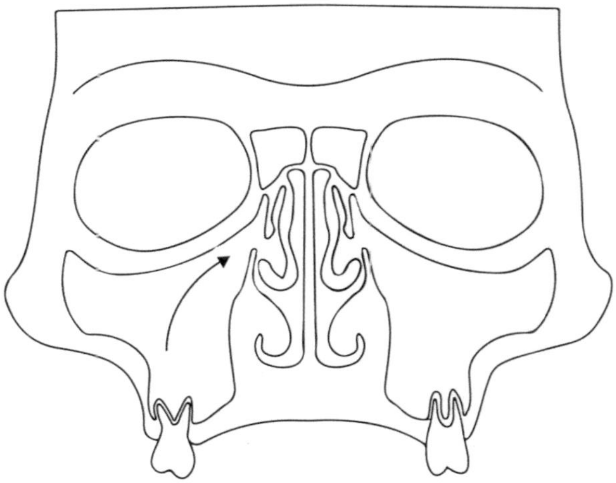

Fig. 2.2 Maxillary sinus drainage: superomedial drainage of the maxillary sinus

Tissue kallikrein and prostaglandin E1 are hypothesised to stimulate mucociliary clearance of the nasal mucosa, while peptides such as neuropeptide Y can decrease this transport (Cervin et al. 1988; Dolata et al. 1989).

Ostium of the Maxillary Sinus

The ostium of the maxillary sinus is located on the highest part of the medial wall of the maxillary sinus. It does not directly open into the nasal fossa but opens into the narrow ethmoidal infundibulum (Prasanna and Mamatha 2010). In most individuals, there is only one ostium for each maxillary sinus; however, an accessory ostium exists in up to 44% of cases (Wilk 1999). The diameter of the ostium is measured as the length of a line connecting the bony portion of the orbital floor to the uncinate process attachment and then to the medial maxillary wall (Basurrah and Kim 2021). To maintain a normal oxygen concentration, the ostium needs to be greater than 2.5 mm (Wilk 1999). Nasal congestion can reduce this ostium diameter. A mean oxygen partial pressure of 116 mmHg is considered normal, decreasing to as low as 75 mmHg in patients with maxillary sinusitis (Wilk 1999). The most important predisposing factor for sinusitis is the occlusion of the ostium. This ostium is one of the passages used in functional endoscopic sinus surgery (Prasanna and Mamatha 2010). Many authors state that the maxillary sinus ostium is found along the course of the ethmoid infundibulum. According to some, the ostium is more frequently found to open into the posterior third of the infundibulum rather than the middle or anterior third. Interestingly, there have been cases reported where this ostium is absent (Kotian et al. 2016).

Obstruction of the Maxillary Sinus Ostium

Drainage of mucus in healthy tissue occurs through the ostiomeatal complex, which reaches the maxillary sinus ostium. From there, the mucus passes through the ethmoidal infundibulum, a small passage that communicates with the nasal cavity. Obstruction of the maxillary sinus does not necessarily result from a primary defect of the maxillary sinus ostium. It can arise from the compression and obstruction of adjacent structures within the ostiomeatal complex, such as the ethmoidal bulla, anterior ethmoid cells, and the uncinate process (Kennedy 1992). Additionally, narrowing of the infundibulum is another factor that can predispose to occlusion and, hence, sinusitis (Akay et al. 2019).

The maxillary sinus ostium is poorly positioned for drainage because it is located at the highest part of the medial wall of the maxillary sinus. Inflammation of the ethmoidal infundibulum is one of the factors that may lead to obstruction. Moreover, Haller cells, which are anatomically continuous with the infundibulum, are important because their infection is known to cause maxillary sinus obstruction (Akay et al. 2019). In addition to the aforementioned factors, colds, allergies, a deviated nasal septum, and chronic infections are also considered causes of maxillary sinus ostium obstruction (Pennmedicine 2024).

References

Akay G, Yaman D, Karadağ Ö, Güngör K (2019) Evaluation of the relationship of dimensions of maxillary sinus drainage system with anatomical variations and sinusopathy: cone-beam computed tomography findings. Med Princ Pract 29:354–363. https://doi.org/10.1159/000504963

Amorosa L, Latini G (2016) Maxillary sinus. Elsevier eBooks, pp 124–134

Ballenger JJ, Ballenger HC (1952) XLIX vacuum frontal sinusitis—absorption of air from the frontal sinus. Ann Otol Rhinol Laryngol 61:542–557. https://doi.org/10.1177/000348945206100226

Basurrah MA, Kim SW (2021) Factors affecting dimensions of the ethmoid infundibulum and maxillary sinus natural ostium in a normal population. Saudi Med J 42:981–985. https://doi.org/10.15537/smj.2021.42.9.20210399

Björn H, Holmberg K, Nylander G (1967) Maxillary sinus in periodontal disease. A clinical and radiographic investigation. Odontol Revy 18:83–114

Cervin A, Bende M, Lindberg S et al (1988) Relations between blood flow and mucociliary activity in the rabbit maxillary sinus. Acta Otolaryngol 105:350–356. https://doi.org/10.3109/00016488809097018

Dolata J, Lindberg S, Mercke U (1989) The effects of prostaglandins E1, E2 and F2 α on mucociliary activity in the rabbit maxillary sinus. Acta Otolaryngol 108:290–297. https://doi.org/10.3109/00016488909125530

Duncavage JA, Becker SS (2011) The maxillary sinus. Thieme

Iwanaga J, Wilson C, Lachkar S et al (2019) Clinical anatomy of the maxillary sinus: application to sinus floor augmentation. Anatomy Cell Biol 52:17. https://doi.org/10.5115/acb.2019.52.1.17

Kennedy D (1992) Prognostic factors, outcomes and staging in ethmoid sinus surgery. https://www.semanticscholar.org/paper/Prognostic-factors%2C-outcomes-and-staging-in-ethmoid-Kennedy/26b4e89bc279b96d9d9250e53eec181b69bb8fe8

Kia'i N, Bajaj T (2023) Histology, respiratory epithelium. StatPearls—NCBI Bookshelf. https://www.ncbi.nlm.nih.gov/books/NBK541061/#:~:text=Respiratory%20epithelium%20is%20ciliated%20pseudostratified

Kotian S, Souza A, Rajagopal K et al (2016) Anatomy of maxillary sinus and its ostium: a radiological study using computed tomography. CHRISMED J Health Res 3:37. https://doi.org/10.4103/2348-3334.172397

Lundberg JO (2008) Nitric oxide and the paranasal sinuses. Anat Rec (Hoboken) 291:1479–1484. https://doi.org/10.1002/ar.20782

Prasanna LC, Mamatha H (2010) The location of maxillary sinus ostium and its clinical application. Indian J Otolaryngol Head Neck Surg 62:335–337. https://doi.org/10.1007/s12070-010-0047-z

Schnoor M, Yin L-M, Sun S (2022) Cell movement in health and disease. Academic Press

Sinus Infections (Sinusitis) (2024) Pen medicine. https://www.pennmedicine.org/for-patients-and-visitors/patient-information/conditions-treated-a-to-z/sinus-infections-sinusitis#:~:text=Colds%20and%20allergies%20may%20cause. Accessed 31 Jul 2024

Stammberger H (1986) Endoscopic endonasal surgery—concepts in treatment of recurring rhinosinusitis. Part I. Anatomic and pathophysiologic considerations. Otolaryngol Head Neck Surg 94:143–147. https://doi.org/10.1177/019459988609400202

Standring S (2015) Gray's anatomy. Churchill Livingstone

Watzek G, Bernhart T, Ulm C (1997) Complications of sinus perforations and their management in endodontics. Dent Clin N Am 41:563–583. References—Scientific Research Publishing. https://www.scirp.org/reference/referencespapers?referenceid=657649

Wilk RM (1999) Physiology of the maxillary sinus. Oral Maxillofac Surg Clin North Am 11:15–19

Imaging

3

Goran Latif Omer, Mahabad Abdalaziz Salih, Kawa Abdullah Mahmood, Sara Maurantonio, Laura Borghesi, Andrea Bravetti, Riccardo Maurizi, Sara Maurantonio, Fiorela Shemsiu, Giulia Marzocchella, and Francesco Maria Passali

Imaging of the Maxillary Sinus

For the evaluation of the paranasal sinuses, and more particularly for that of the maxillary sinus, the use of radiodiagnostic methods is now almost indispensable. The techniques used are ultrasound, X-ray, CT, and MRI.

Ultrasound can be used as a screening method for acute and chronic diseases and in follow-up (Karantanas and Sandris 1997).

Usually, the sinus examination is performed on the axial plane. The transducer of the ultrasound scanner is placed horizontally, inferior to the orbital cavity, on the anterior wall of the maxillary sinus (Bozzato et al. 2022).

Ultrasound has a greater sensitivity for the maxillary sinus than for all the other paranasal sinuses, but in any case, the results learned with this technique should always be correlated with the clinical study and with the endoscopy of the nose or further investigated with other radiological techniques in the case of abnormal results, or of possible pathological significance (Hsu et al. 2018). Several previous studies have shown highly variable sensitivity (32–99%) and specificity (61–100%) of ultrasound compared with results obtained by radiography or other diagnostic investigations (Hsu et al. 2018).

In the clinical interpretation of A-scan, one-dimensional mode ultrasound, the air-mucosal echo (AME) is the first measurable echo. Front wall echo (FWE) is clearly detectable if there is no fluid in the sinus. The posterior wall echo (BWE) is a single echo that indicates the presence of fluid in the maxillary sinus. So, under normal conditions, this posterior echo should not be detected.

G. L. Omer (✉) · M. A. Salih · K. A. Mahmood
Department of Clinical Sciences, College of Medicine, University of Sulaimani, Sulaymaniyah, KRI, Iraq

S. Maurantonio · L. Borghesi · A. Bravetti · R. Maurizi · S. Maurantonio · F. Shemsiu · G. Marzocchella · F. M. Passali
Department of Otorhinolaryngology, University of Rome Tor Vergata, Rome, Italy

© The Author(s), under exclusive license to Springer Nature Switzerland AG 2025

G. L. Omer, S. Di Girolamo (eds.), *Maxillary Sinus: A Comprehensive Guide*, https://doi.org/10.1007/978-3-031-83468-4_3

In an abnormal sinus obstructed with mucus, a complete sinusogram, which indicates that the sinus is filled with fluid, or a partial sinusogram, which is a nonspecific sign, can be found. To increase the specificity of the latter finding, the patient can be evaluated in either a semi-supine or sitting position. If the partial sinusogram is present in both positions, a hydroaerial level is present, which is considered a positive sign of sinusitis; however, if the sinusogram is present only in the sitting position, this test is indicative of mucosal thickening of the sinus (Bell and Gaillard 2008; Lichtenstein 1998, 2007; John et al. 2013; Kamalian et al. 2019) Currently, however, there are no conclusive criteria or guidelines for the study of the sinus using A-mode ultrasound because of the heterogeneous results of various studies (Hsu et al. 2018).

In contrast, B-scan mode ultrasound is two-dimensional; the anterior sinus bone wall (AWMS) is identified at about 1 cm depth, and the posterior sinus wall is identified at about 4 cm depth.

In general, A-scan ultrasound can be used for acute sinus pathology, but the chosen ultrasound method in the clinical setting, especially for chronic pathology, should be B-scan ultrasound (Bozzato et al. 2022). Facial and sinus X-ray is used as a first-level investigation in cases of facial trauma and suspected sinus fractures, particularly for the maxillary sinus, as it is the most anterior and, therefore, the easiest to visualise (Lambert et al. 1997; MüllerRichter et al. 2007; Reffat et al. 2022; Reuben et al. 2005; Unger et al. 1990). This is because X-ray is a very useful method for evaluating the fracture lines of the bone tissue, and it is very quick because it can be used even in an emergency setting. The most commonly used projection for this purpose is the Waters (or occipitomental) Projection, which is a specific type of scan not only for the maxillary sinus but also for the evaluation of the orbit and zygoma (MüllerRichter et al. 2007; Unger et al. 1990). This method can also be used for dental assessment and for odontogenic surgery planning, in correlation with the maxillary sinus, in order to provide preparatory details for dental surgeries, as the roots of the upper teeth can create damage to the floor of the maxillary sinus (Lambert et al. 1997; MüllerRichter et al. 2007; Reffat et al. 2022; Reuben et al. 2005; Unger et al. 1990). Approximately, 20% of infections that occur in the maxillary sinus have odontogenic origins, and it is therefore important to evaluate both the sinus and the underlying dental structures together. Another use of X-ray is for postoperative evaluations, but it is now almost entirely replaced by the massive facial CT scan as it is more accurate. This technique is not used for inflammatory or neoplastic diseases because the obtained results are inaccurate and much less concordant with nasal endoscopy images and CT and MRI results (Lambert et al. 1997; MüllerRichter et al. 2007; Reffat et al. 2022; Reuben et al. 2005; Unger et al. 1990).

For other pathologies, especially for planning sinus surgery, the method is not considered reliable, and it has now been almost completely supplanted by CT. This is because X-rays cannot provide exact information regarding the true morphology, volume, and location of the detected lesions (Hung et al. 2022a, b).

It may be useful, however, to let the radiologist be able to recognise a normal RX image in the three standard projections (occipitofrontal, occipitomental, and lateral projections), showing a radiolucent sinus from an image that is instead altered, with partial or complete obliteration of the sinus, with the presence of a hydroaerial level, or with thickening of the sinus mucosa. However, this method should be compared with other endoscopic and radiologic investigations when suspecting inflammatory or neoplastic disease, as the American College of Radiology (ACR) has revealed a high percentage of inaccurate or incorrect diagnoses of sinusitis using a simple sinus film (Hsu et al. 2018; Puhakka et al. 2000).

Currently, CT is the most widely used technique for the study of the sinuses, as it allows very accurate diagnosis and follow-up for various pathologies. It is used to study acute and chronic inflammatory or infectious conditions and to evaluate any complications induced by them (Bhattacharyya and Fried 2003). It is also almost mandatory for preoperative planning of sinus-nasal surgeries (Busaba and Salman 1999; De Menezes 2016; Lombardo et al. 2018). In the cases explained above, a standard CT without an intravenous contrast medium is usually used.

The CT technique also aids MRI in the study of neoplastic pathology (Busaba and Salman 1999, De Menezes 2016, Lombardo et al. 2018). In this other case, an intravenous contrast agent is necessary.

Even in cases of maxillofacial malformations and extensive or complicated facial trauma, a CT examination can be used directly or as a second-level examination (Campbell et al. 2009; Lambert et al. 1997; MüllerRichter et al. 2007; Reuben et al. 2005). The standard sinus CT protocol is performed in an axial scan (1.5 mm or thinner slices) and coronal and sagittal scans (3-mm or thinner slices) to delineate both the sinus-nasal anatomy and the extent of disease (Fig. 3.1) (Bozzato et al. 2022; Hopkins et al. 2007; Huang et al. 2009; Lund et al. 2000; Radiology 2004; Vaid et al. 2011).

The main purpose of CT is to visualise the possible presence of inflammatory or neoformed tissue and to detect bony lesions in the context of the paranasal cavities. This is possible because this method studies bony lesions, erosions, bone fractures, and calcifications accurately without the need for a contrast medium, and it also studies possible changes in the maxillary mucosa quite well, whether the latter is inflamed, hyperplastic, thickened or degenerated. Other relevant findings that are studied with sinus CT are pneumatisation of the maxillary cavity, obliteration of the COM and antrum of the sinus itself (Hopkins et al. 2007; Huang et al. 2009; Lawson et al. 2008; Lund et al. 2000; Radiology 2004; Vaid et al. 2011).

Two types of CT are mainly used: spiral CT and cone beam CT. The first type involves a higher radiation dose for the patient, but it allows for a more thorough study of soft tissue than the latter. The second is very useful in the study of the maxillofacial area, and it is chosen more frequently for deforming pathologies or traumatic injuries (Campbell et al. 2009).

The choice of radiological technique to be used is, therefore, dependent on the underlying pathology to be studied. For the diagnostic framing of sinus pathologies, the former remains more useful to date, while the latter can be chosen for pathologies of dental relevance (Campbell et al. 2009).In fact, because of the proximity of the sinus floor to the alveolar ridge, the maxillary sinus is particularly relevant for multiple dental procedures, ranging from tooth extraction to implant placement, and

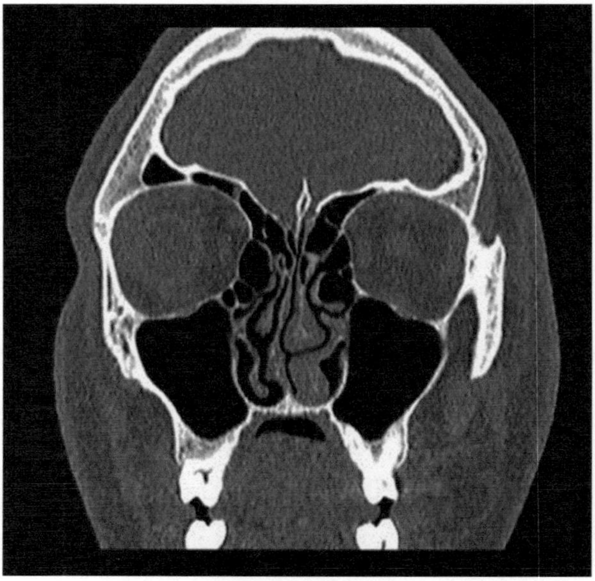

Fig. 3.1 Maxillary sinus CT scan, coronal view

in some surgical planning, it is therefore essential for dentists to have a CB CT scan, rather than a 2D or a spiral CT scan (Yeung et al. 2022).

CT shows the anatomical structure of the maxillary sinus better than all other techniques, making it the method to choose for pre and postoperative study (Fig. 3.2) (Bolger et al. 1991; Bozzato et al. 2022; Huang et al. 2009; Lund et al. 2000; Marino et al. 2020; Radiology 2004; Vaid et al. 2011).

Instead, for the diagnostic study of cancer pathologies, it is necessary to use an intravenous contrast medium or MRI, which has a higher sensitivity for neoplastic pathologies in general (Jégoux et al. 2013).

The latest radiological technique used for diagnosis, operative planning, and follow-up of many diseases affecting the maxillary sinus is MRI (Fig. 3.3). The use of this method is partly complementary or overlapping with the use of CT, while in other cases, it is the primary choice (MüllerRichter et al. 2007; Unger et al. 1990).

This technique is used to study the sinus lining mucosa, all its possible impairments, and the pneumatisation of the paranasal cavities.

It may be required as a complementary study, in addition to images obtained by CT, for complications of acute or chronic inflammatory sinus disease and for greater diagnostic accuracy. MRI provides better soft tissue resolution than CT, allowing better imaging and characterisation of inflammatory involvement of extra-sinus soft tissue and sinonasal masses (Bailey 1992; Chong and Fan 1998; Pulickal et al. 2018).

However, it should be kept in mind that since even mild abnormalities of the maxillary mucosa can be easily detected by MRI, indiscriminate interpretation of

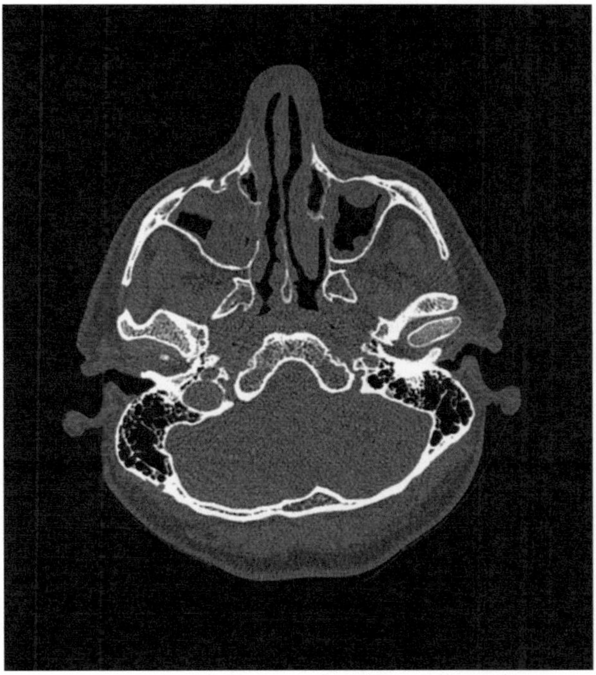

Fig. 3.2 Maxillary sinus CT scan, axial view

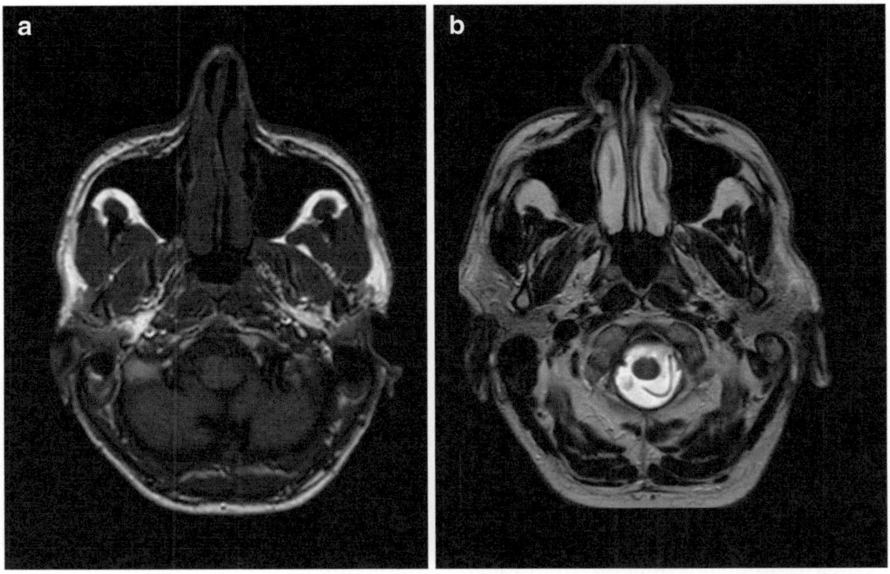

Fig. 3.3 Maxillary sinus MRI T1 (**a**) and T2 weighted (**b**), axial view

the images could lead to overdiagnosis of infectious or chronic inflammatory pathology (Puhakka et al. 2000; Rak et al. 1991). On the other hand, it is the gold standard for the diagnostic and even postoperative follow-up of all neoplastic lesions of the maxillary sinus (Madani et al. 2009; Raghavan and Phillips 2007).

The standard protocol uses thin sections of about 3 mm, including not only the sinuses but also the orbital cavities and skull base (Battal and Zamora 2023). Normal sinus mucosa appears hyperintense in T2-weighted images. Inflamed or transforming sinus mucosa improves in gadolinium-weighted T1 scans (Huyett et al. 2016; Kamalian et al. 2019; Lee et al. 2016; Som and Curtin 2011).

Therefore, in order to obtain meaningful images of the mucosa and the pathologies that afflict it in the context of the maxillary sinus, it is practically always recommended to use a contrast medium. However, it remains useful to combine these scans with CT images, as mentioned above, also for planning the treatment of different pathologies.

Imaging of Pathologies of Maxillary Sinus

The maxillary sinus is a pyramid-shaped structure with its base pointing towards the nasal sidewall and its apex pointing towards the zygomatic process of the maxilla. An ostium, located towards the cranial side, connects the maxillary sinus to the middle meatus of the nasal cavity, thus enabling the clearance of its content (Whyte and Boeddinghaus 2019) (Fig. 3.4).

Different kinds of pathologies may involve it: anatomical conditions such as aplasia or hypoplasia of the maxillary sinus, nonspecific and specific infectious and inflammatory processes, and allergic and tumoral pathologies. Diagnostic imaging techniques are often necessary to reach a correct diagnosis. Inflammatory processes, generically known as sinusitis, are the most frequent sinus pathologies. They are classified into five categories: acute maxillary sinusitis, recurring acute maxillary sinusitis, subacute maxillary sinusitis, chronic maxillary sinusitis, and acute exacerbation of chronic maxillary sinusitis, which may be specific (e.g., fungal) or nonspecific (Pérez-Sayáns et al. 2020). In most cases, they present themselves as rhinosinusitis, which is defined as the inflammation of the nose and sinuses. Rhinosinusitis is mostly a clinical diagnosis; imaging is reserved for those cases of complicated rhinosinusitis, recurrent sinusitis, chronic rhinosinusitis, and immunocompromised patients (Kroll et al. 2017). Moreover, imaging does not always correlate with symptoms. Radiography can detect thickening, air-fluid levels, opacification of the sinuses, anatomic variants, and foreign bodies (Aring and Chan 2016), but it has poor sensitivity and specificity for sinus disease and thus is not usually recommended (Lau et al. 1999). CT of the sinuses has become the gold standard for sinus imaging in the case of complicated sinus disease because of improved visualisation of sinus anatomy. Cone beam CT, a technique that creates three-dimensional images of bony and soft tissue structures of the face, is used primarily in dental imaging to evaluate the structure of the face, nasal cavity, and sinuses (Bromberg and Brizuela 2023). It may be useful in the assessment of

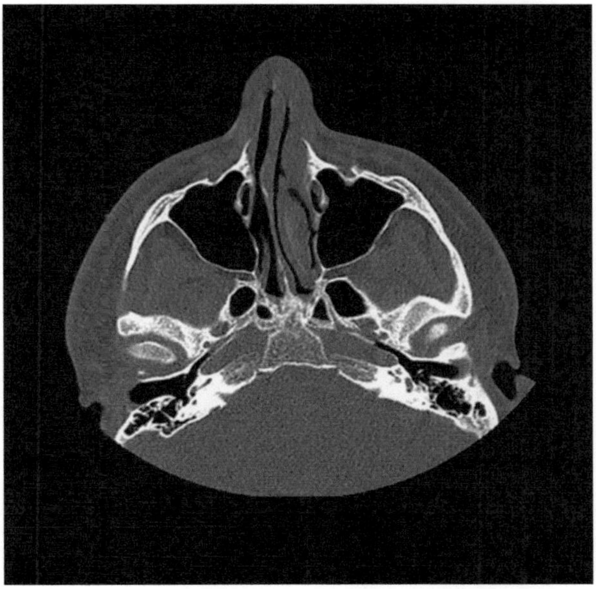

Fig. 3.4 Normal maxillary sinus, axial view

odontogenic sinusitis and maxillary sinus involvement (Kirsch et al. 2017). Magnetic resonance imaging (MRI) with or without intravenous contrast may be used to evaluate sinus disease, but it is not often the first imaging test performed. CT without contrast enhancement is the gold standard of sinus imaging and is often the first performed when complications of rhinosinusitis are suspected, as it affords the best delineation of bone and allows for visualisation of bony integrity and erosion. Findings on CT suggestive of sinusitis include thickened mucosa (>4 mm), air-fluid levels, and opacification of the sinuses (Bromberg and Brizuela 2023). MRI may be indicated when complications such as aggressive intracranial or intraorbital spread of infection or cavernous sinus thrombosis are suspected and for definition of soft tissue masses (Kirsch et al. 2017). T1 weighted MRI is recommended to evaluate abscess or extension of infection post the sinuses, and T2 weighted MRI can differentiate inflammatory mucosa from soft tissue masses. Contrast-enhanced MRI is recommended if cavernous sinus thrombosis is suspected (Frerichs and Brateanu 2020). When complications involving the orbit or cranium are suspected, the American College of Radiology recommends CT with contrast enhancement or MRI without contrast for evaluation (Kirsch et al. 2017). While the American College of Radiology notes that intravenous contrast is generally not needed, IDSA guidelines recommend contrast-enhanced CT with axial and coronal views in the case of suspected complications (Chow et al. 2012). For a chronic rhinosinusitis condition (symptoms lasting more than 12 weeks with objective evidence of inflammation of the mucosa visualised endoscopically or radiographically), a noncontrast CT is indicated as preliminary work before any surgery, as it provides

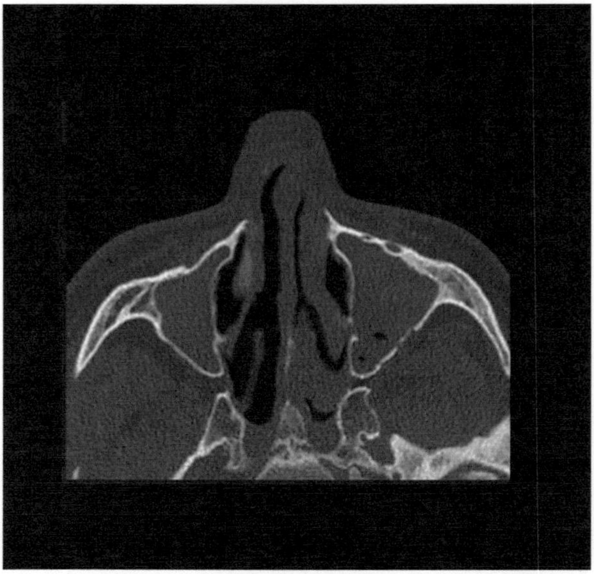

Fig. 3.5 Chronic maxillary sinusitis. Axial enhanced CT scan obtained with soft tissue setting

the best preoperative information, including delineation of complex anatomy, and can be used intraoperatively to guide surgery (Fig. 3.5) (Rosenfeld et al. 2015).

Odontogenic sinusitis refers to bacterial maxillary sinusitis, with or without extension to other paranasal sinuses. It may account for 25–40% of all chronic maxillary sinusitis, occurs unilaterally most commonly (Albu and Baciut 2010; Melén et al. 1986) and represents 45–75% of unilateral maxillary sinus opacification on computed tomography (CT). This kind of sinusitis is secondary to a dental source, with no primary sinonasal inflammation. Although cardinal sinusitis symptoms are common in Odontogenic sinusitis, foul smell is a more specific one. Nasal endoscopy was considered the most important method for confirming sinusitis, with a CT scan adding further support (Fig. 3.6) (Kroll et al. 2017).

Nasal polyps are the second most frequent disease and the most common mass lesion in the nose. They are benign mucosal protrusions into the nasal cavity of multifactorial origin and characterised by chronic mucosal inflammation. A solitary polyp may not be distinguished from a retention cyst on an unenhanced CT and MRI. Unlike cysts, polyps demonstrate marked contrast enhancement. When multiple polyps are present, sinus secretions become entrapped within the crevices between the polyps, as well as on the surfaces of the polyps. On CT scans, they show soft-tissue attenuation; however, depending on the concentration of the entrapped mucosal secretions, the CT attenuation rises, and the chronic sinonasal polyposis may show mixed CT attenuation with areas of increased density, simulating focal or diffuse dystrophic calcifications. One important observation on CT or MRI of NPs is the smooth expansion of nasal fossae and pressure atrophy of

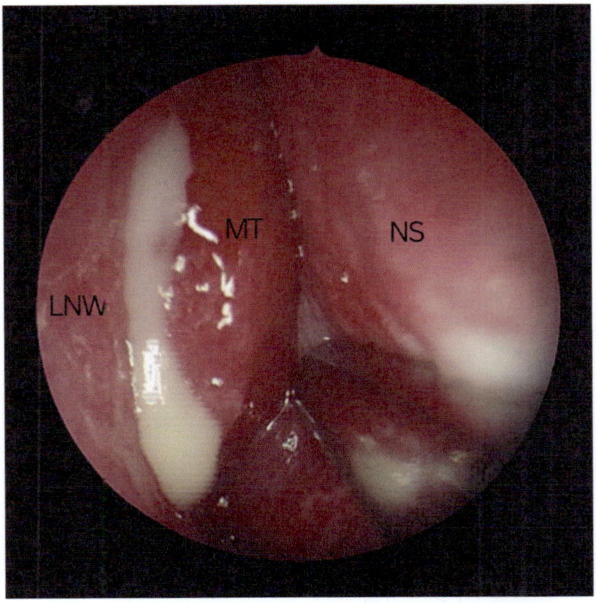

Fig. 3.6 Patient with odontogenic right sinusitis, nasal endoscopy demonstrating purulence and significant oedema in the right middle meatus

the adjacent bony wall of the sinonasal cavities. Bone erosion is not common with polyps. However, in aggressive, long-standing polyposis, there may be significant expansion of the sinuses, as well as bone erosion. Polyps tend to have various signal intensities on MRI pulse sequences. The MRI characteristics of polyps reflect the various stages of polyps (edematous, glandular, cystic, and fibrous) as well as various stages of desiccation of the entrapped mucosal secretions within the crevices between the polyps and on the surfaces of the polyps. This appearance distinguishes them from tumours that do not have variable signal intensity in each MRI sequence (Mafee et al. 2006).

The antro-choanal polyps (ACP) are also part of the polypoid pathology (18.2%). ACPs are benign lesions which emerge in the maxillary sinus mucosa and reach the choana, and the main symptom of these is nasal obstruction (Maldonado et al. 2004).

Imaging in fungal sinusitis depends on the type of the fungal infection suspected. For saprophytic fungal infestations, which are frequently asymptomatic, the diagnosis is made clinically, and no imaging is required for diagnosis. A fungus ball represents a non-invasive fungal presentation that may be evaluated with CT of the sinuses or panoramic dental imaging. It appears to be a hyperattenuated material filling a single sinus (Fig. 3.7) (Frerichs and Brateanu 2020).

A differential diagnosis must be made with mycetomas as a tropical disease. Mucormycosis (Prakash and Chakrabarti 2019) and aspergillosis (Martins and Rosa 2004) are among the most frequent specific entities. The most common causative organism of this disease is Aspergillus fumigatus, a ubiquitous dimorphic fungus

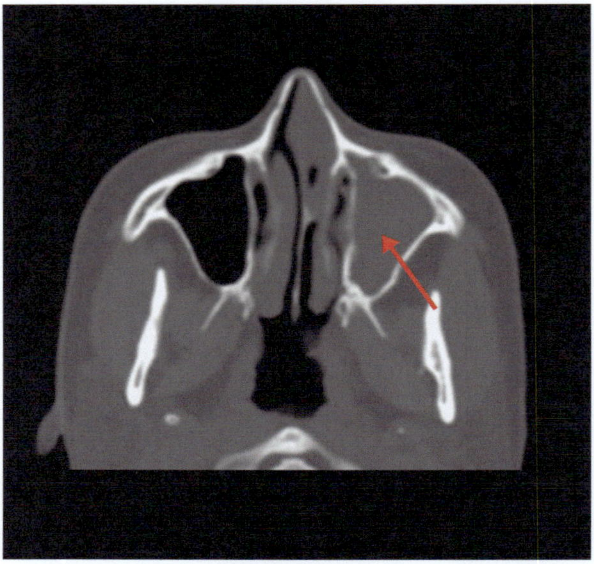

Fig. 3.7 Paranasal sinuses, CT scan axial view, fungus ball in left maxillary sinus (arrow)

that causes several types of lung diseases. In non-invasive aspergillosis, the fungus colonises a pre-existing cavity and forms a fungal ball made up of compact concentric hyphae. Mucormycosis is an angioinvasive fungal infection associated with high morbidity and mortality. This clinical entity can be found in immunosuppressed and also immunocompetent patients (Pérez-Sayáns et al. 2020).

Allergic fungal rhinosinusitis is the most common form of fungal sinus disease and is evaluated with CT or MRI. Classic findings on CT include the double density sign caused by thick fungal mucin surrounded by hyperplastic mucosa. MRI with T1 and T2 weighting can be used to support the diagnosis (Frerichs and Brateanu 2020).

Sinonasal tumours are rare neoplasms divided into benign and malignant tumours. Inverted papilloma is the most benign tumour of the nose and paranasal sinuses. It is preferably located in the lateral nasal wall, and it is characterised by its relapse tendency and its potential transformation into malignant neoplasms (Husain et al. 2012; López et al. 2016). The diagnosis of inverted papilloma may be suggested by the presence of a mass in the middle meatus with unilateral opacification of the antrum and ipsilateral paranasal sinuses. The characteristic of CT is that of a mass continuous from the middle meatus into the adjacent maxillary antrum through a wounded maxillary ostium. The maxillary antrum is the most commonly affected, although the ethmoids, the frontal and occasionally the sphenoid sinus may be involved with or without antral involvement. CT limitation is that the boundaries of the tumour are difficult or

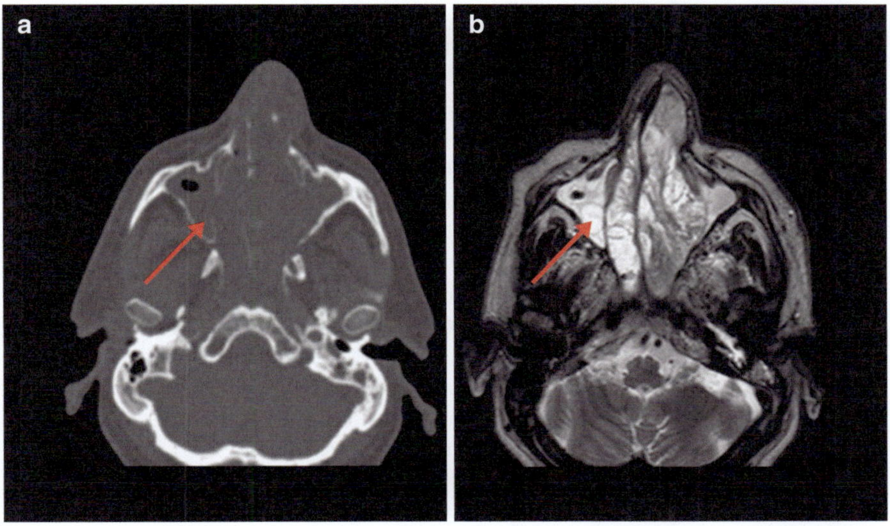

Fig. 3.8 CT scan (**a**) and MRI T2-weighted (**b**), both axial view. Inverted papilloma involving paranasal sinuses originated from the posterior wall of the maxillary right sinus

impossible to distinguish from adjacent soft tissue. The advantage of MRI over CT is in defining the extent of inverted papilloma rather than making the diagnosis. T2 weighted MRI is very accurate in distinguishing papilloma (intermediate signal) from adjacent inflammatory tissue (very high signal). In common with CT, MRI is unable to differentiate foci of coexistent squamous cell carcinoma from inverted papilloma, although it has been suggested that the malignant tumour enhances more homogeneously than the benign one (Roobottom et al. 1995). The combination of bone deformity and sclerosis suggests a slow-growing tumour, such as an inverted papilloma (Fig. 3.8).

The most common malignant tumour types are squamous cell carcinoma, adenocarcinoma, and epidermoid carcinoma. Other histological varieties are lymphomas, mostly histological subtype B. An important histological subtype is adenoid cystic carcinoma, which represents less than 2% of malignant tumours of the head and neck and 5–15% of paranasal sinuses, although it has a high local infiltration capacity (Husain et al. 2012; Trope et al. 2019). Esthesioneuroblastoma is a rare neoplasm that originates from the olfactory neuroepithelium of the nasal cavity. Metastases are rare but can occur. The most common metastases originate in the kidney, breast, thyroid, and prostate, although they have been described as originating in multiple locations (López et al. 2016). In the works of Moffa et al. and Bastier et al., we have evidence of metastasis of clear cell renal carcinoma, which appears to be the histological subtype with the greatest predilection to cause metastasis in the maxillary sinus (Bastier et al. 2018; Moffa et al. 2019).

Mucoceles are (cyst-like) structures covered with epithelium and filled with mucin, produced by the obstruction of the drainage ostium due to their destructive capacity, and usually cause pain (Abdel-Aziz et al. 2016). On CT, the mucocele appears as a homogenous lesion with smooth, clear-cut margins of bone erosions in the sinus walls; the lesion is iso-dense with brain and has no contrast enhancement unless infected(Busaba and Salman 1999; Caylakli et al. 2006; Han et al. 1995; Jayaraj et al. 1999) Maxillary sinus mucocele may expand upwards to the orbit causing proptosis and may affect the visual acuity downwards to the alveolus can even cause loosening of teeth, medially to the nasal cavity displaces the inferior turbinate and causes nasal obstruction, and anteriorly to the cheek causing a unilateral facial swelling (Caylakli et al. 2006; Khong et al. 2004; Martin et al. 2000; Patel et al. 2013).

Retention cysts, on the other hand, have a linear epithelial cystic structure that does not cause destruction, and these are caused by alterations in the homeostatic balance of the mucosa (Fig. 3.9) (Ferreira Júnior and Oliveira 2001).

Paranasal sinus osteoma is the second most common benign tumour of the paranasal sinuses. It is mostly seen in the frontal (70–80%) and ethmoid (20–25%) sinuses and less frequently in the maxillary sinus (5%) and sphenoid sinus (very rare) (Huang et al. 2001). The maxillary sinus osteomas are usually located on the lateral wall of the sinus (Zouloumis et al. 2005). Sometimes, an ethmoid osteoma can cause maxillary sinusitis by blocking the drainage routes of the maxillary sinus (Fig. 3.10).

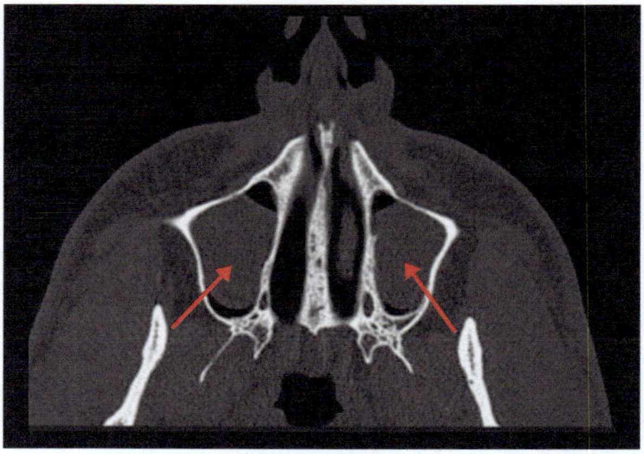

Fig. 3.9 CT scan, axial view of retention cysts (arrows) of both maxillary sinuses

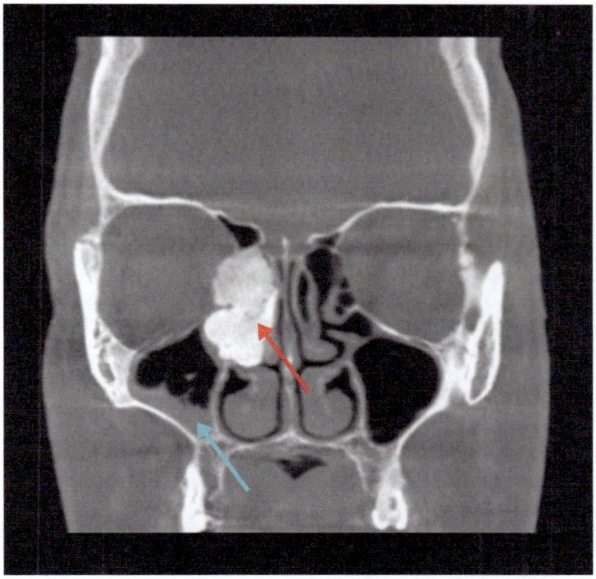

Fig. 3.10 CT scan of paranasal sinuses, coronal view shows an ethmoid osteoma (red arrow) involving the right osteo-meatal complex causing maxillary sinusitis (blue arrow)

References

Abdel-Aziz M, El-Hoshy H, Azooz K et al (2016) Maxillary sinus mucocele: predisposing factors, clinical presentations, and treatment. Oral Maxillofac Surg 21:55–58. https://doi.org/10.1007/s10006-016-0599-5

Albu S, Baciut M (2010) Failures in endoscopic surgery of the maxillary sinus. Otolaryngol Head Neck Surg 142:196–201. https://doi.org/10.1016/j.otohns.2009.10.038

Aring AM, Chan MM (2016) Current concepts in adult acute rhinosinusitis. AAFP. https://www.aafp.org/pubs/afp/issues/2016/0715/p97.html

Bailey BJ (1992) Otolaryngology-head and neck surgery. JAMA 268:395–397. https://doi.org/10.1001/jama.268.3.395

Bastier P-L, Dunion D, De Bonnecaze G et al (2018) Renal cell carcinoma metastatic to the sinonasal cavity: a review and report of 8 cases. Ear Nose Throat J 97:E6–E12. https://doi.org/10.1177/014556131809700902

Battal B, Zamora C (2023) Imaging of skull base tumors. Tomography 9:1196–1235. https://doi.org/10.3390/tomography9040097

Bell D, Gaillard F. Acute sinusitis. Radiopaediaorg. 2008 Oct 31

Bhattacharyya N, Fried MP (2003) The accuracy of computed tomography in the diagnosis of chronic rhinosinusitis. Laryngoscope 113:125–129. https://doi.org/10.1097/00005537-200301000-00023

Bolger WE, Parsons DS, Butzin CA (1991) Paranasal sinus bony anatomic variations and mucosal abnormalities: CT analysis for endoscopic sinus surgery. Laryngoscope 101:56–64. https://doi.org/10.1288/00005537-199101000-00010

Bozzato A, Arens C, Linxweiler M et al (2022) Multicenter observational study to evaluate the diagnostic value of sonography in patients with chronic rhinosinusitis. Diagnostics 12:2065. https://doi.org/10.3390/diagnostics12092065

Bromberg N, Brizuela M (2023) Dental cone beam computed tomography. StatPearls—NCBI Bookshelf. https://www.ncbi.nlm.nih.gov/books/NBK592390/

Busaba NY, Salman SD (1999) Maxillary sinus mucoceles: clinical presentation and long-term results of endoscopic surgical treatment. Laryngoscope 109:1446–1449. https://doi.org/10.1097/00005537-199909000-00017

Campbell PD, Zinreich SJ, Aygun N (2009) Imaging of the paranasal sinuses and in-office CT. Otolaryngol Clin N Am 42:753–764. https://doi.org/10.1016/j.otc.2009.08.015

Caylakli F, Yavuz H, Cagici AC, Ozluoglu LN (2006) Endoscopic sinus surgery for maxillary sinus mucoceles. Head Face Med 2:29. https://doi.org/10.1186/1746-160x-2-29

Chong VF, Fan YF (1998) Comparison of CT and MRI features in sinusitis. Eur J Radiol 29:47–54. https://doi.org/10.1016/s0720-048x(98)00019-9

Chow AW, Benninger MS, Brook I et al (2012) Executive summary: IDSA clinical practice guideline for acute bacterial rhinosinusitis in children and adults. Clin Infect Dis 54:1041–1045. https://doi.org/10.1093/cid/cir1043

da Silva de Menezes JD, Moura LB, Pereira-Filho VA, Hochuli-Vieira E (2016) Maxillary sinus mucocele as a late complication in zygomatic-orbital complex fracture. Craniomaxillofac Trauma Reconstr 9:342–344. https://doi.org/10.1055/s-0036-1582453

Ferreira Júnior O, Oliveira DT (2001) Mucosal cysts of the maxillary sinus: a literature review. Organo Oficial De La Sociedad Espanola De Medicina Oral Y De La Academia Iberoamericana De Patologia Y Medicina Bucal, Medicina Oral

Frerichs N, Brateanu A (2020) Rhinosinusitis and the role of imaging. Cleve Clin J Med 87:485–492. https://doi.org/10.3949/ccjm.87a.19092

Han MH, Chang KH, Lee CH et al (1995) Cystic expansile masses of the maxilla: differential diagnosis with CT and MR. Am J Neuroradiol 16(2):333–338

Hopkins C, Browne JP, Slack R et al (2007) The Lund-Mackay staging system for chronic rhinosinusitis: how is it used and what does it predict? Otolaryngol Head Neck Surg 137:555–561. https://doi.org/10.1016/j.otohns.2007.02.004

Hsu C-C, Sheng C, Ho C-Y (2018) Efficacy of sinus ultrasound in diagnosis of acute and subacute maxillary sinusitis. J Chin Med Assoc 81:898–904. https://doi.org/10.1016/j.jcma.2018.03.005

Huang H, Liu C, Lin K, Chen H (2001) Giant ethmoid osteoma with orbital extension, a nasoendoscopic approach using an intranasal drill. Laryngoscope 111:430–432. https://doi.org/10.1097/00005537-200103000-00010

Huang BY, Lloyd KM, DelGaudio JM et al (2009) Failed endoscopic sinus surgery: Spectrum of CT findings in the frontal recess. Radiographics 29:177–195. https://doi.org/10.1148/rg.291085118

Hung KF, Ai QYH, Leung YY, Yeung AWK (2022a) Potential and impact of artificial intelligence algorithms in dento-maxillofacial radiology. Clin Oral Investig 26:5535–5555. https://doi.org/10.1007/s00784-022-04477-y

Hung KF, Ai QYH, Wong LM et al (2022b) Current applications of deep learning and radiomics on CT and CBCT for maxillofacial diseases. Diagnostics 13:110. https://doi.org/10.3390/diagnostics13010110

Husain Q, Kanumuri VV, Svider PF et al (2012) Sinonasal adenoid cystic carcinoma. Otolaryngol Head Neck Surg 148:29–39. https://doi.org/10.1177/0194599812464020

Huyett P, Lee S, Ferguson BJ, Wang EW (2016) Sinus opacification in the intensive care unit patient. Laryngoscope 126:2433–2438. https://doi.org/10.1002/lary.25971

Jayaraj S, Patel S, Ghufoor K, Frosh A (1999) Mucocoeles of the maxillary sinus. Int J Clin Pract 53:391–393. https://doi.org/10.1111/j.1742-1241.1999.tb11754.x

Jégoux F, Métreau A, Louvel G, Bedfert C (2013) Paranasal sinus cancer. Eur Ann Otorhinolaryngol Head Neck Dis 130:327–335. https://doi.org/10.1016/j.anorl.2012.07.007

John O, Mateer JR, Reardon RF, Joing SA (2013) Ma and Mateer's emergency ultrasound, 3rd edn. McGraw Hill Professional

Kamalian S, Avery L, Lev MH et al (2019) Nontraumatic head and neck emergencies. Radiographics 39:1808–1823. https://doi.org/10.1148/rg.2019190159

Karantanas AH, Sandris V (1997) Maxillary sinus inflammatory disease: ultrasound compared to computed tomography. Comput Med Imaging Graph 21:233–241. https://doi.org/10.1016/s0895-6111(97)00015-3
Khong JJ, Malhotra R, Selva D, Wormald PJ (2004) Efficacy of endoscopic sinus surgery for paranasal sinus mucocele including modified endoscopic Lothrop procedure for frontal sinus mucocele. J Laryngol Otol 118:352–356. https://doi.org/10.1258/002221504323086534
Kirsch CFE, Bykowski J, Aulino JM et al (2017) ACR appropriateness criteria® sinonasal disease. J Am Coll Radiol 14:S550–S559. https://doi.org/10.1016/j.jacr.2017.08.041
Kroll H, Hom J, Ahuja N et al (2017) R-SCAN: imaging for uncomplicated acute rhinosinusitis. J Am Coll Radiol 14:82–83.e1. https://doi.org/10.1016/j.jacr.2016.08.018
Lambert DM, Mirvis SE, Shanmuganathan K, Tilghman DL (1997) Computed tomography exclusion of osseous paranasal sinus injury in blunt trauma patients: the "clear sinus" sign. J Oral Maxillofac Surg 55:1207–1210. https://doi.org/10.1016/s0278-2391(97)90167-1
Lau J, Zucker D, Engels E et al (1999) Diagnosis and treatment of acute bacterial rhinosinusitis: summary. AHRQ Evidence Report Summaries—NCBI Bookshelf. https://www.ncbi.nlm.nih.gov/books/NBK11860/
Lawson W, Patel ZM, Lin FY (2008) The development and pathologic processes that influence maxillary sinus pneumatization. Anat Rec 291:1554–1563. https://doi.org/10.1002/ar.20774
Lee EK, Lee EJ, Kim S, Lee YS (2016) Importance of contrast-enhanced fluid-attenuated inversion recovery magnetic resonance imaging in various intracranial pathologic conditions. Korean J Radiol 17:127. https://doi.org/10.3348/kjr.2016.17.1.127
Lichtenstein DA (2007) General ultrasound in the critically ill. Springer
Lichtenstein D, Biderman P, Mezière G, Gepner A (1998) The "sinusogram", a real-time ultrasound sign of maxillary sinusitis. Intensive Care Med 24:1057–1061. https://doi.org/10.1007/s001340050716
Lombardo N, Ferrise P, Piazzetta G, Motta G (2018) Maxillary sinus mucocele with orbital complications. Ann Ital Chir 7:S2239253X18028190
López F, Devaney KO, Hanna EY et al (2016) Metastases to nasal cavity and paranasal sinuses. Head Neck 38:1847–1854. https://doi.org/10.1002/hed.24502
Lund VJ, Savy L, Lloyd G (2000) Imaging for endoscopic sinus surgery in adults. J Laryngol Otol 114:395–397. https://doi.org/10.1258/0022215001905670
Madani G, Beale TJ, Lund VJ (2009) Imaging of sinonasal tumors. Semin Ultrasound CT MR 30:25–38. https://doi.org/10.1053/j.sult.2008.10.013
Mafee MF, Tran BH, Chapa AR (2006) Imaging of rhinosinusitis and its complications: plain film, CT, and MRI. Clin Rev Allergy Immunol 30:165–186. https://doi.org/10.1385/criai:30:3:165
Maldonado M, Martínez A, Alobid I, Mullol J (2004) The antrochoanal polyp. Rhinology 42:178–182
Marino MJ, Riley CA, Wu EL et al (2020) Variability of paranasal sinus pneumatization in the absence of sinus disease. Ochsner J 20:170–175. https://doi.org/10.31486/toj.19.0053
Martin RJ, Jackman DS, Philbert RF, McCoy JM (2000) Massive proptosis of the globe. J Oral Maxillofac Surg 58:794–799. https://doi.org/10.1053/joms.2000.7268
Martins WD, Rosa EAR (2004) Aspergillosis of the maxillary sinus: review and case report. Scand J Infect Dis 36:758–761. https://doi.org/10.1080/00365540410021036a
Melén I, Lindahl L, Andréasson L, Rundcrantz H (1986) Chronic maxillary sinusitis: definition, diagnosis and relation to dental infections and nasal polyposis. Acta Otolaryngol 101:320–327. https://doi.org/10.3109/00016488609132845
Moffa A, Casale M, Moffa AP et al (2019) Maxillary sinus mass as first presentation of silent metastatic renal cell carcinoma. J Craniofac Surg 30:e135–e137. https://doi.org/10.1097/scs.0000000000005035
MüllerRichter UDA, Kohlhof JK, Driemel O et al (2007) Traumatic dislocation of the globe into the maxillary sinus. Int J Oral Maxillofac Surg 36:1207–1210. https://doi.org/10.1016/j.ijom.2007.05.017

Patel PA, Warren SM, McCarthy JG (2013) Maxillary mucocele with proptosis and visual impairment: a late complication of Le Fort III distraction. J Craniofac Surg 24:2000–2002. https://doi.org/10.1097/scs.0b013e3182a4d72e

Pérez-Sayáns M, Peñaranda JMS, Quintanilla JAS et al (2020) Clinicopathological features of 214 maxillary sinus pathologies. A ten-year single-centre retrospective clinical study. Head Face Med 16:24. https://doi.org/10.1186/s13005-020-00239-x

Prakash H, Chakrabarti A (2019) Global epidemiology of mucormycosis. J Fungi 5:26. https://doi.org/10.3390/jof5010026

Puhakka T, Heikkinen T, Mäkelä MJ et al (2000) Validity of ultrasonography in diagnosis of acute maxillary sinusitis. Arch Otolaryngol Head Neck Surg 126:1482. https://doi.org/10.1001/archotol.126.12.1482

Pulickal GG, Navaratnam AV, Nguyen T et al (2018) Imaging sinonasal disease with MRI: providing insight over and above CT. Eur J Radiol 102:157–168. https://doi.org/10.1016/j.ejrad.2018.02.033

Radiology (ed) (2004) Head and Neck Imaging, 4th edn. Radiology. http://pubs.rsna.org/doi/10.1148/radiol.2331042535. Accessed 31 Jul 2024

Raghavan P, Phillips CD (2007) Magnetic resonance imaging of sinonasal malignancies. Top Magn Reson Imaging 18:259–267. https://doi.org/10.1097/rmr.0b013e31815711b7

Rak KM, Newell JD, Yakes WF et al (1991) Paranasal sinuses on MR images of the brain: significance of mucosal thickening. Am J Roentgenol 156:381–384. https://doi.org/10.2214/ajr.156.2.1898819

Reffat M, Sweed E, AbdulSahib M (2022) Role of MDCT in the detection of paranasal variants and their surgical and clinical impact. Benha Med J 40(Spec Issue, Radiology):129–139. https://doi.org/10.21608/bmfj.2022.95331.1480

Reuben AD, Watt-Smith SR, Dobson D, Golding SJ (2005) A comparative study of evaluation of radiographs, CT and 3D reformatted CT in facial trauma: what is the role of 3D? Br J Radiol 78:198–201. https://doi.org/10.1259/bjr/26977910

Roobottom CA, Jewell FM, Kabala J (1995) Primary and recurrent inverting papilloma: appearances with magnetic resonance imaging. Clin Radiol 50:472–475. https://doi.org/10.1016/s0009-9260(05)83163-0

Rosenfeld RM, Piccirillo JF, Chandrasekhar SS et al (2015) Clinical practice guideline (update): adult sinusitis. Otolaryngol Head Neck Surg 152:S1–S39. https://doi.org/10.1177/0194599815572097

Som PM, Curtin HD (2011) Head and neck imaging. Elsevier Health Sciences

Trope M, Triantafillou V, Kohanski M et al (2019) Adenoid cystic carcinoma of the sinonasal tract: a review of the national cancer database. Int Forum Allergy Rhinol 4:427–434

Unger JM, Gentry LR, Grossman JE (1990) Sphenoid fractures: prevalence, sites, and significance. Radiology 175:175–180. https://doi.org/10.1148/radiology.175.1.2315477

Vaid S, Vaid N, Rawat S, Ahuja AT (2011) An imaging checklist for pre-FESS CT: framing a surgically relevant report. Clin Radiol 66:459–470. https://doi.org/10.1016/j.crad.2010.11.010

Whyte A, Boeddinghaus R (2019) The maxillary sinus: physiology, development and imaging anatomy. Dentomaxillofac Radiol 48:20190205. https://doi.org/10.1259/dmfr.20190205

Yeung AWK, Hung KF, Li DTS, Leung YY (2022) The use of CBCT in evaluating the health and pathology of the maxillary sinus. Diagnostics 12:2819. https://doi.org/10.3390/diagnostics12112819

Zouloumis L, Lazaridis N, Maria P, Epivatianos A (2005) Osteoma of the ethmoidal sinus: a rare case of recurrence. Br J Oral Maxillofac Surg 43:520–522. https://doi.org/10.1016/j.bjoms.2005.01.014

4 Epidemiology and Incidence of Maxillary Sinus Lesions

Goran Latif Omer, Mohammed Gubari, Pier Giorgio Giacomini, Gianluca Velletrani, Rekawt Hama Rashid Kareem, Sahand Soran Ali, Aland Salih Abdullah, Beatrice Francavilla, and Stefano Di Girolamo

Introduction

Many abnormalities occur within the maxillary sinus and are relatively common. Many different aetiologies contribute to these lesions, which are broadly divided into non-neoplastic, neoplastic benign, and neoplastic malignant.

Maxillary Rhinosinusitis

Chronic Rhinosinusitis and Nasal Polyposis

Nasal polyps are lesions that extend into the nasal airway from the ethmoid sinus due to inflammation. It can present with inflammation of the mucosa lasting for more than 12 weeks. Chronic rhinosinusitis with nasal polyposis (CRSwNP) presents with nasal stuffiness, loss of smell, and painful sinuses (Masood et al. 2007).

G. L. Omer (✉) · M. Gubari · S. S. Ali · A. S. Abdullah
Department of Clinical Sciences, College of Medicine, University of Sulaimani, Sulaymaniyah, KRI, Iraq

P. G. Giacomini · G. Velletrani · B. Francavilla · S. Di Girolamo
Department of Otorhinolaryngology, University of Rome Tor Vergata, Rome, Italy

R. H. R. Kareem
Royal Hospital, Sulaymaniyah, KRI, Iraq

© The Author(s), under exclusive license to Springer Nature Switzerland AG 2025
G. L. Omer, S. Di Girolamo (eds.), *Maxillary Sinus: A Comprehensive Guide*, https://doi.org/10.1007/978-3-031-83468-4_4

Acute Infective Rhinosinusitis

Inflammation of the nasal mucosa presents with sudden onset of 2 or more nasal blockages and congestion, nasal discharge, and a decrease in smell or a complete absence of smell, all lasting for less than 12 weeks (ACAAI 2022).

Fungal Maxillary Rhinosinusitis

Allergic Fungal Rhinosinusitis

An intense localised inflammation of the sinuses that is either allergic and/or eosinophilic. This intense inflammation leads to the accumulation of eosinophilic mucus and the characteristic radiographic findings of the disease (Akhondi et al. 2023).

Mucormycosis

A fungal infection that is mostly harmless in immunocompetent; however, in immunocompromised patients such as those with poorly controlled diabetes, haematological malignancies and steroid users, the outcome is deadly.

Fungus Ball

A fungus ball, also known as aspergilloma, is a non-invasive fungal lesion that is composed of a dense collection of fungal hyphae that typically develop in a solitary maxillary sinus.

Chronic Invasive Fungal Sinusitis

This is a subdivision of fungal sinusitis that has histopathological evidence of invasion to surrounding soft tissue.

Granulomatous Invasive Rhinosinusitis

A subtype of invasive fungal sinusitis that typically occurs in immunocompromised individuals and has histopathological evidence of granuloma formations.

Benign Lesions of the Maxillary Sinus

Antrochoanal Polyp

Isolated polypoid lesions of the sinonasal mucosa develop in the maxillary sinus (antrum). These polyps can penetrate and widen the sinus ostium and posterior nasal cavity in the region of the choana.

Retention Cyst

It is an epithelium-lined cyst containing mucous or serous fluid (yellowish or clear). It results from an obstruction of the mucosal serous and/or mucinous glands ducts.

Dentigerous Cyst

This is a type of odontogenic test that always includes a tooth that cannot complete its eruption process. It occurs around the crown due to the fluid accumulation between the layers of the enamel organ.

Maxillary Sinus Cholesterol Granuloma

A cholesterol granuloma (CG) is granulation tissue that results from recurrent haemorrhage. They resemble benign tumours, thus not easily diagnosed and have a cystic cavity filled with a fluid that is chocolate-brown in colour.

Angiofibroma Involving Maxillary Sinus

Nasopharyngeal angiofibroma is a rare benign fibrovascular tumour. Although histologically benign, when it comes to its vascular entities, the tumour is considered aggressive.

Inverted Papilloma

Inverted papilloma is a benign epithelial growth that occurs in the underlying stroma of the nasal cavity and the paranasal sinuses. It is most well-known for its invasiveness, tendency to recur, and relationship with malignancy, which are the three characteristics that differentiate it vastly from other sinonasal tumours.

Osteoblastoma

A rare neoplasm characterised by osteoblast proliferation and formation of bone trabeculae within a vascular and fibrotic connective tissue stroma is referred to as osteoblastoma (Masood et al. 2007).

Fibrous Dysplasia

The replaced fibro-osseous fibrous dysplasia (FD) is defined as a non-malignant bone disease with slow growth and a recurrent character in which the normal cancellous bone structure is replaced by a fibro-osseous tissue. This tissue subsequently leads to overgrowth and distortion of the affected part within the bone.

Ossifying Fibroma

Ossifying fibroma is a benign, non-cancerous tumour. The tumour is composed of bone tissue forming within connective tissue. These tumours most often affect bones in your face, with emphasis on the jawbones, and they also grow slowly.

Maxillary Mucocele

Mucoceles are epithelial lined mucus-containing sacs located within one of the paranasal sinuses, leading to expansion of the involved sinus cavity and remodelling of the sinus walls. It is lined by either pseudostratified or low-columnar epithelium in contradistinction to a cyst that has a distinct, separate membrane.

Schwannoma

Schwannoma(SC), also known as neurilemmoma, is a benign tumour of nerve sheath origin arising from any nerve that is covered with a Schwann cell sheath. These include the cranial nerves (except for optic and olfactory), the spinal nerves, or nerves arising from autonomic nervous systems, especially the sympathetic system.

Osteoma

Osteomas are benign tumours of the head composed of bone. These tumours are non-cancerous but do result in headaches, sinus infections, vision problems, and hearing issues.

Pyogenic Granuloma

Small, raised red bumps of skin with a smooth surface and a bleeding tendency due to its high vascularity.

Malignant Lesions of the Maxillary Sinus

Squamous Cell Carcinoma

A form of cancer that arises from squamous cells. These cells make up the middle and outer layers of the skin. The lesion commonly occurs in areas of the body exposed to sunlight and ultraviolet (UV) light. Although it generally follows an aggressive pattern, squamous cell carcinoma of the maxillary sinus is rare.

Adenoid Cystic Carcinoma

Adenoid Cystic carcinoma is a slow-growing malignant tumour of the salivary gland. The tumour is uncommon, and it is rare for the tumour to occur in the maxillary sinus; however, it does have an inclination for distant metastasis when it does.

Olfactory Neuroblastoma

Olfactory neuroblastoma, also referred to as esthesioneuroblastoma, is a tumour arising from within the nasal cavity. The lesion is known to arise from the neuroepithelium and to have neuroblastic differentiation. It is rare for the lesion to occur in areas such as the sphenoid sinus, sellar region, anterior ethmoid, pituitary gland, and maxillary sinus due to the lack of neuroepithelium.

Maxillary Sinus Lymphoma

Lymphomas are cancers of abnormal white blood cell proliferation beginnings within the lymphatic system. Sinus cavity lymphoma arises from lymphoid cells that are typically found within the bone marrow or submucosa. A mass of soft tissue can be identified within the sinus.

Other Pathologies of Maxillary Sinus

Silent Sinus Syndrome

Silent sinus syndrome (SSS), also known as imploding antrum syndrome, is a very rare condition, usually represented by asymptomatic spontaneous collapse of the sinus walls and floor of the orbit. Silent sinus syndrome (SSS) and chronic maxillary sinus atelectasis (CMA) have been used interchangeably in the past; the fundamental difference between CMA and SSS is the absence of sinusitis symptoms and facial pain.

Maxillary Sinus Agenesis

Embryologically, the development of the maxillary sinus begins in the tenth week. At about the 16th week, the primordial structure of the maxillary sinus arises from the inferior aspect of the ethmoidal infundibulum. Maxillary sinus agenesis refers to the lack of maxillary sinus due to the absence of its primordial tissue.

Missed Maxillary Sinus Ostium Syndrome

The phenomenon occurs whenever the natural maxillary sinus ostium is missing. This happens when the most anterior part of the uncinate process is not completely removed, which consequently obscures the site of the natural maxillary sinus ostium. This obstruction inhibits the middle meatal antrostomy from interacting with the natural ostium, leading to recirculation.

Maxillary Sinus Fracture

It occurs in patients who sustain facial trauma, generally from road traffic accidents, sports or assault. To prevent morbidity and mortality, these fractures require immediate assessment.

Maxillary Sinus Foreign Body

Cases of foreign bodies entering the sinuses are rare. This is why whenever unusual symptoms appear, the thought that a foreign object may be in the maxillary sinus does not always come to mind. However, if sinusitis does not go away for a long time, it is worth taking an X-ray to see if it is caused by a foreign body.

Oroantral Fistula

An unnatural communication is present between the oral cavity and the maxillary sinus. This fistula is epithelialised and occurs when the oroantral communication doesn't spontaneously involute but rather remains and gets epithelialised.

Cleft Palate

An opening that is present in the roof of the mouth of a newborn baby. This results in communication between the oral cavity and the nose.

Purpose of Epidemiology

Through epidemiology, the long-term health of the community can be improved, and the lives of many can be saved. Epidemiology can prevent and possibly even reverse unwanted health outcomes (Writer 2019). One way this is done is through population screening. Screening is when usually non-invasive and simple tests are used to test an apparently healthy population with the aim of identifying those individuals who either pose a risk factor for the disease or those who may have an early stage of the disease but are still asymptomatic (Faculty of Public Health 2024).

To diagnose pathologies of the maxillary sinus, both radiography and histopathological analysis are required. Radiographs are the tool generally used for screening maxillary sinus anomalies. This is because although they have harmful radiations, they are still less invasive than biopsy and histopathological analysis.

Prevalence of Maxillary Sinus Lesions

Studies evaluating the prevalence of the different maxillary sinuses tend to utilise radiographic means to screen either high-risk population groups or retrospectively evaluate hospital or clinic records of patients who have already undergone imaging of the sinuses. Different studies yield different results regarding the most common pathologies. Studies have shown unspecified sinusitis to be the most common, occurring in 44.4% of the individuals, followed by polyps in 18.2% and malignant tumours in 9.8% (Pérez-Sayáns et al. 2020). Others have demonstrated mucosal thickening as the most frequent lesion of the maxillary sinus, accounting for 35.1% of the lesions. Other common lesions were opacification, occurring in 16.6%, and polypoidal-mucosal thickening, present in 7.2% (Raghav et al. 2014). Drumond et al. conducted a spiral CT scan study to evaluate 762 cases for maxillary sinus abnormalities. Similar to the previous studies, mucosal thickenings with 324 (21/5%) cases were found to be the most common pathologies. This was followed by polypoid lesions with 164 (10.76%) cases, chronic sinusitis with 114 (7.48%) cases and odontogenic sinusitis with 35 (2.29%) cases. On the contrary, bone injuries with only 10 (0.65%) cases, foreign bodies with 2 (0.13%) cases and oroantral fistula with only 1 (0.06%) cases were the least common pathologies of the maxillary sinus (Drumond et al. 2016).

Furthermore, Drumond et al. also evaluated for the side most affected by maxillary sinus lesions. Among the 762 patients with their CT scans analysed, 457 (59.97%) of them had abnormal CT scan findings. Among these 457 abnormal patients, 190 (41.57%) had abnormalities present in both maxillary sinuses, whereas 139 (30.41%) patients had anomalies on the right side alone, and 128 (28.01%) had anomalies on the left alone. Not all lesions of the maxillary sinus affect the same anatomical locations. When considering isolated locations within the sinus, the inferior surface of the sinus was the most common, with (24.26%) of the cases. However, combined lesions or lesions affecting more than one surface of the sinus were the most common overall, occurring in 57.34% of the cases. This was followed by the medial with 41 (6.33%) and the lateral with 37 (5.72%) cases. The posterior surface with only 8 (1.24%) cases was the least common surface (Drumond et al. 2016).

Risk Factors of Maxillary Sinus Lesions

Many studies have evaluated the association between gender and different maxillary sinus pathologies; however, although some mild differences do exist, the majority have found no significant association (Tassoker 2019).

Other studies have evaluated concha bullosa, maxillary sinus septa, and nasal septal deviation as potential risk factors contributing to maxillary sinus pathologies. None of the factors had a statistically significant correlation with maxillary sinus pathologies (p-value > 0.05) [A4]. Furthermore, a risk factor found to have a significant association with maxillary sinus anomalies was lesions adjacent to the maxillary sinus. The study showed that adjacent lesions increased the likelihood of a maxillary sinus pathology by 5.24 times on the right and 4.67 times on the left (Tassoker 2019).

Regarding cancers of the maxillary sinus, it shares its risk factors with other cancers occurring in the nasal and paranasal cavities (National Cancer Institute 2023).

Demographic Factors

- Sex: Men are two times more likely to encounter cancers of the paranasal and nasal cavities.
- Age: The majority (80%) of patients are older than 55 years.
- Race: White people are much more likely to be impacted than black people.

Occupational Factors

- Wood dust.
- Dust from textiles.

- Leather dust.
- Flour.
- Nickel and chromium dust.
- Mustard and radium gas.

Others

- Smoking: Smoking is specifically associated with squamous cell carcinoma of the maxillary sinus.
- Human papillomavirus (HPV).
- Genetic factors.
- Prior radiation treatment.
- Glues.
- Formaldehyde.
- Organic solvents.

Certain genes have been studied and found to have a role in the development of different maxillary sinus lesions. Among these genes, the IRAK 4 gene has been found to make an individual more susceptible to gram-positive infections and individuals with this mutation have demonstrated a weakened leukocytic response to toll-like receptors (TLR). This susceptibility to infections subsequently makes the individual more prone to odontogenic sinusitis (Pereira et al. 2014).

Another pathology that can involve the maxillary sinus is cleft lip/palate. The pathology has a multifactorial aetiology. Both genetics and environment are involved in the pathophysiology of cleft lip and palate (Betin-Noriega et al. 2023).

Genes Involved in the Aetiology of Cleft Lip and Palate

- T-box transcription factor-22 (TBX22).
- Poliovirus receptor-like-1 (PVRL1).
- Interferon regulatory factor-6 (IRF6).

Environmental Factors Associated with Cleft Lip and Palate

- Smoking.
- Alcohol use.
- Deficiency of folic acid and other vitamins.
- Steroids.
- Anticonvulsants.

Regarding mucosal thickenings, studies have found that elevated height of the ostium, decreased length or width of the infundibulum, periapical lesions, and periodontal involvement are all factors associated with an increase in the thickening. Moreover, foreign material presence is also correlated with mucosal abnormalities along with atrophic alveolar processes (Edens et al. 2016).

Another common pathology of the maxillary sinus is sinusitis. Inflammation of the maxillary sinus mucosa has many risk factors (Akhondi et al. 2023).

Risk Factors of Maxillary Sinusitis

- Upper respiratory tract infection.
- Allergic rhinitis.
- Due to the close proximity to the maxillary posterior teeth, 10% of the cases of maxillary sinusitis are due to spread from odontogenic sources.

Common Pathogens Involved in Bacterial Maxillary Sinusitis

- Streptococcus pneumoniae.
- Haemophilus influenzae.

Risk Factors for Fungal Maxillary Sinusitis (Leland et al. 2022)

- Diabetes.
- Chemotherapy.
- Corticosteroids.
- Any other cause of immunosuppression.

Common Organisms Responsible for Fungal Maxillary Sinusitis

- Aspergillus.
- Mucor and Rhizopus (Mucormycosis).

Geographical Distribution of Maxillary Sinus Lesions

Based on the aetiology, lesions of the maxillary sinus might occur more commonly in certain geographical regions than others. Developing third-world countries with high pollution have a greater prevalence of maxillary sinusitis. This is because the relationship between air pollution and both the incidence/prevalence and the severity of maxillary sinusitis has been well established (Choi 2024). Regarding fungal sinusitis, countries such as Sudan, Pakistan, and India have a higher incidence of granulomatous invasive sinusitis, which often arises as a complication of chronic fungal sinusitis. Regarding mucormycosis, countries in Asia account for the majority of its traumatic cases, whereas for cases that occur due to immunosuppression, the majority of the cases are in developed countries (Leland et al. 2022).

Outcomes and Prognosis

The prognosis of maxillary sinus lesions varies widely based on the type and the stage or extent of the lesion. For malignant tumours, the cure rate is up to 80%, provided that the tumour is still in its early stages. The overall 5-year survival rate is approximately 40%; however, this decreases to less than 20% for patients who present with an unresectable tumour and have already been treated with radiotherapy (Kara et al. 2015). These survival rates fluctuate based on many tumour characteristics and the type of therapy received.

Prognosis of Some of the Benign Maxillary Sinus Lesions

- Antrochoanal polyp: 15% recurrence rate in children, higher in patients solely treated endoscopically.
- Retention cyst: Spontaneous regression and disappearance are between 17.6% and 38%.
- Dentigerous cyst: Complete removal of the cyst yields a good prognosis (Lin et al. 2014).
- Maxillary sinus cholesterol granuloma: Following resection, very little recurrence occurs.
- Angiofibroma: Since the tumour is benign, the prognosis is considered good; however, disease recurrence can occur with advanced forms of the tumour. Rarely transforms into malignant tumours.
- Inverted Papilloma: The 5-year survival of inverted papilloma is 98.6%; with dysplasia, it is 100%, and with carcinoma, it is 66% (Bokhari et al. 2012).
- Osteoblastoma: Proper surgical excision of the tumour with a thorough long-term follow-up yields a good prognosis (Bhattacharya et al. 2013).
- Ossifying fibroma: An ossifying fibroma can regrow months or years after surgery. Children are more prone than adults to have a tumour recurrence.
- Maxillary mucocele: After complete surgical excision, the prognosis is excellent.
- Schwannoma: It is very rare for recurrence to occur after successful enbloc removal of the tumour.

Prognosis of some of the Malignant Maxillary Sinus Lesions

- Squamous cell carcinoma: Due to its aggressive nature and the fact that the lesion becomes advanced by the time the disease becomes symptomatic and is diagnosed, the survival rate decreases, and the prognosis is unfavourable.
- Adenocystic carcinoma: Compared to other adenocystic carcinoma within the head and neck region, the long-term overall prognosis of maxillary sinus adenocystic carcinoma is worse. This worse prognosis of the lesion within the maxillary sinus could be attributed to its subclinical invasion and late detection.
- Olfactory Neuroblastoma: The overall survival rate of olfactory neuroblastoma is 55–90%; however, this varies based on many factors, primarily the stage of the disease (Masood et al. 2007). The involvement of the nodes, which occurs in approximately 20% of all patients, is the greatest factor in predicting the prognosis.
- Maxillary sinus lymphoma: The majority are non-Hodgkin's lymphoma, where the prognosis is good if detected early; however, if the patient is older than 60 and the tumour is stage 3 or 4, the prognosis will likely be unfavourable (Lenkeit et al. 2023).

Prognosis of Rhinosinusitis of the Maxillary Sinus

- Chronic rhinosinusitis with nasal polyposis: There is limited data available on the long-term outcomes.
- Acute infective rhinosinusitis: The majority of the cases will either be treated with antibiotics or will resolve spontaneously on their own.
- Allergic fungal rhinosinusitis: The short-term prognosis is good; however, the recurrence rate is high.
- Mucormycosis: Mucormycosis is frequently a potentially fatal infection with an overall mortality rate of 54% for all causes.
- Fungus Ball: Generally, complications of fungal balls are rare; however, there have been reports of infections becoming invasive after significant immunosuppression. Recurrence is uncommon.
- Granulomatous invasive rhinosinusitis: Prognosis is favourable following either radical surgery or even antifungal therapy, provided that the lesion is diagnosed early.

Prognosis of Other Pathologies of the Maxillary Sinus

- Silent sinus syndrome: Whenever surgery is performed to provide ideal drainage, further volume loss will be arrested. However, any deformity at the time of surgery will be permanent and may require surgical correction, especially if diplopia is present.
- Missed maxillary sinus ostium syndrome: Unless surgically treated, patients will have persistent and recurrent sinus complaints.
- Maxillary sinus fracture: The prognosis is hard to predict since it depends on the extent of injuries and the other structures that are also affected by the fracture. Generally, anosmia, severe fracture displacement, complete vision loss and long-term malunion of the fracture location are among the common complications (Hacker 2024).

Public Health Implications

Like any other pathologies, those of the maxillary sinus pose a burden on both the patients and the healthcare system. This burden is more noticed in chronic lesions and illnesses of the sinus, such as chronic rhinosinusitis with nasal polyposis. Apart from the physical weight of long-term illness, they also pose a financial and possibly even psychological burden on the patient. Regarding the healthcare system, the cost of managing chronic illnesses is enormous and is only increasing. This could be partly due to the overall growth of age in the population. Furthermore, many of the pathologies in the maxillary sinus, such as nasal polyposis, have an increased tendency to recur after they're managed, increasing the burden of the disease. This is what makes prevention strategies essential. Many of the chronic illnesses have identifiable risk factors and can be prevented. Common modifiable risk factors include tobacco smoking and an unhealthy diet. Furthermore, in the maxillary sinus, viruses such as human papillomavirus and occupational risk factors such as nickel and radon gas should be avoided as they increase the likelihood of cancer development. Another significant yet avoidable lesion in the maxillary sinus is maxillary sinus fracture. These fractures are usually present in individuals frequently undergoing physical brawls. Raising awareness of the different risk factors that make an individual susceptible to maxillary sinus pathology and how to work to prevent the development of these pathologies is crucial. Moreover, the maxillary sinus and, specifically, its pathologies are understudied, and there seems to be a lack of information available on their aetiology and epidemiology. Therefore, we advocate for more research to look into these lesions with the hopes of better understanding their aetiology, epidemiology, and positive risk factors.

Conclusion

Many different pathologies can impact the maxillary sinus; some are acute and self-limiting, whereas some are long-term and debilitating. Mucosal thickening and polypoid lesions are the most frequent, and the pathologies generally impact more than one surface of the sinus. Due to the limited information in the literature on pathologies of the maxillary sinus, little is known about their epidemiology, aetiology, and pathophysiology. More research is necessary to be conducted in this area and to raise public awareness of the modifiable risk factors for the lesion.

References

ACAAI (2022) Chronic rhinosinusitis with nasal polyps—ACAAI patient. ACAAI Patient. https://acaai.org/allergies/allergic-conditions/chronic-rhinosinusitis-with-nasal-polyps/

Akhondi H, Woldemariam B, Rajasurya V (2023) Fungal sinusitis. StatPearls—NCBI Bookshelf. https://www.ncbi.nlm.nih.gov/books/NBK551496/

Betin-Noriega C, Valle SEU-D, Saldarriaga-Naranjo CI et al (2023) Analysis of risk variables for association with maxillary sinus mucosal thickenings: a cone-beam computed tomography-based retrospective study. Surg Radiol Anat 45:417–429. https://doi.org/10.1007/s00276-023-03090-2

Bhattacharya A, Adwani D, Arora R, Bhagat B (2013) Non-Hodgkin's lymphoma of maxillary sinus: an unusual presentation. Ann Maxillofac Surg 3:95. https://doi.org/10.4103/2231-0746.110079

Bokhari K, Hameed MS, Ajmal M, Togoo RA (2012) Benign osteoblastoma involving maxilla: a case report and review of the literature. Case Rep Dent 2012:1–4. https://doi.org/10.1155/2012/351241

Choi KY (2024) Malignant tumors of the sinuses treatment & management: approach considerations, complications, outcome and prognosis. https://emedicine.medscape.com/article/847189-treatment?form=fpf

Drumond J, Allegro B, Novo N et al (2016) Evaluation of the prevalence of maxillary sinuses abnormalities through spiral computed tomography (CT). Int Arch Otorhinolaryngol 21:126–133. https://doi.org/10.1055/s-0036-1593834

Edens MH, Khaled Y, Napeñas JJ (2016) Intraoral pain disorders. Oral Maxillofac Surg Clin North Am 28:275–288. https://doi.org/10.1016/j.coms.2016.03.008

Faculty of Public Health (2024) Principles, methods, applications and organisation of screening for early detection, prevention, treatment and control of disease | Health knowledge. Faculty of Public Health. https://www.healthknowledge.org.uk/public-health-textbook/disease-causation-diagnostic/2c-diagnosis-screening/principles-methods-applications. Accessed 31 Jul 2024

Hacker K (2024) The burden of chronic disease. Mayo Clin Proc Innov Qual Outcomes 8:112–119. https://doi.org/10.1016/j.mayocpiqo.2023.08.005

Kara Mİ, Yanık S, Altan A et al (2015) Large dentigerous cyst in the maxillary sinus leading to diplopia and nasal obstruction: case report. J Istanb Univ Fac Dent 49:46. https://doi.org/10.17096/jiufd.10506

Leland EM, Vohra V, Seal SM et al (2022) Environmental air pollution and chronic rhinosinusitis: a systematic review. Laryngoscope Investig Otolaryngol 7:349–360. https://doi.org/10.1002/lio2.774

Lenkeit CP, Lofgren DH, Shermetaro C (2023) Maxillary sinus fracture. StatPearls—NCBI Bookshelf. https://www.ncbi.nlm.nih.gov/books/NBK557455/

Lin G, Akkina S, Chinn S et al (2014) Sinonasal inverted papilloma: prognostic factors with emphasis on resection margins. J Neurol Surg B Skull Base 75:140–146. https://doi.org/10.1055/s-0033-1363169

Masood A, Moumoulidis I, Panesar J (2007) Acute rhinosinusitis in adults: an update on current management. Postgrad Med J 83:402–408. https://doi.org/10.1136/pgmj.2006.054767

National Cancer Institute (2023) Paranasal sinus and nasal cavity cancer treatment. Cancer.gov. https://www.cancer.gov/types/head-and-neck/patient/adult/paranasal-sinus-treatment-pdq

Pereira I, Vaz P, Almeida RF et al (2014) Genetic susceptibility to maxillary sinus pathology development in the presence of an odontogenic cyst. Revista Portuguesa De Estomatologia, Medicina DentáRia E Cirurgia Maxilofacial 55:110–114. https://doi.org/10.1016/j.rpemd.2014.04.003

Pérez-Sayáns M, Peñaranda JMS, Quintanilla JAS et al (2020) Clinicopathological features of 214 maxillary sinus pathologies. A ten-year single-centre retrospective clinical study. Head Face Med 16:24. https://doi.org/10.1186/s13005-020-00239-x

Raghav M, Karjodkar FR, Sontakke S, Sansare K (2014) Prevalence of incidental maxillary sinus pathologies in dental patients on cone-beam computed tomographic images. Contemp Clin Dent 5:361. https://doi.org/10.4103/0976-237x.137949

Tassoker M (2019) What are the risk factors for maxillary sinus pathologies? A CBCT study. Oral Radiol 36:80–84. https://doi.org/10.1007/s11282-019-00382-5

Writer S (2019) What is epidemiology?—MPH online. MPH Online. https://www.mphonline.org/importance-of-epidemiology/

5 Maxillary Rhinosinusitis

Goran Latif Omer, Vivek Sasindran, Mithra Sara, Gianluca Velletrani, Beatrice Francavilla, Sveva Viola, Arianna Alagna, Stefano Di Girolamo, Francesco Maria Passali, Fouad Ahmed Abdullah, Gianluca Scialla, Marco Perla, Sahand Soran Ali, and Aland Salih Abdullah

Chronic Rhinosinusitis and Nasal Polyposis

Chronic Rhinosinusitis (CRS) is an inflammation of the sinus or nasal passages occurring for more than 12 weeks at a time (Fig. 5.1). It may present as chronic sinusitis with nasal polyps (CRSwNP phenotype), chronic sinusitis without nasal polyps (CRSsNP phenotype), and chronic sinusitis with allergic fungal Rhinosinusitis (Kwon and O'Rourke 2023). This disease is more prevalent in patients with chronic conditions such as environmental allergies, asthma, or chronic obstructive pulmonary disease.

Epidemiology

This disease affects 5–12% of the general population and has a profound impact on quality of life. This might be an overestimation because of overlap with other diseases, such as allergic rhinitis. Patients with particular conditions develop sinusitis

G. L. Omer (✉) · S. S. Ali · A. S. Abdullah
Department of Clinical Sciences, College of Medicine, University of Sulaimani, Sulaymaniyah, KRI, Iraq

V. Sasindran · M. Sara
KM Cherian Institute of Medical Sciences, Chengannur, Kerala, India

G. Velletrani · B. Francavilla · S. Viola · A. Alagna · S. Di Girolamo · F. M. Passali
G. Scialla· M. Perla
Department of Otorhinolaryngology, University of Rome Tor Vergata, Rome, Italy

F. A. Abdullah
Royal Hospital, Sulaymaniyah, KRI, Iraq

© The Author(s), under exclusive license to Springer Nature Switzerland AG 2025
G. L. Omer, S. Di Girolamo (eds.), *Maxillary Sinus: A Comprehensive Guide*, https://doi.org/10.1007/978-3-031-83468-4_5

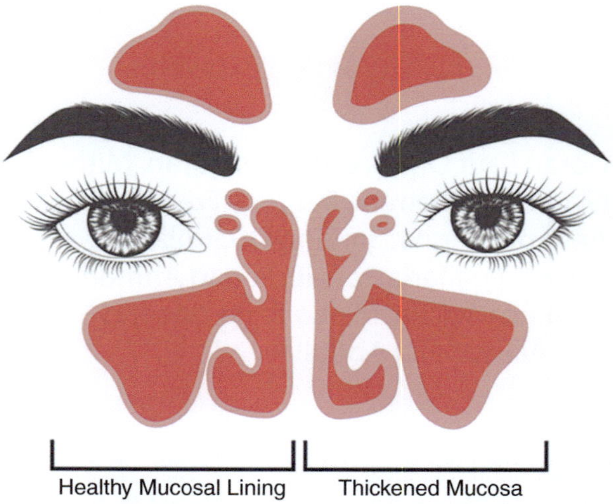

Fig. 5.1 Chronic rhinosinusitis: thickening of the sinus lining due to chronic inflammation

more often—for example, 25–30% of allergic patients, 43% of asthmatic patients, 37% of patients with transplants, and 54–68% of patients with AIDS. Even with the development of nasal endoscopy and imaging, we still do not know the precise prevalence of chronic sinusitis; problems with definitions and a lack of knowledge of the pathophysiology and natural history of this disease could explain this. However, it seems that almost 15% of the population suffers from chronic sinusitis, with the highest prevalence occurring in children (Van Cauwenberge and Watelet 2000).

Based on epidemiological studies, the prevalence of CRSwNP was estimated at 2.1% in France, 4.4% in Finland, and approximately 4.2% in the United States. According to EPOS-based surveys conducted in China, the prevalence of CRSwNP was estimated at 2.2–8%. Furthermore, the prevalence of nasal polyps was reported more frequently among urban residents than rural ones (Wojas et al. 2021).

The 1992, 1997, and 2007 NHIS results consistently show CRS to be more common in female subjects (59%) than in male subjects in the United States. Similar results were reported in the Canadian survey. However, the Global Allergy and Asthma European Network reported no significant variations in CRS prevalence by gender. Although there was no difference in CRS prevalence according to age in a study from Germany, CRS prevalence is reportedly higher in adults aged 18–64 years in the United States and Europe. CRS is geographically more common in the Midwest and the South of the United States than in the Northeast and is least common in the West. The lower incidence of CRS in Canada is consistent with these data and supports the hypothesis of a North-South gradient whereby CRS seems to be less prevalent in cooler countries. A similar lower prevalence in cooler areas is seen in Scandinavian countries versus a higher prevalence in the more humid weather of Amsterdam and Poland. Interestingly, a comparative study between North Scotland and South Caribbean showed no difference in the prevalence of CRS in these two regions despite the difference in climates (Halawi et al. 2013).

Dysbiosis of Sinus Microbiota in Chronic Rhinosinusitis

Analysis of the normal state of the microbiome in sinus cavities is crucial because there is a clear role for commensals in pathogen exclusion and the modulation of the healthy host–microbial immune response. The deeper nasal cavity and sinuses have unique local microenvironments (pH, Po2, and so forth) and host immune properties. Disruption of stable microbiota may contribute to the exacerbation of chronic inflammatory disease in the absence of acute infection. Many opportunistic pathogens are found at low abundance in healthy sinuses and, therefore, have the potential to create disease after an acute alteration in the stable baseline microbial community (i.e., dysbiosis). Dysbiosis can lead to benign microbial communities becoming pro-inflammatory or invasive or allowing the overgrowth of pathogens. Disruption of healthy commensal interactions with the local immune system seems to be a critical determinant of CRS progression. Linear discriminant analysis identified the genus Corynebacterium as a potential biomarker that was significantly increased in abundance in CRS patients; however, this genus was also omnipresent in healthy subjects from other studies. Bacterial supplementation and modulation of the microbiota through prebiotics or probiotics and equivalents are opportunities for thoughtful and ethical clinical research. Whether probiotics directly target inflammatory processes within the sinonasal epithelium or aim to restore normal upper airway microbiota by mucus transfer, novel strategies to address pathogens in CRS are needed (Cho et al. 2020a, b).

Clinical Features and Patterns

Chronic Rhinosinusitis is diagnosed when at least two of the following four symptoms are present and occur for more than 12 weeks:

1. Purulent drainage: Green or yellow nasal discharge.
2. Facial/dental pain: Fullness or pressure-like pain.
3. Nasal obstruction: This can cause difficulty breathing from one or both nasal passages or lead to mouth breathing.
4. Hyposmia: A decreased sense of smell, often included in other symptoms.

The most common symptoms can be seen in Fig. 5.2. Other symptoms include ear pain, snoring, halitosis, cough, fatigue, and headache. The duration of symptoms is a key factor in diagnosing this disease as well as distinguishing between chronic sinusitis and recurrent sinusitis. In the CRSwNP phenotype, small nasal polyps may not cause symptoms; however, large growths or groups of nasal polyps can lead to breathing problems. Many people with nasal polyps also have asthma, and inflamed sinuses caused by nasal polyps can exacerbate asthma symptoms. When nasal polyps are associated with bronchial asthma and allergic reactions to aspirin or NSAIDs, this constitutes a syndrome called Vidal Wright Syndrome.

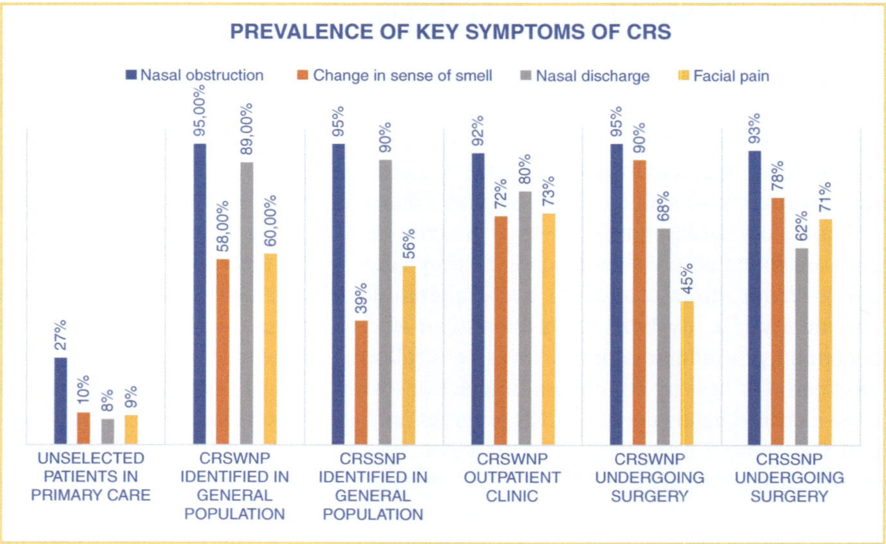

Fig. 5.2 Prevalence of cardinal symptoms of CRS. *CRS* chronic rhinosinusitis, *CRSsNP* chronic rhinosinusitis without nasal polyps, *CRSwNP* chronic rhinosinusitis with nasal polyps (Miglani et al. 2022)

CRSwNP is frequently associated with olfactory dysfunction, obstructive symptoms, steroid responsiveness, and the need for multiple surgeries. However, nasal polyp tissue often contains elevated levels of Type 2 inflammatory biomarkers like IL-4, IL-5, and IgE, whereas the type characterised by the absence of nasal polyps is associated with elevations in IFN-γ, IL-8, and neutrophilia. Over 75% of patients with CRSwNP experience reduced sleep quality, and worse sleep quality correlates with more severe disease, which can also affect psychological well-being and mental health. Patients may experience anxiety, phobias, hopelessness, embarrassment, and depression.

The EPOS2020 steering group has chosen to look at CRS in terms of primary and secondary and to divide each into localised and diffuse diseases based on anatomic distribution. In primary CRS, the disease is considered by endotype dominance, either type 2 or non-type 2. From a clinical standpoint, the primary localised form can be further subdivided into two phenotypes: allergic fungal Rhinosinusitis (AFRS) for type 2 and isolated sinusitis for non-type 2. For the diffuse form, the predominant clinical phenotypes are eosinophilic CRS (eCRS), CRSwNP, AFRS, and central compartment allergic disease (CCAD) for type 2, while non-eCRS is the predominant phenotype for non-type 2. For secondary CRS, the division is again based on localised and diffuse disease but then considered by four categories dependent on local pathology (localised form) and mechanical/inflammatory/immunological factors (diffuse form) (Norwood et al. 2023).

Definition of Chronic Rhinosinusitis in Children

The prevalence of CRS in paediatric patients is now estimated to be up to 4%. Both passive and active cigarette smoking are associated with chronic rhinitis and Rhinosinusitis in children, though a clear and definitive causal relationship between allergic rhinitis and CRS has not been established. Evidence suggests that adenoids may act as a reservoir for pathogenic bacteria rather than as a source of obstruction. A large database study suggests a significant familial risk associated with paediatric CRS, but studies on monozygotic twins have not shown that both siblings always develop polyps, indicating that environmental factors are as likely as genetic ones to influence the occurrence of nasal polyps.

Chronic Rhinosinusitis (with or without nasal polyps) in children is defined as the presence of two or more symptoms, one of which should be either nasal blockage/obstruction/congestion or nasal discharge (anterior/posterior nasal drip):

- +/− facial pain/pressure
- +/− cough.

For ≥12 weeks.

There is no high-level evidence to support the efficacy of either short-term or long-term antibiotics or the efficacy of intranasal steroids in the treatment of CRS in children. There are a few clinical trials demonstrating the efficacy of saline irrigations in paediatric patients. The EPOS steering group supports the use of saline in light of its excellent safety record in children. Adenoidectomy is effective in younger children with symptoms, while FESS is safe and effective for the treatment of older children with CRS refractory to medical therapy or previous adenoidectomy (Fokkens et al. 2020).

Diagnosis

We have detailed many, but not all, of the sinonasal entities that may mimic nasal polyps. When evaluating a patient with nasal polyps, it is important to obtain a good history, physical examination, and nasal endoscopy, as these will guide the differential diagnosis. If a mass is found on nasal endoscopy to be unilateral or if there are associated cranial neuropathies, one's level of concern should be raised for an alternative diagnosis rather than benign nasal polyps. As with masses of the head and neck, a biopsy should be performed to confirm the diagnosis. However, one should consider imaging prior to biopsy, as improper biopsy of an encephalocele or vascular anomaly, for example, could be catastrophic.

Typically, a CT scan is the primary imaging modality, as it determines the extent of the mass and delineates any bony breakdown. If a neoplasm or encephalocele is suspected, an MRI can assess the extent of soft tissue involvement and any local extensions, such as intracranial or intraorbital invasion. Lastly, in the workup for patients with CRS that is recalcitrant to medical management, one should consider potential alternative diagnoses. Clinical suspicion should be raised in patients whose polyps are unilateral, unresponsive to medical management, or associated with cranial neuropathies (London and Reh 2016).

Meanwhile, CRS is a relatively common disease in children, but its symptoms are often subtle and nonspecific, which may result in overlooking a correct diagnosis. When CRS is suspected, confirmation may be obtained through imaging criteria or nasal fibroendoscopy. In imaging, computed tomography (CT) is the first-choice technique for the evaluation of CRS and provides an anatomic roadmap when surgery is required. Magnetic resonance imaging (MRI) of the sinuses, orbits, and brain should be performed whenever extensive or multiple complications of sinusitis are suspected. For middle ear disorders, CT is the first choice because it detects opacification of the middle ear cavity and mastoid cells, the presence of fluids or debris, and allows for evaluation of the ossicular chain and the cortical bone of the mastoid. Another important diagnostic consideration is the need to look for disorders frequently associated with CRS, such as obstructive sleep apnoea syndrome (OSAS), which has recognised risk factors including adenotonsillar hypertrophy, craniofacial anomalies, obesity, and neuromuscular disorders. Other associated disorders requiring investigation are recurrent or persistent otitis media and difficult asthma (Leo et al. 2012).

Sinonasal polyposis is most commonly encountered in adults and is rare in children. Polyps are formed by the influx of fluid into the lamina propria of the sinonasal Schneiderian mucosa. It is important to understand the Meltzer grading system, which is as follows:

- **Grade 0**: No visible polyposis.
- **Grade 1**: Single polyp confined to the middle meatus.
- **Grade 2**: Multiple polyps in the middle meatus.
- **Grade 3**: Polyps extending beyond the middle meatus.
- **Grade 4**: Nasal cavity obstruction.

When assessing radiographic features, it is important to note several details in CT imaging, including:

- Extensive mucosal polyps are occupying and obliterating the nasal cavity and paranasal sinuses (usually hypodense, but they may be hyperdense due to increased protein content or fungal infection).
- Associated local benign bone remodelling or erosion (as opposed to mucocele, where the entire sinus is expanded), including:
  - Enlargement of infundibulum.
  - Attenuation of the ethmoid sinus walls and nasal septum.
  - Occasionally sparing the inferior nasal meatus.
  - Truncation of the middle turbinate.
- Opacified ethmoid sinuses with convex lateral walls and gas-fluid levels.
- Concurrent fungal sinus infection may be present (Bell and Abdel-Halim 2014).

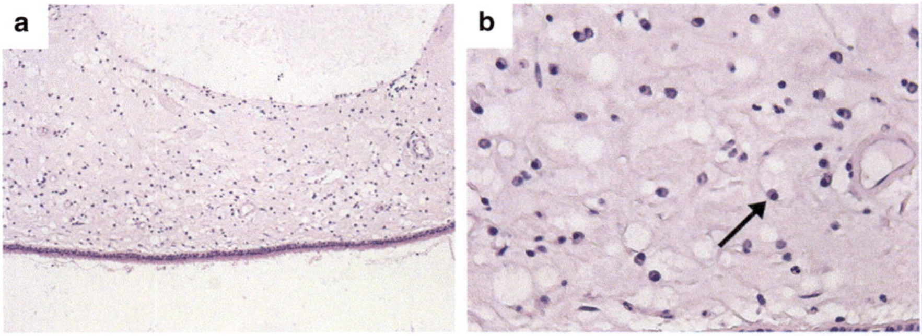

Fig. 5.3 Non-eosinophilic chronic rhinosinusitis with nasal polyposis: ciliated respiratory epithelium can be observed in this image (**a**: 4×, **b**: 10×), overlying a mucoid stroma infiltrated by both acute and chronic inflammatory cells, including neutrophils and plasma cells (Black Arrow)

In the case of sinonasal polyposis, it is important to exclude differential diagnoses:

- **Sinonasal retention cyst**:
  - Can be indistinguishable.
  - Usually, it spares the nasal cavity.
- **Allergic fungal sinusitis**:
  - Commonly associated with polyps.
  - Hyperdense central areas.
  - MRI may show low T1 and T2 signals.
- **Granulomatosis with polyangiitis**:
  - Centred in the nasal cavity (Bell and Abdel-Halim 2014).

As previously mentioned, a biopsy is performed after imaging to confirm the diagnosis (Fig. 5.3).

Control of Disease

In EPOS 2012, the concept of control was introduced. The primary goal of any treatment, especially in chronic diseases, is to achieve and maintain clinical control, which can be defined as a disease state in which the patient does not have symptoms or the symptoms do not impact quality of life. Based on different validation studies, the EPOS 2020 steering group believes that the current EPOS 2012 control criteria might overestimate the percentage of patients being uncontrolled. For example, a typical migraine headache should not be considered when evaluating control in CRS. Given the importance of the concept of disease control from both a clinical and research perspective, there remains a need for a gold standard to assess disease control in CRS. Assessment of current clinical control of CRS:

Controlled: All of the following criteria must be met:

- **Nasal blockage:** Not present or not bothersome.
- **Rhinorrhoea/Post nasal drip:** Little and mucousy.
- **Facial pain/Pressure:** Not present or not bothersome.
- **Smell:** Normal or only slightly impaired.
- **Sleep disturbance or fatigue:** Not present.
- **Nasal endoscopy (if available):** Healthy or almost healthy mucosa.
- **Rescue treatment (in the last 6 months):** Not needed.

Partly Controlled: At least one of the following criteria is present:

- **Nasal blockage:** Present on most days of the week.
- **Rhinorrhoea/Post-nasal drip:** Mucopurulent on most days of the week.
- **Facial pain/Pressure:** Present on most days of the week.
- **Smell:** Impaired.
- **Sleep disturbance or fatigue:** Present.
- **Nasal endoscopy (if available):** Diseased mucosa.
- **Rescue treatment (in the last 6 months):** Need of 1 course of rescue treatment.

Uncontrolled: Three or more of the following criteria are present:

- **Nasal blockage:** Present on most days of the week.
- **Rhinorrhoea/Post-nasal drip:** Mucopurulent on most days of the week.
- **Facial pain/Pressure:** Present on most days of the week.
- **Smell:** Impaired.
- **Sleep disturbance or fatigue:** Present.
- **Nasal endoscopy (if available):** Diseased mucosa.
- **Rescue treatment (in the last 6 months):** Symptoms persist despite rescue treatment(s).

Treatment of CRS

EPOS 2020 provides a comprehensive, evidence-based systematic review of the management of CRS, which has been incorporated into an integrated care pathway. A significant shift in the management of CRS has occurred since EPOS 2012 (Fokkens et al. 2020). The primary treatment modalities for chronic Rhinosinusitis (CRS) are corticosteroids, antibiotics, and surgery. Antibiotics are likely effective in a subset of patients, but the various phenotypes and endotypes that make up CRS have thus far been poorly defined (Ghogomu and Kern 2016). Early surgery, as well as biologics, may also be more efficacious and cost-effective in some phenotypes. Historically, nasal polyps and chronic sinusitis were seen as distinct entities, with prevailing hypotheses suggesting that nasal polyps were caused by some form of allergy, while chronic sinusitis was driven by persistent infection. In contrast to antibiotics, the use of topical and oral corticosteroids for the management of CRS is supported by a higher level of evidence. In patients with chronic Rhinosinusitis without nasal polyps (CRSsNP), a meta-analysis showed that, compared to placebo, intranasal corticosteroids lead to improvements in symptom scores. In patients with nasal polyps, the data supporting the benefit of steroids is even stronger (Li and Peters 2015). A meta-analysis in 2012 revealed that topical steroids improved symptom scores and reduced polyp size, with the overall benefit being greater in patients who had previously undergone sinus surgery. Systemic steroids may avoid or delay the need for surgical intervention, but they are associated with significant risks that limit their long-term use, including avascular necrosis of the femoral head, decreased bone density leading to vertebral fractures, cataracts, glaucoma, and diabetes. From this population-based perspective, the use of oral corticosteroids for CRS should be viewed as a fairly aggressive medical intervention and should only be rational if the benefits can be maintained using intranasal corticosteroids for at least several months (Snidvongs et al. 2013).

Studies have shown increased expression of cysteinyl leukotriene (CysLT) receptors in nasal polyps, suggesting a potentially larger role in the pathogenesis of aspirin-tolerant nasal polyps. Medications targeting leukotrienes come in two forms: an LT-receptor antagonist (montelukast) or a 5-lipoxygenase inhibitor (zileuton). Compared to topical steroids, overall symptom improvement is fairly similar, but polyp recurrence rates tend to be higher in patients on montelukast. When added to topical steroids, montelukast may confer some additional symptomatic benefits for CRSwNP patients (Chao et al. 2006).

The EPOS document recommends against the routine use of this class of drugs in CRSwNP, while the International Consensus Statement on Rhinosinusitis (ICOR) states that it is an option, particularly in patients who do not tolerate topical steroids. Viral and bacterial infections can lead to secondary mucociliary dysfunction, supporting the hypothesis that this is a key factor contributing to CRS in general. For this reason, saline irrigations (both hypertonic and isotonic saline) appear to be beneficial and safe, though there are risks of infection associated with the failure to use sterile water and to clean the irrigation bottles.

The goals of modern endoscopic sinus surgery (ESS) in the management of CRS include the following: relief of nasal airway and sinus ostial obstruction, debridement of inflamed tissue, and provision for greater access for topical medications to the sinus mucosa. While exceptions exist (e.g., mucocele), surgery is generally an option only after a trial of medical therapy to control symptoms (Ghogomu and Kern 2016). CRSwNP is characterised by a type 2-predominant eosinophilic endotype in most patients. The presence of high levels of total IgE and IL-5 in the nasal tissues and secretions of patients with CRSwNP, along with increased recognition of their respective roles in inflammation, has led to the testing of mAbs specifically targeting IgE (Omalizumab) or IL-5 (mepolizumab) in trials. These therapeutic agents reduced signs and symptoms of CRSwNP. Recently, a new study reported that dupilumab, an IL-4Rα inhibitor that blocks IL-4 and IL-13 signalling, was well tolerated, reduced polyp size, and rapidly improved smell in patients with CRSwNP. It's important to underline the reduction of multiple inflammatory biomarkers, including total IgE and markers of eosinophilic inflammation, in both nasal secretions and polyp tissues of patients with CRSwNP treated with dupilumab (Jonstam et al. 2019). The acceptance of dupilumab for the treatment of CRSwNP by the US Food and Drug Administration has significantly changed the treatment options for type 2 CRS, and it is expected that other monoclonal antibodies will follow (Fokkens et al. 2020).

Comparative effectiveness research between endoscopic sinus surgery (ESS) and biologic therapy for CRSwNP is a nascent field as new therapeutic modalities become clinically available. ESS and dupilumab offer comparable improvement in smell identification at 24 weeks of treatment. Compared to omalizumab, ESS offers superior SNOT-22 improvements. ESS offers significantly greater reductions in polyp size compared to omalizumab and mepolizumab therapies (Miglani et al. 2022). In dealing with the recalcitrant nature of CRSwNP, surgical techniques have simultaneously become more nuanced and aggressive. Bony resection in anatomically unfavourable areas such as the frontal, maxillary, and sphenoid outflow regions, replacing diseased or denuded mucosa with healthy grafts or flaps at the neo-ostia, and introducing drug-eluting biomaterials to newly opened sinus outflow tracts are highlights in the recent advancements in sinus surgery for CRSwNP. The Draf 3 or modified endoscopic Lothrop procedure has become a standard technique and has been demonstrated to improve quality of life and decrease polyp recurrence. A number of mucosal grafting or mucosal flap techniques have been described to cover exposed bone of the neo-ostium, and evidence shows that this improves healing and the diameter of the Draf 3. Partial middle turbinectomy, while controversial, appears to help decrease polyp recurrence in long-term follow-up studies. Modified endoscopic medial maxillectomy improves access to the maxillary sinus mucosa, facilitates debridement and, particularly in the cystic fibrosis nasal polyp patient, improves overall management of the disease. The sphenoid drill-out procedure provides wider access for topical steroid irrigations and may also improve the management of CRSwNP (Norwood et al. 2023).

In the standard functional endoscopic sinus surgery (FESS) procedure, the amount of dissection is often determined by the extent of disease, with the goal of preserving as much normal mucosa as possible while restoring ventilation and reestablishing mucociliary clearance. A subset of patients with chronic Rhinosinusitis with nasal polyposis, however, may continue to have persistent mucosal inflammation and aggressive polyp regrowth despite standard FESS and maximal pharmacologic therapy, leading to recurrent and recalcitrant disease. Advanced endoscopic surgery techniques such as the modified endoscopic medial maxillectomy, endoscopic modified Lothrop procedure (known as a Draf 3 frontal sinusotomy), and nasalisation or radical ethmoidectomy are extensive surgical procedures designed to maximise disease clearance while providing sizeable drainage pathways for effective post-operative surveillance and topical delivery of medications. Studies have shown a decreased risk of revision surgery as well as a longer time interval for revision surgery in patients with refractory CRSwNP who have undergone extensive sinus surgery for polyps (Southwood et al. 2016).

The introduction of biologics in the management of chronic Rhinosinusitis with nasal polyposis (CRSwNP) has provided new therapeutic options, with dupilumab representing the first approved biological agent. Biologics have revolutionised the management of chronic Rhinosinusitis (CRS), a condition characterised by persistent inflammation of the sinuses affecting 5–12% of the general population. Traditional treatments for CRS include pharmacological interventions such as nasal corticosteroids, nasal douches, systemic antibiotics, and systemic corticosteroids, as well as surgical interventions like endoscopic sinus surgery (ESS). Despite these treatments, many patients experience persistent symptoms, prompting the development and use of biologics—advanced therapies that target specific inflammatory pathways involved in CRS. Among the biologics, omalizumab, mepolizumab, reslizumab, and dupilumab have shown promising results. Omalizumab, an anti-IgE monoclonal antibody, binds to free IgE and prevents it from interacting with its receptors on mast cells and basophils, thereby inhibiting the allergic inflammatory cascade. Studies (Damask et al. 2021) have shown that omalizumab significantly reduces nasal polyp size, decreases sinus opacification, and improves symptoms such as nasal congestion and loss of smell, as measured by the Sino-Nasal Outcome Test (SNOT-22).

Mepolizumab and reslizumab, both targeting IL-5, are designed to reduce eosinophilic inflammation, which is a hallmark of severe CRSwNP. Clinical trials have demonstrated that these biologics effectively reduce eosinophil levels in the blood and tissues, leading to a decrease in nasal polyp size and improvement in sinus symptoms and quality of life (Lombardo et al. 2020; Cavaliere et al. 2024; Santomasi et al. 2023). Specifically, mepolizumab has been shown to significantly reduce the need for surgery and systemic corticosteroids, providing a sustainable treatment option for patients with refractory CRSwNP (Fokkens et al. 2022; Bachert et al. 2022; Han et al. 2021). Dupilumab, which targets the IL-4 and IL-13 pathways, has been particularly effective in patients with CRSwNP. By inhibiting these key cytokines involved in T2 inflammation, dupilumab not only reduces nasal polyp size but also improves overall nasal and sinus symptoms, including nasal congestion and loss of smell. Additionally, dupilumab has been shown to decrease the need for systemic corticosteroids and reduce the frequency of sinus infections. Its efficacy has led to its approval by the U.S. FDA for the treatment of CRSwNP, highlighting its importance in the therapeutic landscape of CRS (De Corso et al. 2022; Ottaviano et al. 2022).

The use of biologics is guided by criteria outlined in guidelines such as EPOS 2020. These criteria recommend biologics for patients with bilateral nasal polyps who meet at least three of the following: need for systemic corticosteroids or contraindications to systemic steroids, significantly impaired quality of life, loss of smell, comorbid asthma, and evidence of type 2 inflammation. This targeted approach ensures that biologics are used in patients who are most likely to benefit from them, particularly those who have not responded adequately to traditional therapies. Furthermore, the impact of biologics extends beyond symptom control and quality of life improvements. By targeting specific inflammatory pathways, biologics have the potential to alter the disease course of CRS, leading to more sustained remissions and possibly reducing the long-term need for surgical interventions. Patients treated with biologics like dupilumab experience fewer recurrences of nasal polyps and less frequent exacerbations of sinusitis. In addition to their use in CRSwNP, ongoing research is exploring the potential benefits of biologics in other forms of CRS and related inflammatory conditions. This includes studies on their efficacy in patients with CRSsNP and those with overlapping allergic and non-allergic rhinitis, as well as in paediatric populations. These investigations aim to expand the indications for biologics and optimise their use in various subsets of CRS patients (Cergan et al. 2023).

EPOS 2020 provides a full, evidence-based systematic review of the management of CRS that has been incorporated into an integrated care pathway. A significant shift in the management of CRS has occurred since EPOS 2012. Many forms of localised CRS, in general, either type 2 or non-type 2, are not responsive to medical treatment and need surgery. For that reason, patients with unilateral disease have to refer to secondary care for further diagnosis with a CT scan (urgent if there is suspicion of a tumour). For diffuse, bilateral CRS, local corticosteroids and saline remain the mainstay of the treatment. Furthermore, the integrated care pathway advises checking treatable traits, avoiding exacerbating factors, and advising against the use of antibiotics. In secondary care, nasal endoscopy can confirm the disease, point to secondary CRS (e.g., vasculitis/immune disorder, in which case the presence of bleeding/crusting, severe pain, tissue loss, and involvement of other organs is important), and further differentiate between localised and diffuse disease. In addition, emphasis is put on optimum techniques of medication delivery and compliance. If treatment with nasal steroids and saline is insufficient, additional workup with a CT scan and endotyping is relevant. Depending on the endotype indication, treatment can be tailored to a more type 2 or non-type two profiles. International guidelines differ regarding whether long-term antibiotics and oral steroids should be included as part of adequate medical therapy (AMT), reflecting conflicting evidence in the current literature and concerns with regard to side effects. There is a lot of debate on the appropriate moment for CRS surgery. In a recent study for adult patients with uncomplicated CRS, it was agreed that ESS could be appropriately offered when the CT Lund-Mackay score was ≥1 and there had been a minimum trial of at least 8 weeks' duration of a topical intranasal corticosteroid plus a short course of systemic corticosteroid (CRSwNP) or either a short course of a broad spectrum/culture-directed systemic antibiotic or the use of a prolonged course of systemic low-dose anti-inflammatory antibiotic (CRSsNP) with a post-treatment total SNOT-22 score ≥ 20. These criteria were considered the minimal threshold, and clearly, not all patients who meet the criteria should have surgery, but their application should reduce unnecessary surgery and practice variation. A subsequent study applied these criteria retrospectively to patients recruited to a multicenter cohort study and found that patients where surgery was deemed 'inappropriate' reported significantly less improvement in their quality of life postoperatively. It is important to emphasise that CRS is a chronic disease, and ESS is a step in the management that is primarily aimed at creating better conditions for local treatment. After surgery, continuous appropriate medical treatment is mandatory. If surgery in combination with appropriate medical treatment fails, additional therapy can be considered. Options are the use of aspirin treatment after aspirin desensitisation (ATAD), longer (tapering) treatment with OCS, long-term antibiotics, and/or biologicals when indicated (Fokkens et al. 2020).

The introduction of biologics in the management of chronic Rhinosinusitis with nasal polyposis (CRSwNP) has allowed for new therapeutic options, and dupilumab represents the first approved biological agent. A bicentric study in a real-life setting of treatment with dupilumab for severe uncontrolled CRSwNP in Italy is particularly interesting. A total of 83 patients included in the study (43 males, 40 females; mean age 55.8 years) were monitored. The study observed improvements in the reduction of nasal polyposis and nasal obstruction, respectively, measured through NPS and PNIF. The study highlights an improvement in quality of life and olfaction, as measured respectively by two questionnaires: SSIT-16 and SNOT-22. In accordance with EPOS 2020 guidelines, before starting dupilumab, most of these patients (89.9%) underwent at least one previous surgery, while the few cases who did not undergo previous FESS were those not fit for surgery. These patients included in the study did not find relief with the common therapeutic strategies, showing persistence or recurrence of the disease, and for this reason, they have recently been identified as having "severe uncontrolled CRSwNP." Several authors have highlighted that the pathophysiology in this type of CRSwNP is mostly driven by type 2 inflammation, with eosinophilia, associated T-helper cell cytokines 2, and IgE formation. Based on their preliminary observations, dupilumab has demonstrated broad efficacy in the management of patients with CRSwNP, with benefits in terms of improved quality of life, reduction of nasal polyps, and disease-related symptoms, especially for the sense of smell. The indications of biological agents can be seen in Fig. 5.4. Only a low percentage of patients suffered from transient side effects, which included irritation and pain at the injection site, fever, asthenia, headache, and joint pain. Most cases reported a transient increase in blood eosinophils with spontaneous resolution. Further studies are needed to confirm our results and to establish new biomarkers able to identify endotypes and predict the response to biological treatment in CRSwNP (Bellocchi et al. 2023).

The Burden of Acute and Chronic Rhinosinusitis

Few studies have measured the impact of ARS on quality of life; this may reflect the short-lived duration of illness, with patients usually returning to their pre-morbid health status. CRS is associated with a wide range of symptoms across sinonasal, aural, sleep, and general domains. The majority of studies evaluating the prevalence and severity of symptoms analyse responses in patients referred to secondary care or those undergoing sinus surgery, therefore selecting those with symptoms more resistant to treatment in primary care. A survey of patients seen in ENT outpatient clinics and those electing sinus surgery shows that cardinal symptoms are reported as the most severe and prevalent. Nasal obstruction and alteration in the sense of smell and taste are both the most severe and prevalent symptoms in CRSwNP, while in CRSsNP, facial pain and nasal discharge are reported as equally severe as altered smell and taste, with nasal obstruction again being the most severe. Fatigue and waking up tired are also highly prevalent and bothersome. When CRS patients (not differentiated by polyps status) were asked what symptoms they felt were the most

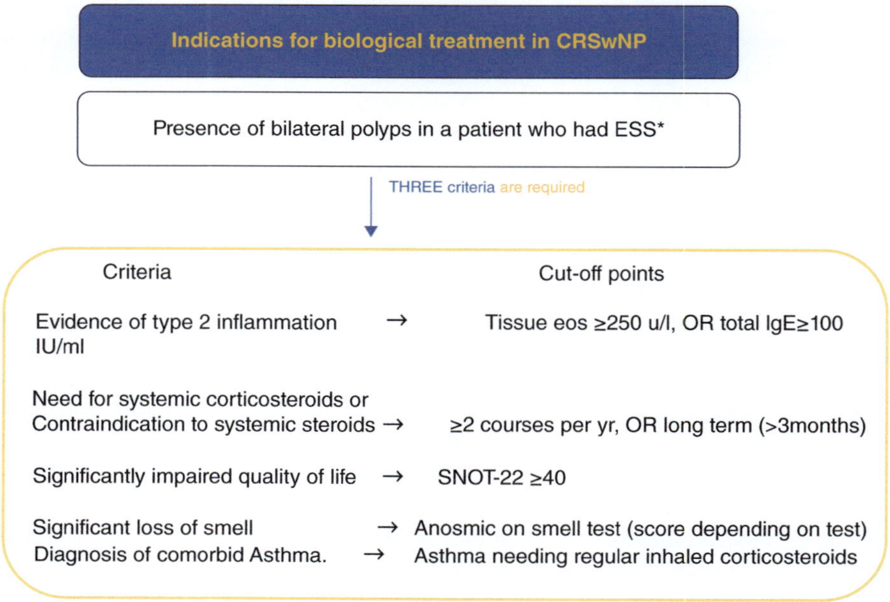

Fig. 5.4 Indications for biological treatment in CRSwNP (Miglani et al. 2022)

important to experience improvement in after surgery, nasal obstruction was rated as "extremely" or "very" important by 93% of patients, followed by smell/taste, thick nasal discharge, need to blow nose, postnasal discharge, and sleep symptoms (range 61–72%). In patients presenting to ENT clinics, the presence of cardinal symptoms has a positive predictive value of 39.9, with high sensitivity but low specificity for a diagnosis of CRS. CRS has been shown to impact patients' health-related quality of life. Symptom severity may be in part determined by the severity of the disease but is further modified by intrinsic patient features (gender, ethnicity, religious, and cultural beliefs), coexisting illnesses and extrinsic features such as socioeconomic factors and support systems.

Research concerning the socioeconomic impact of Rhinosinusitis is a nascent field. CRSw/sNP is a common condition with long-term ramifications with regard to both medical and surgical treatments, associated total cost, and the impact of disease on patient productivity and quality-adjusted life years (Fokkens et al. 2020).

Acute Infective Rhinosinusitis

Introduction

Rhinosinusitis is a common condition in which the mucosa of the paranasal sinuses and the nasal cavity become inflamed (Siddiqui et al. 2021). This condition is broadly divided into acute and chronic Rhinosinusitis. While it was previously thought that chronic Rhinosinusitis occurs due to anatomical abnormalities of the upper airway, it is now primarily considered an inflammatory condition. In contrast, acute Rhinosinusitis usually has an infectious aetiology (Cho et al. 2020a, b). For Rhinosinusitis to be classified as acute, the inflammation of the nasal mucosa must last less than 4 weeks (Ah-See 2015). The term subacute rhinosinusitis has been proposed for inflammation lasting longer than 4 weeks but less than 12 weeks (Meltzer et al. 2004). Most cases of acute infective Rhinosinusitis result from a viral upper airway infection; however, both bacteria and fungi can also be involved (Cho et al. 2020a, b). The clinical presentation of acute Rhinosinusitis includes rhinorrhea, nasal congestion, facial pain, hyposmia, and sneezing. Diagnosis does not always require radiological or bacteriological examinations and can often be made based solely on the clinical picture (Ah-See 2015). Since the majority of cases are self-limiting, the management of acute Rhinosinusitis mainly focuses on symptom control using saline nasal spray, nasal corticosteroids, decongestants, and allergy medications, among other treatments (Acute sinusitis 2023).

Epidemiology

The epidemiology of acute Rhinosinusitis indicates that every adult is expected to experience two episodes of viral Rhinosinusitis each year, while school-age children may have up to seven episodes annually. The aetiology is predominantly viral (Courey and Pletcher 2016). In approximately 0.5–2.0% of cases, a secondary bacterial infection may complicate the condition (Meltzer and Hamilos 2011).

Aetiology and Pathophysiology

Although most cases follow a viral upper respiratory tract infection, acute Rhinosinusitis can also have bacterial or fungal aetiologies (Cho et al. 2020a, b). Common viral agents include rhinovirus, influenza virus, and parainfluenza virus, while common bacterial agents include *Streptococcus pneumoniae*, *Haemophilus influenzae*, *Moraxella catarrhalis*, *Staphylococcus aureus*, *Streptococcus aureus*, and anaerobic bacteria. After the inflammation of the nasal mucosa, negative atmospheric pressure can build up within the sinuses, leading to a decrease in oxygen partial pressure. This, along with increased mucus production, can impair ciliary motility in the sinuses, resulting in mucus accumulation and subsequent occlusion of the osteo-meatal complex, which facilitates the growth of pathogenic organisms. Factors predisposing individuals to Rhinosinusitis include previous upper respiratory infections, anatomic variations that promote obstruction, allergic rhinitis, nasal dryness, irritant inhalation, dental infections, trauma, or procedures (Masood et al. 2007). Among bacterial causes, *Haemophilus influenzae* is a common pathogen that can produce toxins damaging mucosal cells and impairing ciliary motility (Lindberg 1994). Other bacteria, such as coliform bacilli, *Proteus*, *Bacteroides*, and anaerobic streptococci, are more frequent in odontogenic sinusitis (Masood et al. 2007).

Although the aetiologies vary, it can be challenging for physicians to differentiate between acute viral Rhinosinusitis, acute bacterial Rhinosinusitis, and simple upper respiratory infections (Patel and Hwang 2018).

Clinical Features and Patterns

Physical signs of acute Rhinosinusitis include rhinorrhoea, nasal congestion, facial pain, hyposmia, and sneezing (Ah-See 2015). Additionally, it may be accompanied by malaise, headache, fever, and cough. Clinical features can vary based on the site of infection. For maxillary sinus infections, patients may report toothache and tenderness over the molar teeth. Inflammation of the frontal sinus can result in pain in that area. Initially, drainage may be serious, but it typically transforms into mucopurulent drainage that usually resolves within 10 days. If the clinical picture deteriorates rather than gradually resolves after 5 days, a superinfection with a bacterial agent is likely (Ah-See 2015). There are no distinct clinical or radiological characteristics to differentiate viral Rhinosinusitis from acute bacterial Rhinosinusitis.

Diagnosis

As previously mentioned, neither radiographical nor bacteriological investigations are necessary for diagnosing acute Rhinosinusitis, as it can often be determined based solely on clinical presentation (Ah-See 2015). A clinical examination may involve assessing tenderness in the nose and face. Although the clinical picture is usually sufficient, tools such as nasal endoscopy, imaging studies like CT scans (Figs. 5.5 and 5.6), and laboratory samples from the sinuses and nose can be utilised to confirm the diagnosis or rule out other diseases (Acute sinusitis 2023).

Differential Diagnosis

Symptoms such as facial and dental pain, along with rhinorrhoea, overlap with many other conditions, including:

- Common cold.
- Allergic and non-allergic rhinitis.
- Primary dental pathology.

For clinical presentations predominantly characterised by facial pain, conditions such as temporomandibular joint pain and neuralgias should also be considered (Patel and Hwang 2018).

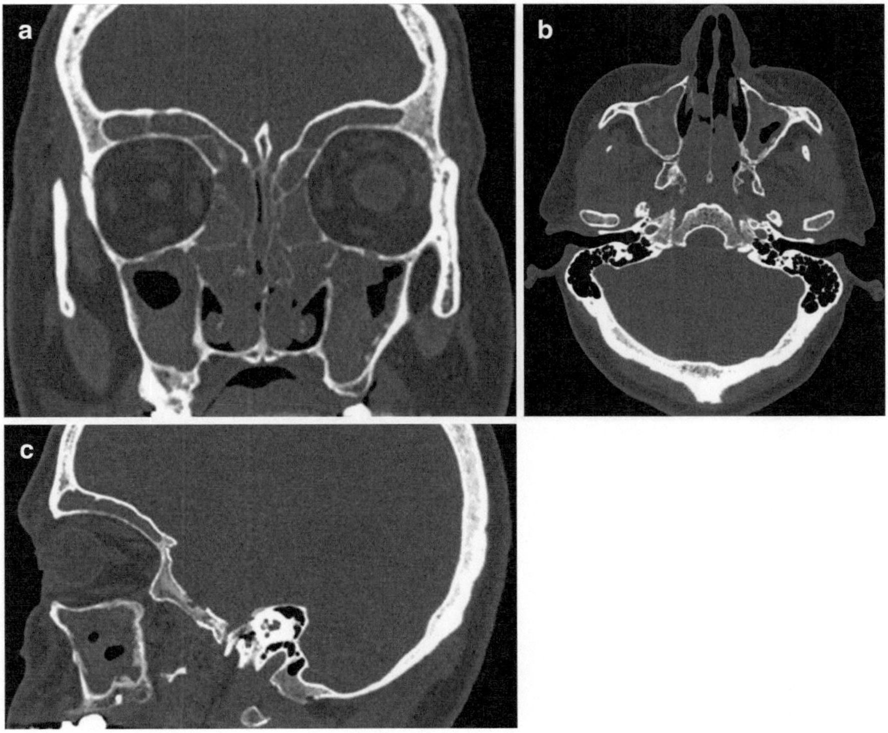

Fig. 5.5 Evidence of diffuse and extensive mucosal thickening and opacifications involving all paranasal sinuses bilaterally, extending through the osteo-meatal complexes into the nasal cavities, merging with the turbinates, and reaching and obstructing the posterior choanae (**a**) Coronal, (**b**) Axial, (**c**) Sagittal

Management

Since most patients improve on their own, the main therapeutic aim for acute infective Rhinosinusitis is to alleviate symptoms. For this reason, pain relievers such as acetaminophen and ibuprofen can be provided. Furthermore, allergy medications, decongestants, nasal corticosteroids, and saline nasal sprays can all play a role in management (Acute sinusitis 2023). Although antimicrobials, specifically antibiotics, can aid in management, it is essential not to overuse them due to the financial burden they impose on the healthcare system and their role in facilitating the emergence of antibiotic-resistant bacteria (Kunin 1993). The majority of cases of acute infective Rhinosinusitis are due to viral agents, rendering antibiotics ineffective. Even in cases caused by bacterial pathogens, since most cases of acute bacterial Rhinosinusitis are self-resolving, antibiotics are generally reserved for severe cases with persistent or worsening symptoms (Mayo Clinic 2023). First-line antibiotics prescribed for acute bacterial Rhinosinusitis include either amoxicillin alone or

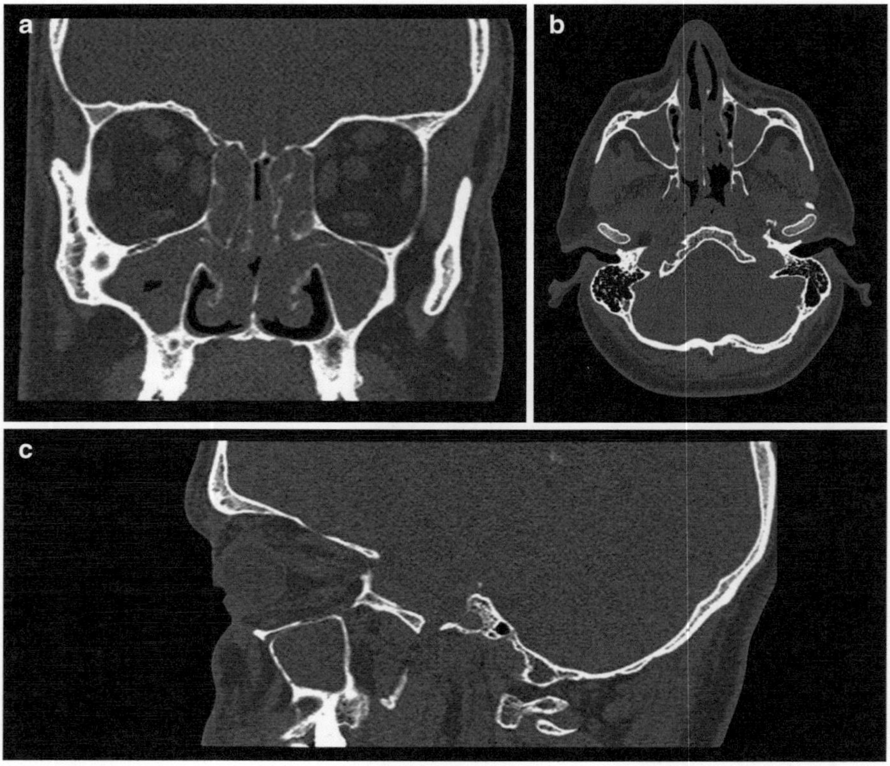

Fig. 5.6 Evidence of diffuse and extensive mucosal thickening and opacifications involving all paranasal sinuses bilaterally, extending through the osteo-meatal complexes into the nasal cavities and merging with the turbinates (**a**) Coronal, (**b**) Axial, (**c**) Sagittal

amoxicillin-clavulanate. For patients with penicillin allergies, doxycycline can be prescribed, or a combination of clindamycin with either cefixime or cefpodoxime may be used (Rosenfeld et al. 2015).

Prognosis

Sinusitis can potentially develop beyond the borders of the paranasal sinuses and result in life-threatening conditions by spreading into the orbit and central nervous system. In instances of orbital spread, complications such as preseptal cellulitis, orbital cellulitis, subperiosteal abscess, orbital abscess, and cavernous sinus thrombophlebitis can occur. Furthermore, if not properly managed, the infection can also spread into the central nervous system, leading to meningitis, epidural abscess, brain abscess, and subdural empyema (Patel and Hwang 2018). Patients with acute bacterial Rhinosinusitis are also at risk of developing chronic Rhinosinusitis.

However, these complications are not very common; according to a meta-analysis of randomised clinical trials, up to two-thirds of patients with acute rhinosinusitis experience spontaneous resolution of their symptoms (Ah-See 2015).

References

Acute sinusitis. (2023) Acute sinusitis—diagnosis and treatment—Mayo Clinic. https://www.mayoclinic.org/diseases-conditions/acute-sinusitis/diagnosis-treatment/drc-20351677

Ah-See K (2015) Sinusitis (acute rhinosinusitis). StatPearls. https://www.ncbi.nlm.nih.gov/pmc/articles/PMC4400653/

Bachert C, Hellings PW, Lund VJ, Fokkens WJ, Hopkins C, Mayer B, Chan RH, Smith SG, Sousa AR, Alfonso-Cristancho R, Yang S (2022) Mepolizumab improves quality of life and reduces activity impairments in patients with CRSwNP. Rhinology 60(6):474–478. https://doi.org/10.4193/Rhin22.053

Bell D, Abdel-Halim A-R (2014) Sinonasal polyposis. Radiopaedia.org. https://doi.org/10.53347/rid-31864

Bellocchi G, Loperfido A, Passali FM et al (2023) Biologics in severe uncontrolled chronic rhinosinusitis with nasal polyps: a bicentric experience. Acta Biomed 94:e2023227. https://doi.org/10.23750/abm.v94i5.14745

Cavaliere C, Loperfido A, Ciofalo A, Di Michele L, Begvarfaj E, Bellocchi G, Bugani M, de Vincentiis M, Greco A, Millarelli S, Plath M, Sculco E, Masieri S (2024) Real-life evidence of mepolizumab treatment in chronic rhinosinusitis with nasal polyps: a multicentric study. J Clin Med 13(12):3575. https://doi.org/10.3390/jcm13123575

Cergan R, Berghi ON, Dumitru M, Vrinceanu D, Manole F, Serboiu CS (2023) Biologics for chronic rhinosinusitis—a modern option for therapy. Life (Basel) 13(11):2165. https://doi.org/10.3390/life13112165

Chao SS, Graham SM, Brown CL, Kline JN, Hussain I (2006) Cysteinyl leukotriene 1 receptor expression in nasal polyps. Ann Otol Rhinol Laryngol 115(5):394–397. https://doi.org/10.1177/000348940611500513

Cho D-Y, Hunter RC, Ramakrishnan VR (2020a) The microbiome and chronic rhinosinusitis. Immunol Allergy Clin N Am 40:251–263. https://doi.org/10.1016/j.iac.2019.12.009

Cho SH, Ledford D, Lockey RF (2020b) Medical management strategies in acute and chronic rhinosinusitis. J Allergy Clin Immunol Pract 8:1559–1564. https://doi.org/10.1016/j.jaip.2020.02.020

Courey MS, Pletcher SD (2016) Upper airway disorders. In: Flint PW, Haughey BH, Lund VJ, Niparko JK, Richardson MA, Robbins KT, Thomas JR, Lesperance MM (eds) Cummings Otolaryngology – Head and Neck Surgery. 6th ed. Elsevier, Philadelphia, pp 877–896.e5

Damask CC, Ryan MW, Casale TB, Castro M, Franzese CB, Lee SE, Levy JM, Lin SY, Lio PA, Peters AT, Platt MP, White AA (2021) Targeted molecular therapies in allergy and rhinology. Otolaryngol Head Neck Surg 164(1_suppl):S1–S21. https://doi.org/10.1177/0194599820965233

De Corso E, Settimi S, Montuori C, Corbò M, Passali GC, Porru DP, Lo Verde S, Spanu C, Penazzi D, Di Bella GA, Nucera E, Bonini M, Paludetti G, Galli J (2022) Effectiveness of dupilumab in the treatment of patients with severe uncontrolled CRSwNP: a "real-life" observational study in the first year of treatment. J Clin Med 11(10):2684. https://doi.org/10.3390/jcm11102684

Fokkens W, Lund V, Mullol J (2020) European position paper on rhinosinusitis and nasal polyps 2020. Rhinology 58:1–464. https://doi.org/10.4193/rhin20.600

Fokkens WJ, Mullol J, Kennedy D, Philpott C, Seccia V, Kern RC, Coste A, Sousa AR, Howarth PH, Benson VS, Mayer B et al (2022) Mepolizumab for chronic rhinosinusitis with nasal polyps (SYNAPSE): in-depth sinus surgery analysis. Allergy 77(12):3752–3762. https://doi.org/10.1111/all.15434

Ghogomu N, Kern R (2016) Chronic rhinosinusitis: the rationale for current treatments. Expert Rev Clin Immunol 13:259–270. https://doi.org/10.1080/1744666x.2016.1220833
Halawi AM, Smith SS, Chandra RK (2013) Chronic rhinosinusitis: epidemiology and cost. Allergy Asthma Proc 34:328–334. https://doi.org/10.2500/aap.2013.34.3675
Han JK, Bachert C, Fokkens W, Desrosiers M, Wagenmann M, Lee SE, Smith SG, Martin N, Mayer B, Yancey SW, Sousa AR, Chan R, Hopkins C (2021) Mepolizumab for chronic rhinosinusitis with nasal polyps (SYNAPSE): a randomised, double-blind, placebo-controlled, phase 3 trial. Lancet Respir Med 9(10):1141–1153. https://doi.org/10.1016/S2213-2600(21)00097-7
Jonstam K, Swanson BN, Mannent LP et al (2019) Dupilumab reduces local type 2 pro-inflammatory biomarkers in chronic rhinosinusitis with nasal polyposis. Allergy 74:743–752. https://doi.org/10.1111/all.13685
Kunin CM (1993) Resistance to antimicrobial drugs—a worldwide calamity. Ann Intern Med 118:557. https://doi.org/10.7326/0003-4819-118-7-199304010-00011
Kwon E, O'Rourke MC (2023) Chronic sinusitis. StatPearls—NCBI Bookshelf. https://www.ncbi.nlm.nih.gov/books/NBK441934/
Leo G, Triulzi F, Incorvaia C (2012) Diagnosis of chronic rhinosinusitis. Pediatr Allergy Immunol 23:20–26. https://doi.org/10.1111/j.1399-3038.2012.01320.x
Li N, Peters AT (2015) Chronic rhinosinusitis management beyond intranasal steroids and salin solution. Allergy Ashtma Proc 36(5):339–343. https://doi.org/10.2500/aap.2015.36.3866
Lindberg S (1994) Morphological and functional studies of the mucociliary system during infections in the upper airways. Acta Otolaryngol 114:22–25. https://doi.org/10.3109/00016489409124318
Lombardo N, Pelaia C, Ciriolo M, Della Corte M, Piazzetta G, Lobello N, Viloa P, Pelaia G (2020) Real-life effects of benralizumab on allergic chronic rhinosinusitis and nasal polyposis associated with severe asthma. Int J Immunopathol Pharmacol 34:2058738420950851. https://doi.org/10.1177/2058738420950851
London NR, Reh DD (2016) Differential diagnosis of chronic rhinosinusitis with nasal polyps. Adv Otorhinolaryngol 79:1–12. https://doi.org/10.1159/000444957
Masood A, Moumoulidis I, Panesar J (2007) Acute rhinosinusitis in adults: an update on current management. Postgrad Med J 83:402–408. https://doi.org/10.1136/pgmj.2006.054767
Mayo Clinic (2023) Acute sinusitis – diagnosis and treatment. https://www.mayoclinic.org/diseases-conditions/acutesinusitis/diagnosis-treatment/drc-20351677
Meltzer EO, Hamilos DL (2011) Rhinosinusitis diagnosis and management for the clinician: a synopsis of recent consensus guidelines. Mayo Clin Proc 86:427–443. https://doi.org/10.4065/mcp.2010.0392
Meltzer EO, Hamilos DL, Hadley JA et al (2004) Rhinosinusitis: establishing definitions for clinical research and patient care. J Allergy Clin Immunol 114:155–212. https://doi.org/10.1016/j.jaci.2004.09.029
Miglani A, Soler ZM, Smith TL et al (2022) A comparative analysis of endoscopic sinus surgery versus biologics for treatment of chronic rhinosinusitis with nasal polyposis. Int Forum Allergy Rhinol 13:116–128. https://doi.org/10.1002/alr.23059
Norwood TG, Grayson JW, Woodworth BA (2023) Advances in sinus surgery for nasal polyps. Am J Rhinol Allergy 37:162–167. https://doi.org/10.1177/19458924221147783
Ottaviano G, Saccardo T, Roccuzzo G, Bernardi R, Di Chicco A, Pendolino AL, Scarpa B, Mairani E, Nicolai P (2022) Effectiveness of dupilumab in the treatment of patients with uncontrolled severe CRSwNP: a "real-life" observational study in naïve and post-surgical patients. J Pers Med 12(9):1526. https://doi.org/10.3390/jpm12091526
Patel ZM, Hwang PH (2018) Acute Bacterial Rhinosinusitis. Springer eBooks, pp 133–143
Rosenfeld RM, Piccirillo JF, Chandrasekhar SS et al (2015) Clinical practice guideline (update): adult sinusitis. Otolaryngol Head Neck Surg 152:S1–S39. https://doi.org/10.1177/0194599815572097
Santomasi C, Buonamico E, Dragonieri S, Iannuzzi L, Portacci A, Quaranta N, Carpagnano GE (2023) Effects of benralizumab in a population of patients affected by severe eosinophilic asthma and chronic rhinosinusitis with nasal polyps: a real life study. Acta Biomed 94(1):e2023028. https://doi.org/10.23750/abm.v94i1.13474

Siddiqui Z, Tahiri M, Gupta A et al (2021) The management of paediatric rhinosinusitis. Int J Pediatr Otorhinolaryngol 147:110786. https://doi.org/10.1016/j.ijporl.2021.110786
Snidvongs K, Kalish L, Sacks R, Sivasubramaniam R, Cope D, Harvey RJ (2013) Sinus surgert delivery method influence the effectiveness of topical corticosteroid for chronic rhinosinusitis: systematic review and meta-analysis. Am Rhinol Allergy 27(3):221–223. https://doi.org/10.2500/ajra.2013.27.3880
Southwood JE, Loehrl TA, Poetker DM (2016) Advances in surgery: extended procedures for sinonasal polyp disease. Adv Otorhinolaryngol 79:148–157
Van Cauwenberge P, Watelet JB (2000) Epidemiology of chronic rhinosinusitis. Thorax 55(Suppl 2):S20–S21
Wojas O, Arcimowicz M, Furmańczyk K et al (2021) The relationship between nasal polyps, bronchial asthma, allergic rhinitis, atopic dermatitis, and non-allergic rhinitis. Postepy Dermatol Alergol 38:650–656. https://doi.org/10.5114/ada.2020.94400

Fungal Maxillary Rhinosinusitis

6

Goran Latif Omer, Gianluca Velletrani, Riccardo Maurizi, Beatrice Francavilla, Andrea Gravina, Stefania Tilotta, Maria Grazia Maglie, Davide Balletta, Gianluca Scialla, Marco Perla, Sahand Soran Ali, Stefano Di Girolamo, and Aland Salih Abdullah

Allergic Fungal Rhinosinusitis

Introduction

Allergic fungal rhinosinusitis (AFRS) is a distinct type of chronic rhinosinusitis that is relatively new, often misdiagnosed, and incompletely understood. It has characteristic clinical, radiographic, and histopathologic findings. Understanding this unique disease is important as it leads to efficient diagnosis and treatment of this curable condition.

Epidemiology

Allergic fungal rhinosinusitis generally affects immunocompetent individuals with atopy. Although it can arise at any age, it tends to present at a younger age (Callejas and Douglas 2013; Hoyt et al. 2016). AFRS is more common in warm and high-humidity countries, probably because such climates are more conducive to fungal presence. The incidence of AFRS is higher in regions with specific environmental conditions:

Supplementary Information The online version contains supplementary material available at https://doi.org/10.1007/978-3-031-83468-4_6.

G. L. Omer (✉) · S. S. Ali · A. S. Abdullah
Department of Clinical Sciences, College of Medicine, University of Sulaimani, Sulaymaniyah, KRI, Iraq

G. Velletrani · R. Maurizi · B. Francavilla · A. Gravina · S. Tilotta · M. G. Maglie
D. Balletta · G. Scialla · M. Perla · S. Di Girolamo
Department of Otorhinolaryngology, University of Rome Tor Vergata, Rome, Italy

© The Author(s), under exclusive license to Springer Nature Switzerland AG 2025

G. L. Omer, S. Di Girolamo (eds.), *Maxillary Sinus: A Comprehensive Guide*,
https://doi.org/10.1007/978-3-031-83468-4_6

- **Southern United States:** High humidity and temperatures in states such as Texas and Louisiana create an ideal environment for fungal growth. Consequently, AFRS is more commonly reported in these areas.
- **Southeast Asia and the Middle East:** Countries in these regions also exhibit higher prevalence rates due to similar climatic conditions.
- **Africa and India:** The tropical and subtropical climates in these regions are conducive to fungal proliferation, contributing to higher AFRS incidence.

The sex predominance seems to vary (Nomura et al. 2013; Tyler and Luong 2018; Yoon et al. 2017).

Seasonal variations seem to influence fungal growth:

- **Spring and Summer:** Higher temperatures and increased humidity during these seasons promote fungal spore proliferation, leading to an increase in AFRS cases.
- **Autumn:** In some regions, autumnal changes in vegetation and increased rainfall can also elevate fungal spore counts, exacerbating AFRS symptoms.

In conclusion, several risk factors have been associated with an increased likelihood of developing AFRS: geographical location, immunocompetence, genetic factors, atopy, and asthma. Further research into the epidemiological trends of AFRS can provide deeper insights into its pathogenesis and inform public health strategies to mitigate its impact (González-Alcaide et al. 2020).

Pathophysiology

AFRS has complex and multiple aetiologies involving different pathways. The lower airways, through the respiratory epithelium, represent the first line of defence against pathogens. In AFRS, the epithelium is altered due to chronic inflammation, which facilitates the alteration of fungal immunity (Tieu et al. 2009; Wiesner and Klein 2017). Additionally, histatin levels are lower than in other CRSwNP subtypes, suggesting a reduced ability to clear fungi from the sinuses (Tyler and Luong 2018). Fungal colonisation promotes the loss of epithelial barrier integrity, apoptosis of epithelial cells, and the release of proinflammatory cytokines, thymic stromal lymphopoietin, IL-25, and IL-33 (Dykewicz et al. 2018; Hoyt et al. 2016). The elevation of these interleukins activates type 2 innate lymphoid cells and TH2 cells, releasing IL-5, which causes eosinophilia, and IL-4 and IL-13, which provoke mucus and IgE production (Dykewicz et al. 2018; Tyler et al. 2021). Elevated local fungal antigen levels stimulate the activation of the fungal IgE receptor on mast cells, leading to degranulation and the release of inflammatory mediators, causing oedema and obstruction (Tyler and Luong 2018; Luong et al. 2022). Some studies show that Staphylococcus aureus colonisation is more common in AFRS than in CRSwNP (Clark et al. 2012), possibly because fungi alter the epithelial barrier, facilitating staph colonisation (Dutre et al. 2013).

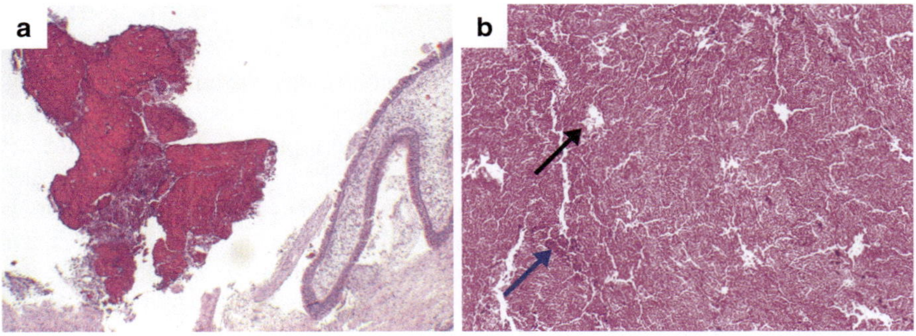

Fig. 6.1 Fungal rhinosinusitis: Aggregates of eosinophilic mucin composed of cellular debris can be seen in this image (**a**: 4×, **b**: 40×) along with epithelial and polymorphonuclear cells (Blue arrow) and degranulated eosinophil

Histology

As shown in Fig. 6.1, analyzing the sinus discharge, microscopic examination shows allergic mucin with prominent eosinophils, necrotic cellular debris, Charcot-Leyden crystals, fungal hyphae, and a background of amorphous eosinophilic mucin (Dykewicz et al. 2018). Haematoxylin and eosin stains reveal a mixed inflammatory infiltrate composed of eosinophils, plasma cells, and lymphocytes, sometimes with fungal elements and calcifications. Gomori methenamine silver or Fontana Mason stains show sparse fungal hyphae that are not well identified on haematoxylin and eosin staining (Uri et al. 2013). Since fungi are frequently present in ambient air, the growth of fungi in culture alone, without clinical, imaging, and laboratory criteria, is not diagnostic, as it might represent saprophytic contamination (Dykewicz et al. 2018).

Clinical Features

AFRS should be considered in a patient with symptoms of CRS that are resistant to conventional medical therapy (Dykewicz et al. 2018). The presentation of AFRS may range from subtle to dramatic signs and symptoms. Nasal congestion, anosmia, rhinorrhoea, posterior pharyngeal drainage, and the presence of thick "peanut butter-like" mucin are the most common symptoms. The more dramatic symptoms are bony erosions, facial deformities, visual disturbances (Al-Radadi and Alnoury 2011; Marple et al. 1999), pressure-induced intracranial neuropathies, or intracranial abscesses (Holbrook et al. 2011; Illing et al. 2015). The result of the bony erosion is not caused by the fungi (Nussenbaum et al. 2001) but more probably by the polyposis with the increment of pressure and atrophy.

Diagnosis and Imaging

The diagnosis of AFRS is based on clinical features, nasal examination, imaging, and laboratory studies. AFRS should be considered in patients with symptoms of CRS resistant to conventional medical therapy. The typical features of AFRS are anosmia, nasal congestion, rhinorrhoea, and the presence of thick mucin, with various colours ranging from light to tan brown, also known as peanut butter-like mucin (Marple 2006). On anterior rhinoscopy, the nasal cavity may appear full of thick and brown mucus with mucosal crusting (Hoyt et al. 2016). In rhino-fibroscopy, this scenario can be more evident, along with significant polyposis (Hoyt et al. 2016). Patients with AFRS are often atopic. The evidence of sensitisation can be identified through positive skin testing or serum-specific IgE tests. The imaging studies are based on CT scans and magnetic resonance imaging (MRI). In contrast with CRS, AFRS is more often unilateral and may be limited to only a few sinuses. AFRS CT findings are heterogeneous opacities with areas of hyperattenuation. It is often described as the "starry sky" because of the aspect of this attenuation, which is usually at the centre. In MRI, mucosal oedema can be appreciated on T2 sequences as hypointensities because of the presence of eosinophilic mucin (with high protein and low water content) (Chua et al. 2023).

Treatment and Management

The main treatment of AFRS is surgical. Functional endoscopic sinus surgery (FESS) aims to debride all the fungal and eosinophilic mucin and open all the involved sinuses widely to facilitate the penetration of topical medications (Fokkens et al. 2012; Marple and Mabry 2000). Most clinical studies have proved that only medical therapy is insufficient to alleviate symptoms, while surgical debridement alone or in combination with medical therapy improves clinical outcomes (Fokkens et al. 2012). Topical and oral corticosteroids are the main medical therapy due to their anti-inflammatory effect: they promote polyp regression and decrease oedema around the sinus. Before surgery, oral corticosteroids decrease symptoms and help improve the view during debridement (Dykewicz et al. 2018). After surgery, systemic corticosteroids decrease disease recurrence (Schubert et al. 2004; Tan et al. 2018). Antifungals, due to the role of the fungus in this disease, seem to be the most logical drug to administer, but most studies find little or no evidence for their efficacy (Bachert et al. 2014). The use of immunotherapy is very controversial in the management of AFRS. Many studies have reported that immunotherapy improves the quality of life and is useful as an adjunct therapy (Bassichis et al. 2001; Mabry et al. 1998; Mabry and Mabry 1997). However, these studies don't have well-characterised controls.

Prognosis

Allergic fungal rhinosinusitis (AFRS) is a chronic recurrent disease that poses significant challenges for long-term management and prognosis. The prognosis of AFRS depends on various factors, including treatment effectiveness, patient adherence to therapy, environmental controls, and management of comorbid conditions. Analysing each influencing aspect is crucial for understanding prognosis (Dykewicz et al. 2018).

Recurrence and Chronicity

AFRS is characterised by its chronic nature and carries a high risk of recurrence, often necessitating revision surgery (Dykewicz et al. 2018). Despite comprehensive treatment strategies involving medical and surgical interventions, many patients experience recurrent symptoms due to residual fungal debris, persistent environmental exposure to fungi, and non-adherence to prescribed treatments.

Impact on Quality of Life

Persistent symptoms such as nasal obstruction, facial pain, and recurrent infections significantly impact patients' quality of life. Chronic symptoms can lead to sleep disturbances, psychological distress, and limitations in social and occupational functioning.

Factors Influencing Prognosis

Several factors influence the long-term prognosis of AFRS:

- **Adherence to Treatment**: Consistent use of intranasal corticosteroids, saline irrigations, and prescribed systemic treatments is critical.
- **Environmental Controls**: Measures to reduce mould exposure and manage allergens are essential.
- **Surgical Interventions**: Effective sinus surgery and post-surgical monitoring are crucial to prevent recurrence.
- **Management of Comorbid Conditions**: Optimising treatment for asthma and allergic rhinitis and modulating the immune response are important considerations.
- **Patient Education and Support**: Educating patients about AFRS treatment adherence and providing support through counselling or support groups can improve outcomes.

Long-Term Outcomes

With comprehensive management, many AFRS patients experience significant symptom relief and improved quality of life. Effective management reduces symptom severity recurrence rates and enhances daily functioning.

Mucormycosis

Introduction

Mucormycosis is a severe fungal infection known as "the most acutely fatal fungal infection" by many researchers (Flint et al. 2020). Although it is typically harmless in immunocompetent individuals, its manifestations are deadly in the immunocompromised, including people with poorly controlled diabetes, haematological malignancies, and those using steroids or other immunosuppressant drugs. Therefore, mucormycosis is regarded as an opportunistic disease. The infection is caused by a fungal order called *Mucorales*, which includes more than 260 species. Among these, *Rhizopus oryzae* is believed to cause approximately 70% of mucormycosis cases (Ibrahim et al. 2012; Stone et al. 2021; Walther et al. 2019). Fungal spores are inhaled and deposited in the nose and paranasal sinuses, from where they can spread to neighbouring areas, including the orbit, mastoid air cells, and the brain. Additionally, due to the fungi's exceptional ability to invade arteries, further damage and thrombosis occur, causing necrosis even in areas with a rich blood supply, such as the maxillary sinus (Dhingra and Dhingra 2013; Kumar et al. 2013).

Epidemiology

Mucormycosis cases have been recorded worldwide, with incidence rates ranging from 0.005 to 1.7 per million people (Mucormycosis 2023). The incidence appears to differ between developed and developing nations. In developed countries, the condition is most common among individuals with diabetes mellitus, haematological malignancies receiving chemotherapy, and those who have received allogeneic stem cell transplantation, although it remains relatively uncommon. In contrast, mucormycosis cases, though sporadic, are more frequent in people with uncontrolled diabetes or trauma in underdeveloped nations, particularly in India, where it is estimated at 140 cases per million people—almost 80 times greater than the incidence in developed countries (Petrikkos et al. 2012); Mucormycosis 2023). Obtaining a detailed picture of the epidemiology of this disease is challenging due to difficulties in diagnosing mucormycosis clinically, with many cases remaining undiagnosed because of challenges in collecting samples from deep tissue and the low sensitivity of diagnostic tests (Petrikkos et al. 2012); Prakash and Chakrabarti 2019).

According to Roden et al., 39% of mucormycosis cases are initially sinus infections, making them the most common type compared to pulmonary, gastrointestinal, cutaneous, etc. (Roden et al. 2005). Furthermore, Turner et al. identified diabetes mellitus as the most common predisposing factor in mucormycosis-associated Acute Invasive Fungal Rhinosinusitis (AIFRS). Recently, cases of rhino-sinu-orbito-cerebral mucormycosis in patients with iron overload have also been reported (Chang et al. 2014; Sataloff 2015). In patients with haematological malignancies, mucormycosis develops in 4 out of 100 cases, with acute myeloid leukaemia (AML) being most commonly involved (62%) (Bhandari et al. 2023).

Aetiology

The order *Mucorales*, part of the phylum *Mucoromycota*, includes 261 species in 55 genera. Apart from those that cause infections, some species in this order have been used as fermenting agents in African and Asian food for many centuries, others in the production of various European cheeses, and still others in biotechnology for the biotransformation of pharmaceutically important compounds such as steroids (Walther et al. 2019).

Fungi of the *Mucoraceae* family, including *Rhizopus*, *Mucor*, and *Absidia*, are responsible for mucormycosis. However, in approximately 70% of cases, the most common organism isolated is *Rhizopus oryzae*, which is also the most virulent (Flint et al. 2020; Ibrahim et al. 2012; Wackym and Snow 2016). These species are typically saprophytic in humans and only cause severe illness in the presence of predisposing factors. They also grow more abundantly in hot, humid climates, particularly in tropical regions and during the summer (Bhandari et al. 2023).

Pathophysiology

When fungal spores are inhaled, they may germinate and develop hyphae if the host is unable to phagocytise them, leading to invasion of the mucosal tissues (Crist et al. 2018). Acidic conditions promote *Mucor* growth, and as the fungus develops, it spreads by vascular invasion, resulting in thrombosis, ischemic infarction, and necrosis (Flint et al. 2020). Typically, an infection begins in the nose, spreads to the paranasal sinuses, and then progresses to the orbit and cavernous sinuses. The inflammatory process can quickly spread to the infratemporal fossa and along the intracranial and infraorbital fissures. Additionally, as a result of ascending infection along the Eustachian tube and tensor tympani, the middle ear and mastoid can be affected (Chang et al. 2014; Flint et al. 2020). The moist environment of the nasal cavity and paranasal sinuses encourages fungal development and invasion, leading to infection of mucosa and bone depending on the severity of the disease, host immunity, and persistence. The maxillary sinus often experiences early fungal implantation, forming a "fungal ball", a non-invasive collection of dense fungal mycelia, inflammatory cells, fibrin, mucus, and tissue debris (Bhandari et al. 2023;

Bois et al. 2017). The middle meatus, septum, and middle turbinate are the most frequently affected sites. Bone invasion is typical in untreated cases and can penetrate all nearby tissues. Mucormycosis has a distinct aetiology that contributes to its rapid growth. When fungal hyphae invade vessel walls, they damage the endothelium, leading to blood clots that obstruct blood vessels, causing ischemia and necrosis of the surrounding tissue. This necrotic tissue serves as a nidus for the growth of organisms, which then invade neighbouring tissues via blood vessels (Bhandari et al. 2023). While normal human serum can inhibit *Rhizopus* growth, serum from diabetic ketoacidosis patients may promote it due to altered transferrin binding, which facilitates iron access for the fungi. Patients receiving deferoxamine, an iron chelator, are at higher risk for mucormycosis as it makes iron available in a form suitable for fungal growth, thus increasing fungal virulence (Flint et al. 2020). Iron chelators also inhibit the formation of free radicals by iron-catalysed peroxidase, which normally helps kill fungi, and mask the antifungal activity of Amphotericin B, a primary treatment for mucormycosis (Bhandari et al. 2023).

As previously mentioned, fungal rhinosinusitis due to mucormycosis primarily affects patients with diabetes mellitus. The condition causes bone necrosis even in highly vascular areas such as the maxillary sinus, as thrombi created by *Mucor* hyphae diminish tissue vascularity, resulting in necrosis. Diabetes-induced peripheral vascular disease (microangiopathy and atherosclerosis) exacerbates local tissue ischemia and susceptibility to infections, leading to necrosis of the maxilla due to persistent hyperglycemia and thrombosis of the internal maxillary artery or descending palatine artery caused by mucormycotic infection.

Histology

Mucorales hyphae are characterised by irregular 90° branching, few or no septa, 7–20 μm wide and 100–200 μm long when viewed under a microscope (Wackym and Snow 2016; Crist et al. 2018). Cultures of *Mucor* species can reach the top of the culture plate in just 24 h due to the rapid growth of the fungus. Therefore, if a diagnosis is suspected, it is crucial to act on that suspicion promptly (Flint et al. 2020). Microscopic assessment should include morphology, width, branching angle, and septation, and occasionally, hyphae can be seen invading blood vessels. Histopathology helps rule out differential diagnoses, and biopsy techniques vary depending on the anatomical location, either directly or endoscopically, in cases involving the paranasal sinuses. Even if only yeast forms are seen on histology, treatment should not be excluded based on the absence of hyphae if risk factors and clinical findings suggest mucormycosis.

Clinical Features

Initial symptoms are nonspecific; however, a one-sided headache behind the eyes and lethargy are the most common (Bhandari et al. 2023). Typically, patients present with fever, nasal ulcerations, periorbital or facial oedema, visual changes, headache, and facial pain (Pai et al. 2021). Patients with nasal involvement often present with ulceration, necrosis, or purulent or serosanguinous discharge. The most typical initial sites of involvement are the lateral nasal wall and turbinates. Cyanosis and black necrosis are followed by oedema and erythema (Ballenger and Snow 2003). Additionally, mucormycosis can cause oral lesions characterised by palatal ulcerations or black, necrotic masses. The palate is a frequent site for initial infection (Pai et al. 2021). Orbital extension can lead to proptosis, periorbital oedema retro-orbital or periorbital pain, amaurosis, diplopia, and blurred vision (Ballenger and Snow 2003; Bhandari et al. 2023). Cranial involvement may result in focal neurologic deficits, cranial neuropathies, and coma. Anaesthesia of an affected area, most frequently of the nasal mucosa or cheeks, which occurs before the development of ischemic necrosis of the nasal cavity, may provide an early indication of mucormycosis (Ballenger and Snow 2003; Flint et al. 2020). On physical examination, common findings include nasal and orbital cellulitis, later-stage nasal bridge and cheek skin oedema and reddening, which eventually turns black due to cell death, and noticeable black eschar on the palatine or nasal mucosa. In severe cases, epistaxis may be observed. Palatal ulceration might be visible upon intraoral inspection. Conjunctival chemosis, nystagmus, and a fixed pupil are additional ophthalmological symptoms that may be present. Patients with cerebral involvement and vascular impairment might be in a coma or exhibit stroke-like symptoms. During a neurological examination, palsies of the second through seventh cranial nerves may be noted (Bhandari et al. 2023).

Diagnosis and Imaging

Due to the nonspecific nature of initial symptoms, the diagnosis of mucormycosis is often delayed. A high index of suspicion is necessary for the presence of risk factors (Bhandari et al. 2023). Green et al. first reported the radiographic findings of mucormycosis in the sinuses, identifying three key features: nodular mucosal thickening, absence of fluid levels, and patchy destruction of bone walls (Chang et al. 2014). As shown in Fig. 6.2, computed tomography may reveal mucoperiosteal oedema with bone damage. Magnetic resonance imaging is useful for assessing intracranial or intraorbital extension (Dave et al. 2021). Nasal endoscopy may reveal mucosal necrosis, a sign of mucormycosis, and, in rare instances, actual fungal sporulation (Flint et al. 2020). CT or MRI scanning clearly demonstrates the relationship between nasal, sinus, and orbital disease and tissue loss due to necrosis, a combination of features so characteristic of mucormycosis that it should be considered in the presence of these findings (Chang et al. 2014). However, it should be noted that radiological evaluations are not entirely unique to mucormycosis, as other invasive diseases may yield false-positive or false-negative results; thus, even a normal sinus CT may not rule out an invasive condition (Bhandari et al. 2023). The diagnosis of mucormycosis is confirmed by histopathological identification of non-septate hyphae from a biopsy of necrotic tissue and by a culture of the fungus on Sabouraud glucose agar, stained with PAS (Periodic Acid-Schiff) or Grocott's modified silver methenamine (Auluck 2007; Bhandari et al. 2023; Crist et al. 2018). For patients

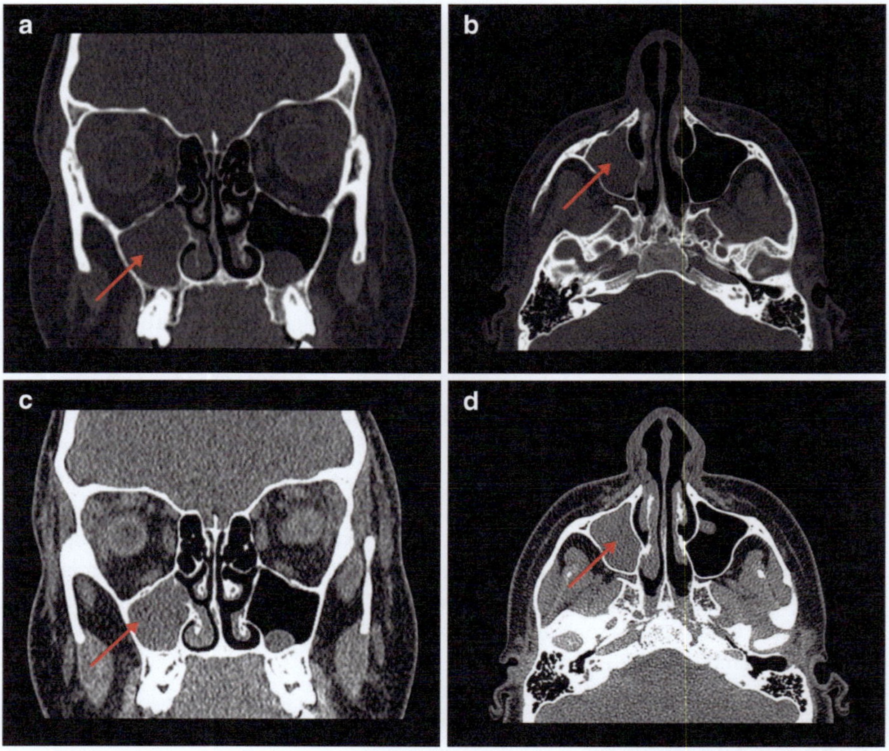

Fig. 6.2 Complete opacification of the right maxillary sinus (arrow, **a** and **c**: coronal views, **b** and **d**: axial views), no sinus expansion, no bone erosion or destruction, and no local invasive/aggressive features

with immunosuppression and respiratory symptoms, a chest CT scan should be performed to check for pulmonary mucormycosis. This condition presents similarly to pneumonia, making diagnosis challenging. Chest radiologic findings may include pleural effusion, nodules, consolidation, and ground-glass infiltrates. Broad non-septate hyphae might be visible in bronchoalveolar lavage (Hernández and Buckley 2023).

Treatment/Management

Mucormycosis requires vigorous treatment due to its rapid spread and high invasiveness. However, definitive treatment and a step-by-step management strategy are not yet established. Comprehensive clinical trials are needed to determine the best management techniques and confirm effective therapies. When mucormycosis is suspected, amphotericin B should be administered immediately. Treatment with amphotericin B for 4–6 weeks is essential to eradicate the infection (Bhandari et al. 2023). Systemic amphotericin B remains the preferred definitive therapy, typically administered intravenously (IV) at doses ranging from 0.25 mg/kg/day to a maximum of 1.5 mg/kg every other day. The primary dose-limiting adverse effect is nephrotoxicity, which can be mitigated by sodium loading. Initial doses often cause fever, chills, nausea, and hypotension. Amphotericin B lipid complex, which uses liposomes to administer amphotericin B, can reduce or eliminate these toxicities. Due to their affinity for the reticuloendothelial system, these liposomes can avoid the toxic effects of amphotericin B on other organs (Flint et al. 2020). Although liposomal amphotericin B is more expensive, it is safer and may be more effective than other formulations, particularly in cancer patients with mucormycosis (Watkinson and Clarke 2018). Nasal irrigations and nebuliser treatments can be used to administer antifungal medications intranasally as an additional supplement to systemic dosing. Such topical therapy may have advantages over other treatments, which outweigh their minor risks (Sataloff 2015). It is important to note that antifungal azoles are ineffective against mucormycosis (Wackym and Snow 2016). In addition to antifungals, warfarin may be used to prevent clotting, as patients with mucormycosis can experience arterial and venous clotting (Bhandari et al. 2023). Medical treatment alone does not improve prognosis significantly. The cornerstone of treatment is urgent, aggressive surgical excision of the entire lesion, which should be performed immediately (Grant and Skilbeck 2014), as shown in Fig. 6.3. Extensive surgical debridement down to the level of bleeding tissue is required, often guided by frozen-section analysis, allowing for more thorough removal of infected tissues (Myers and Snyderman 2018; Crist et al. 2018). Surgery may alter the configuration of affected body parts, and multiple operations might be necessary. The type of surgical technique, such as a maxillectomy or ethmoidectomy, depends on the location and extent of involvement. Severe cases may require complete maxillectomy for significant palate ulceration and oroantral fistula formation, whereas partial maxillectomy may suffice for minor bone erosion and swelling. Affected tissue must be adequately removed, with excision of healthy tissue extending beyond 1 cm. In cases with significant orbital involvement, orbital exenteration is necessary, though the orbital floor can be preserved if the orbital contents are unaffected. Debridement and craniotomy are required for intracranial involvement (Bhandari et al. 2023). Postoperative hyperbaric oxygen therapy may improve survival by providing direct fungicidal effects, enhancing host phagocytic activity, and reducing local acidosis, which inhibits fungal growth (Myers and Snyderman 2018; Pai et al. 2021). Management of underlying conditions should involve consulting relevant specialists. For example, diabetic ketoacidosis should be treated with insulin and oral hypoglycaemic agents, and immunosuppressive medications used in chemotherapy and steroids should be discontinued or reduced. Granulocyte colony-stimulating factors can be used to enhance immunity (Bhandari et al. 2023). Due to the rarity of mucormycosis, significant studies comparing various treatment regimens directly in a randomised fashion are lacking (Grant and Skilbeck 2014).

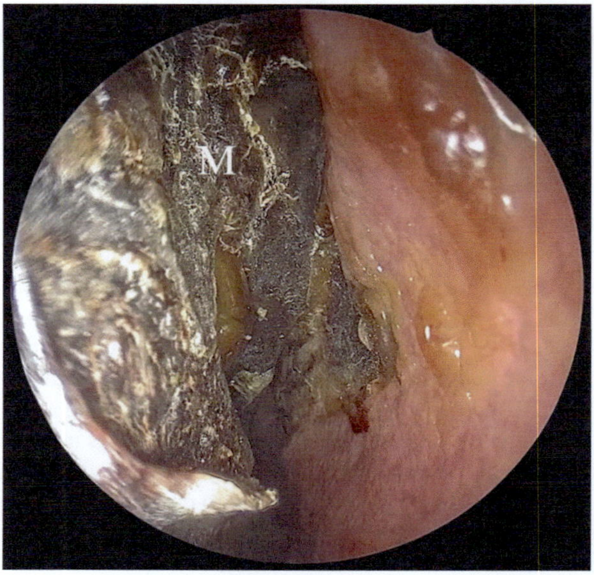

Fig. 6.3 This is an intraoperative video of a patient undergoing Endoscopic Sinus Surgery for mucormycosis. In the thumbnail (right side nasal cavity), black fungus can be seen in the nasal cavity, which is mucormycosis (M) (Audio and Video 6.1)

Differential Diagnosis

Clinicians must maintain a high index of suspicion to differentiate rhinocerebral mucormycosis from other disorders with overlapping symptoms and similar locations.

Bacterial Sinusitis and Allergic Fungal Sinusitis

Early-stage mucormycosis may be mistaken for bacterial sinusitis. If mucormycosis is identified, antibiotics for bacterial sinusitis should be discontinued. A history of recurrent allergic rhinitis, nasal polyps, and elevated IgE levels suggests allergic fungal sinusitis. Allergic fungal sinusitis can cause proptosis and may present as a large rhinocerebral mass. Unlike the invasive rhinocerebral form, allergic fungal sinusitis does not cause fungal invasion (Bhandari et al. 2023).

Aspergillosis

Aspergillosis can invade nasal tissues, particularly in patients with weakened immune systems due to immunosuppressive medications (Dhingra and Dhingra 2013). Aspergillosis shares similarities with rhinocerebral mucormycosis, including CNS invasion but does not typically present with black eschar upon gross inspection (Bhandari et al. 2023). *Aspergillus* hyphal elements may appear swollen and similar to mucormycosis due to frozen-section artefacts. The differentiation is usually made on permanent histopathologic sections, where *Aspergillus* species show narrower hyphae with regular septations and 45° branching (Flint et al. 2020). Itraconazole is effective against aspergillosis, while amphotericin B is used to treat mucormycosis.

Nasal and Paranasal Malignancies

Malignancies, such as squamous cell carcinoma, can mimic mucormycosis due to their high invasiveness. Findings of nasal malignancy and haemorrhage can lead to misdiagnosis. Malignancies typically present with a chronic course and affect older individuals, whereas mucormycosis often has a shorter duration and is more common in younger populations. Mucosal thickening of the paranasal sinuses is also more common with mucormycosis (Anjum et al. 2020).

Wegener's Granulomatosis

This condition affects the upper airways, lungs, kidneys, and skin and can present with tumour-like vegetations in the oral cavity, resembling palate ulcers seen in mucormycosis (Dhingra and Dhingra 2013). However, Wegener's granulomatosis features strawberry gingivitis, which is absent in mucormycosis (Anjum et al. 2020).

Other Causes of Cavernous Sinus Thrombosis

Other conditions that present with one-sided headache, proptosis, increased intracranial pressure, and other features common to mucormycosis should be ruled out (Bhandari et al. 2023).

Prognosis

Mucormycosis is frequently a potentially fatal infection. An analysis of reported cases of mucormycosis revealed an overall mortality rate of 54%. The fatality rate varies depending on the underlying medical condition, the type of fungus, and the body site affected. For instance, the mortality rate is 46% for sinus infections, 76% for pulmonary infections, and 96% for disseminated mucormycosis (Mycetoma 2024a, b). Despite vigorous therapy, the prognosis is typically poor. Early diagnosis and timely treatment significantly improve prognosis (Bhandari et al. 2023). Since the introduction of combined treatment with amphotericin B and surgery, more than 80% of patients can be expected to survive a condition that was previously almost always fatal (Grant and Skilbeck 2014). A combination of surgical debridement and antifungal medication has been shown to yield a higher survival rate (70%) compared to surgery alone (57%) or medical therapy alone (61%). One study found that 85% of patients survived when treated within 5 days after diagnosis, compared to 49% when therapy was started after the sixth day of diagnosis. Patients with predisposing factors and cerebral involvement have a higher mortality rate than those without these risk factors (Bhandari et al. 2023). The prognosis is considerably better if the disease has not spread beyond the sinus; mortality rates for local sinonasal disease have been reported to be less than 10% (Grant and Skilbeck 2014). One study found no survival difference between patients with orbital involvement who underwent exenteration and those who did not. However, patients with orbital involvement had a higher overall mortality rate (33% vs. 14%) (Myers and Snyderman 2018). Furthermore, a recent assessment revealed that 12 out of 14 individuals with orbital involvement died from the condition, and the only two who survived had undergone orbital exenteration (Myers and Snyderman 2018). Once it is confirmed that the disease has been completely cured, reconstructive surgery is necessary, as post-surgical deformity and visual impairment are highly likely. Ongoing medical treatment requires tight glycaemic control, thorough drug monitoring, and vigilance for disease recurrence. A patient's prognosis is significantly worsened if they have hemiplegia, bilateral sinus involvement, facial necrosis, nasal deformity, concomitant renal disease, or are taking deferoxamine (Grant and Skilbeck 2014).

Fungal Ball in Maxillary Sinus

Introduction

The categorisation, diagnosis, and treatment of rhinosinusitis caused by fungi have improved over the past 30 years, in part due to advancements in endoscopic technology and imaging capabilities. Rhinosinusitis is essentially divided into invasive and non-invasive types based on the presence or absence of microscopic evidence of fungal hyphae within the tissues. Aspergilloma, or "fungus ball," is one of the non-invasive fungal sinus diseases that is becoming more widely recognised (Grosjean and Weber 2007). A fungal ball is a non-invasive, dense collection of fungal hyphae that typically develops in a solitary maxillary sinus. However, it can occasionally involve other sinuses, such as the ethmoids or sphenoids, and may be associated with conditions like concha bullosa. While most individuals are asymptomatic, some experience persistent mucopurulent rhinorrhoea. Surgery is used to remove the fungus from the affected sinus, and because the procedure is non-invasive, no further treatment is usually necessary. Although complications are rare and recurrence is only about 1%, there have been reports of infections becoming invasive in immunocompromised individuals (Garcia-Rubio and Alcazar-Fuoli 2018; Lund et al. 2013).

Epidemiology

Fungal balls occur in immunocompetent individuals and are often discovered unexpectedly during the treatment of chronic rhinosinusitis (Hathiram and Khattar 2009). In clinical practise, the paranasal fungal ball, typically located in the maxillary sinus, is the most common type of non-invasive fungal rhinosinusitis (Wu et al. 2021). A French retrospective study of 173 cases found that 87.8% had fungal balls in the maxillary sinus (Dufour et al. 2006). Maxillary sinus fungal balls primarily affect older individuals, as shown in an American retrospective study with an age range of 28–86 years, averaging 64 years (Hathiram and Khattar 2009; Wu et al.

2021). No paediatric cases have been documented. Most studies report a female incidence of about 64%, indicating a significant female preponderance (Wu et al. 2021). The reason for this female predominance is unknown, though a hormonal association has been proposed (Garcia-Rubio and Alcazar-Fuoli 2018). The prevalence of paranasal sinus fungal balls (PSFB) in the general population is not well-defined. Recent studies show a rising incidence of PSFB since the mid-2000s. Data from 713 individuals who received treatment for paranasal sinus fungal balls at a single facility between 2005 and 2018 revealed that the percentage of PSFB cases in all Endoscopic Sinus Surgery cases was 5.5% in 2005 but increased to more than 10% after 2008. These findings may not reflect annual incidence precisely but suggest a growing trend, possibly due to increased disease awareness, improved diagnostic tools, broader use of antibiotics, and an ageing population (Wu et al. 2021).

Aetiology

Aspergillus species are among the most common causes of fungal balls, forming an Aspergilloma, which consists of *Aspergillus* hyphae aggregated in a mass along with fibrin, mucus, and cellular debris (Garcia-Rubio and Alcazar-Fuoli 2018). Of the 669 PSFB samples collected by Liu et al., 151 (22.6%) contained fungi, with *Aspergillus* spp. (72.8%) being the most common (Wu et al. 2021). *Aspergillus* species are typically found in soil, decaying plants, seeds, and grains, where they thrive as saprophytes. Humans can occasionally be affected by *Aspergillus* species, which are present year-round in various environments. However, only a few species are known to cause significant opportunistic infections in humans (Mousavi et al. 2016). In the case of fungal balls, *Aspergillus fumigatus* is the most common pathogen (Garcia-Rubio and Alcazar-Fuoli 2018). The term "Mycetoma", previously used instead of "fungal ball", was generally applied to describe chronic, deep granulomatous bacterial (Actinomycetoma) or fungal infections (Eumycetoma) (Garcia-Rubio and Alcazar-Fuoli 2018; Mycetoma 2024a, b).

Pathophysiology

The pathophysiology of fungal ball formation is not fully understood, but the progression is generally gradual and benign. Patients may experience symptoms for months or years before diagnosis. A fungal ball forms when fungal hyphae and spores become lodged in a paranasal sinus, and conditions favour their growth. Pathological conditions that interfere with normal mucociliary clearance or block the sinus ostium, such as acute or chronic rhinosinusitis, contribute to this process. This blockage causes fungal spores to germinate in the sinus cavity, leading to further hyphal growth and continued obstruction (Hathiram and Khattar 2009). Previous surgery or mucosal damage may also play a role. Additionally, maxillary fungal balls have been associated with prior dental work, particularly dental fillings and iatrogenic oroantral communications. Sealers used in endodontic therapy, such as those containing zinc oxide, can promote fungal growth, although this may take years after the initial procedure. Studies have shown a significant correlation between prior dental operations and fungal balls, with rates reaching 89.2% in affected patients. Therefore, panoramic dental imaging is recommended for individuals suspected of having fungal balls (Deutsch et al. 2019).

Histology

Histologically, fungal balls are characterised by entangled masses of fungi or fungi embedded in fibrinous, necrotic exudate without mucosal inflammatory response. There is no tissue invasion or granulomatous reaction in the surrounding tissue. At low magnification, a fungal ball might be confused with eosinophilic (allergic) mucin found in allergic fungal rhinosinusitis, as both can appear "layered." However, high magnification reveals numerous fungal species, which helps differentiate them (Montone 2016).

Clinical Features

Patients with fungal balls typically do not exhibit immunocompromise or a high prevalence of atopy, which would otherwise be necessary to explain the development of this syndrome (Hathiram and Khattar 2009). A fungal ball may be asymptomatic or present with symptoms similar to those of chronic rhinosinusitis. Common symptoms include nasal obstruction, purulent nasal secretions, a foul smell, and facial pain. Less frequent symptoms include convulsions, epistaxis, proptosis, fever, coughing, and impaired vision. Symptoms often persist for extended periods, sometimes for months or even years (Bosi et al. 2012). Approximately, 10% of patients have nasal polyps, which are a nonspecific reaction to various inflammatory conditions. Rarely, a fungal ball may alter bone structure, enlarging the affected sinus and changing its architecture. It can also cause bone erosion. In rare cases, a fungal ball may become invasive if the host's immune system declines during the infection. Generally, it does not penetrate tissue; however, an acute or chronic inflammatory infiltrate may be present in the adjacent mucosa, even if granulomas are not visible (Hathiram and Khattar 2009).

Diagnosis and Imaging

When dealing with unilateral sinusitis or sinusitis that does not respond to previous antibiotic treatments, the possibility of a fungal ball should be considered. This diagnosis is supported by radiological evidence, primarily from CT scans. However, the definitive diagnosis depends on histopathology and the macroscopic features of the surgical specimen. Cultures are only helpful in 23–50% of cases and often yield negative results. Among these, *Aspergillus* fumigatus is found in more than 90% of cases (Bosi et al. 2012). Common CT findings for fungal balls include heterogeneous partial or often total opacification of the affected sinus, with intralesional calcifications and sclerosis of the opacified sinus wall, as shown in Fig. 6.4. While these characteristics are not pathognomonic, they strongly suggest a fungal ball diagnosis. Other sinus opacities are less heterogeneous than those of a fungal ball. Approximately, 90% of partially or completely opacified sinuses show heterogeneous opacification, while homogeneous opacification is seen in only 10% of cases. On non-contrast CT scans, a sinus fungal ball typically appears hyperattenuated due to the dense fungal hyphae and metabolic deposits. The high-density opacities of the fungal ball may be due to the solid mass of tangled fungal hyphae and metabolic deposits. If metallic hyperdensity is observed on a CT scan, metal metabolites from the fungus are likely present. Reports indicate that the fungus ball contains calcium phosphate and calcium sulfate, particularly in the necrotic centre, corresponding to areas of high attenuation. Essential metallic elements for fungal growth and metabolic activation include copper, zinc, iron, and calcium. Zinc and calcium can cause microcalcifications or areas of metallic density on CT images. The diagnostic criteria for fungus balls based on sinus opacification and areas of hyperattenuation have

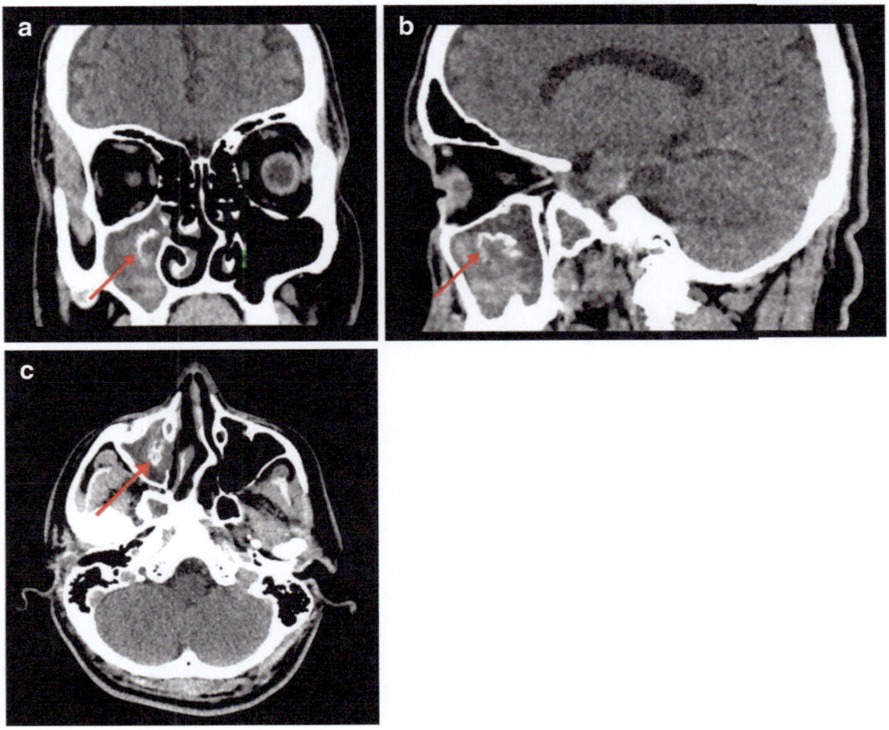

Fig. 6.4 Total dense opacification of the right maxillary sinus with stippled central calcification (arrows, **a**: Coronal, **b**: Sagittal, **c**: Axial view) associated with obstruction of the maxillary sinus. No sinus wall erosion or destruction

reported a sensitivity of 62% and a specificity of 99% for CT imaging. Preoperative diagnosis can be challenging if intralesional calcification spots are absent on CT scans of the sinuses (Lee and Lee 2020).

Summary of Diagnostic Criteria for Fungal Balls (Garcia-Rubio and Alcazar-Fuoli 2018)

- Sinus opacification with or without heterogeneity.
- Dense concentration of fungus hyphae distinct from the sinus mucosa.
- Mucopurulent, clay-like, or cheesy material inside the sinus cavity.
- Chronic nonspecific mucosal inflammation.
- Absence of eosinophils, granulomas, or allergic mucin as predominant features.
- Histopathology shows no evidence of mucosal fungus invasion.

Treatment/Management

Surgery is the primary treatment for removing the fungus from the affected sinus, an example of which can be seen in Fig. 6.5. Since the disease is non-invasive by definition, no additional treatment is typically necessary (Garcia-Rubio and Alcazar-Fuoli 2018). Surgical intervention is needed for symptomatic patients with sinus opacification and bone erosion, but whether surgery is appropriate for

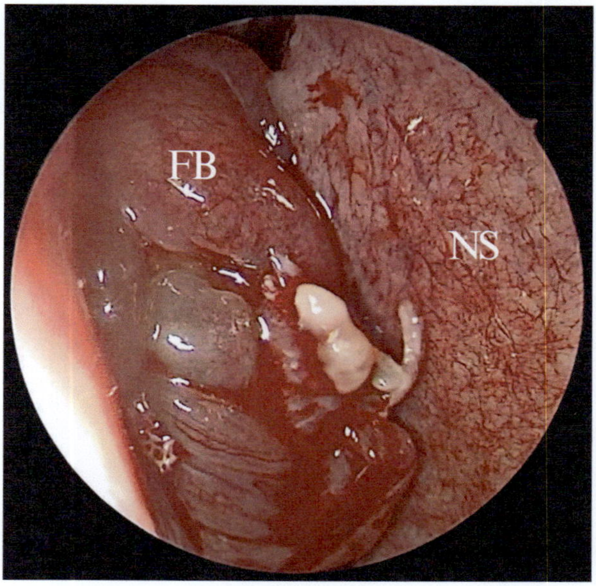

Fig. 6.5 This is an intraoperative video of a patient undergoing endoscopic sinus surgery (ESS) for a fungal ball. As can be seen in the thumbnail (right side nasal cavity), granulation tissue has almost entirely blocked the right side nasal cavity. (*NS* nasal septum, *FB* fungal ball) (Audio 6.2 and Video 6.2)

asymptomatic patients remains debatable. If the patient has asthma, surgery should be performed to prevent potential exacerbation of asthma attacks by the fungal ball (Hathiram and Khattar 2009). The medical literature describes two surgical methods for fungal ball removal from the maxillary sinus: the historical Caldwell-Luc procedure, which involves opening the canine fossa to access the maxillary sinus, and endoscopic surgery, which is considered the gold standard. Paranasal sinus endoscopy aims to restore normal drainage and ventilation of the sinus by accessing its ostium. Debridement can be performed if mucous polyps are present near the original meatus. Additionally, a wide antrostomy can be created by removing a significant portion of the posterior fontanelle and establishing a potential secondary ostium in the region of the maxillary ostium (Bosi et al. 2012).

Prognosis

Generally, complications from fungal balls are rare; however, there have been reports of infections becoming invasive following significant immunosuppression (Garcia-Rubio and Alcazar-Fuoli 2018). Recurrence is uncommon but has been documented, even up to 2 years after surgery. In Klossek's series, the recurrence rate was 4%, while Ferriero reported a slightly higher rate of 7%. Many of these recurrences can be managed with straightforward irrigation or suctioning in an outpatient setting or with conservative endoscopic surgery, making regular follow-up crucial (Hathiram and Khattar 2009).

Chronic Invasive Fungal Sinusitis

Introduction

Fungal rhinosinusitis encompasses a range of disease processes that vary in clinical presentation, histologic appearance, and biological significance. Hora (1965) first recognised two categories of fungal rhinosinusitis based on tissue invasion by fungi: non-invasive, which clinically resembles chronic bacterial sinusitis, and invasive, which behaves like a malignant neoplasm, eroding bone and spreading into adjacent tissues. However, Hora's report did not provide histologic evidence of invasion (Hora 1965).

In the late 1990s, deShazo et al. proposed a new classification for invasive fungal rhinosinusitis based on clinical condition, immune status, histopathology, and fungus isolation, similar to the current classification. This classification includes acute (fulminant), granulomatous, and chronic types (deShazo et al. 1997).

Fungal rhinosinusitis can be categorised as follows:

- **Acute:** Aggressive, with symptoms lasting less than 30 days.
- **Chronic:** Indolent, with symptoms lasting more than 90 days (Chakrabarti et al. 2009a, b).

Non-invasive sinonasal fungal diseases include saprophytic fungal infestation, fungal ball, and allergic fungal rhinosinusitis. The invasive forms of fungal rhinosinusitis include acute, chronic, and chronic granulomatous types. While non-invasive fungal rhinosinusitis is serious and requires surgical and medical intervention, the invasive forms more often result in significant morbidity and mortality, particularly if left untreated (Montone 2016). Both forms of fungal sinusitis should be treated with surgical debridement and systemic antifungal therapy (Montone 2016).

Chronic Invasive Fungal Sinusitis (CIFS)

Chronic invasive fungal sinusitis (CIFS) is an invasive fungal infection characterised by a slow-growing process with fungal organisms invading the sinonasal mucosa, often with rare angioinvasion. This slowly destructive process most commonly affects the ethmoid and sphenoid sinuses but may involve any paranasal sinus. The disease typically persists for more than 12 weeks. In contrast to granulomatous invasive fungal rhinosinusitis, CIFS is characterised by a dense accumulation of hyphae, occasional vascular invasion, and sparse inflammatory infiltrate, with involvement of local structures. It is commonly associated with conditions such as AIDS, diabetes mellitus, solid organ transplantation, and long-term corticosteroid use. Cultures of tissue are positive in over 50% of cases, with *Aspergillus fumigatus* being the most commonly isolated agent. CIFS can be distinguished from other invasive forms of fungal sinusitis by its chronic course, dense hyphal accumulation resembling a mycetoma, and association with orbital apex syndrome, diabetes mellitus, and corticosteroid treatment. Biopsy and orbital exploration typically reveal vascular invasion by fungal elements and only sparse chronic inflammatory infiltrate.

Epidemiology and Risk Factors

CIFS is a rare and distinct subtype of invasive fungal sinusitis, and precise incidence data in the general population is lacking (Pasquini 2016). There is no evidence of its prevalence in specific geographic areas. Recent studies reveal a higher prevalence in immunocompromised patients, such as those with AIDS, undergoing organ transplantation, suffering from diabetes mellitus, or receiving long-term corticosteroid treatment (D'Anza et al. 2016).

Aetiology and Pathophysiology

Although *Aspergillus* species were initially identified as the primary causative organisms of chronic invasive fungal rhinosinusitis, CIFS can now be caused by a variety of organisms, including Mucor, Alternaria, Curvularia, Bipolaris, Candida,

Drechslera, Sporothrix schenckii, and Pseudallescheria boydii. *Aspergillus* and Mucor are the most commonly found organisms (Deutsch et al. 2019). Fungi are significant aeroallergens in many areas, with airborne spore counts sometimes thousands of times higher than those of pollen. The host defence mechanisms against fungi are not fully understood, but the pathophysiology of fungal sinusitis likely involves compromised sinus aeration, altered immune responses to fungi, and other factors (deShazo et al. 1997).

Clinical Presentation

Chronic invasive fungal rhinosinusitis usually occurs in individuals who are apparently healthy, although many have a history of chronic rhinosinusitis symptoms, upper respiratory allergies, or nasal polyposis. Nonspecific symptoms such as nasal obstruction, facial pain, rhinorrhoea, headaches, and epistaxis are common. In immunocompetent patients, these chronic symptoms might mimic other types of chronic sinusitis, leading to treatment delays or misdiagnosis (Alotaibi et al. 2020). If neglected and left untreated, the disease can invade neighbouring structures and lead to severe manifestations, including proptosis, altered mental status, seizures, and intracranial complications (Thurtell et al. 2013).

Symptoms related to invasive disease may develop over months or years once the orbit or skull base is involved:

- **Erosion into the orbit:** May produce proptosis, more common in the granulomatous type.
- **Invasion of the maxillary floor:** This may cause palatal erosions.
- **Erosion of the cribriform plate** may result in chronic headaches, seizures, decreased mental status, or focal neurological findings.
- **Extension through the sphenoid sinus:** This may lead to orbital apex syndrome or cavernous sinus syndrome.
- **Extension to the pterygopalatine fossa** May cause cranial nerve deficits.

Orbital apex syndrome is characterised by decreased vision and ocular immobility due to a mass in the superior portion of the orbit, resulting from bony erosion and fungal spread from the ethmoid sinus. This condition may be misdiagnosed as inflammatory pseudotumor, leading to premature corticosteroid therapy before appropriate orbital exploration and biopsy are conducted. Catastrophic complications such as mycotic aneurysm, internal carotid artery rupture, and cavernous sinus thrombosis have been reported (Corvisier et al. 1987).

The condition may start as a sinus mycetoma and become invasive, potentially due to immunosuppression associated with diabetes mellitus or corticosteroid treatment. In rhinoscopy examination, severe nasal congestion, polypoid mucosa, and a soft tissue mass covered by mucosa or ulcerated with overlying debris or dried secretions may be observed (Stringer and Ryan 2000).

Diagnosis

Fungal sinusitis should be considered in all patients with chronic sinusitis, especially if certain clinical features suggest the diagnosis. Non-invasive forms of fungal sinusitis often present as intractable sinusitis that fails to respond to repeated courses of antibiotics and may require multiple operations before the diagnosis is confirmed. Invasive fungal sinusitis typically occurs in immunocompromised patients and is characterised by acute onset of symptoms such as fever, cough, nasal mucosal ulceration or eschars, epistaxis, and headache. Commonly associated conditions include malignant diseases, leukaemia, other causes of neutropenia, diabetes, hemochromatosis, and protein-calorie malnutrition. More chronic forms of invasive disease may present with proptosis or orbital apex syndrome.

Radiological diagnosis of fungal sinusitis can be challenging with plain X-rays. Aspergillosis may affect one or more sinuses, often presenting as nodular mucosal thickening and the absence of air/fluid levels in homogeneously cloudy maxillary and ethmoidal sinuses, with or without bony destruction. The presence of hyperdense fungal concretions on plain X-rays is almost pathognomonic for fungal sinusitis. These concretions may be calcium deposits within a central necrotic region of the fungal mycelium or represent zinc oxide from the endodontic treatment of molar and premolar teeth (Beck-Mannagetta and Necek 1986).

A more reliable diagnosis can be made with CT scans (Figs. 6.6 and 6.7), which are better for identifying bony destruction. CT imaging is the assessment of any intracranial spread or orbital involvement. Typically, a heterogeneous opacity of the antrum is seen with focal areas of high signal on non-contrast views (Zinreich et al. 1988). Sinus wall expansion and/or destruction may be evident in the invasive form of aspergillosis. A CT scan showing bony erosion should alert clinicians to the possibility of invasive fungal disease, but definitive diagnosis requires histological confirmation of mucosal or bony invasion. CT plays a crucial role in determining the extent of the disease prior to any necessary definitive surgery.

Magnetic resonance imaging (MRI) has been found to be more sensitive than CT in diagnosing fungal sinusitis, though only a small number of cases have been studied (Zinreich et al. 1988). MRI with contrast can provide additional information on deeper invasion, meningeal enhancement, or cavernous sinus involvement.

Differentiating between malignant neoplasms and chronic invasive fungal rhinosinusitis using radiologic findings can be difficult or impossible. The definitive distinction between invasive and non-invasive fungal rhinosinusitis, and between these

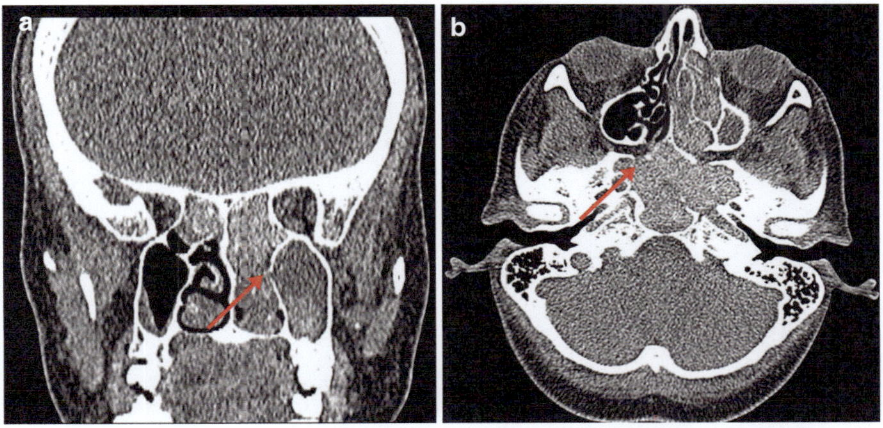

Fig. 6.6 Evidence of diffuse mucosal thickening and total opacifications (**a**: Coronal, **b**: Axial view), which involve the left maxillary, left frontal, and both sphenoid sinuses as well as the left ethmoidal air cells and nasal cavity, in which they are merging with the hypertrophied turbinates and obstructing the osteo-meatal complexes and posterior choana. The nasopharynx is clear. The sinus opacifications are mainly hyperdense material suggesting fungal elements. The sphenoid sinuses also have marked expansion with multifocal erosions and sinus wall destructions at their roof, floor and lateral walls

and neoplasms, is best made histologically. Early tissue diagnosis is crucial, showing evidence of invasion of neurovascular structures. Chronic invasive fungal rhinosinusitis typically has a lower inflammatory response compared to acute invasive fungal rhinosinusitis and may present with a less dense population of inflammatory cells. Histologically, the chronic invasive type is characterised by a dense accumulation of hyphae, sometimes with vascular invasion, a chronic or sparse inflammatory reaction, and the presence of *A. fumigatus* with direct destruction of adjacent tissues. The presence of fibrosis is not consistently clear (Chakrabarti et al. 2009a, b).

Initial blood tests should include a full blood count to assess for neutropenia or signs of haematological malignancies, renal function, blood glucose, capillary ketones, iron levels, and tests for infectious diseases such as HIV. These tests help identify underlying causes for susceptibility to invasive fungal sinusitis (ICFS). The poor prognosis associated with ICFS suggests that it should be treated as aggressively as acute (fulminant) invasive fungal sinusitis.

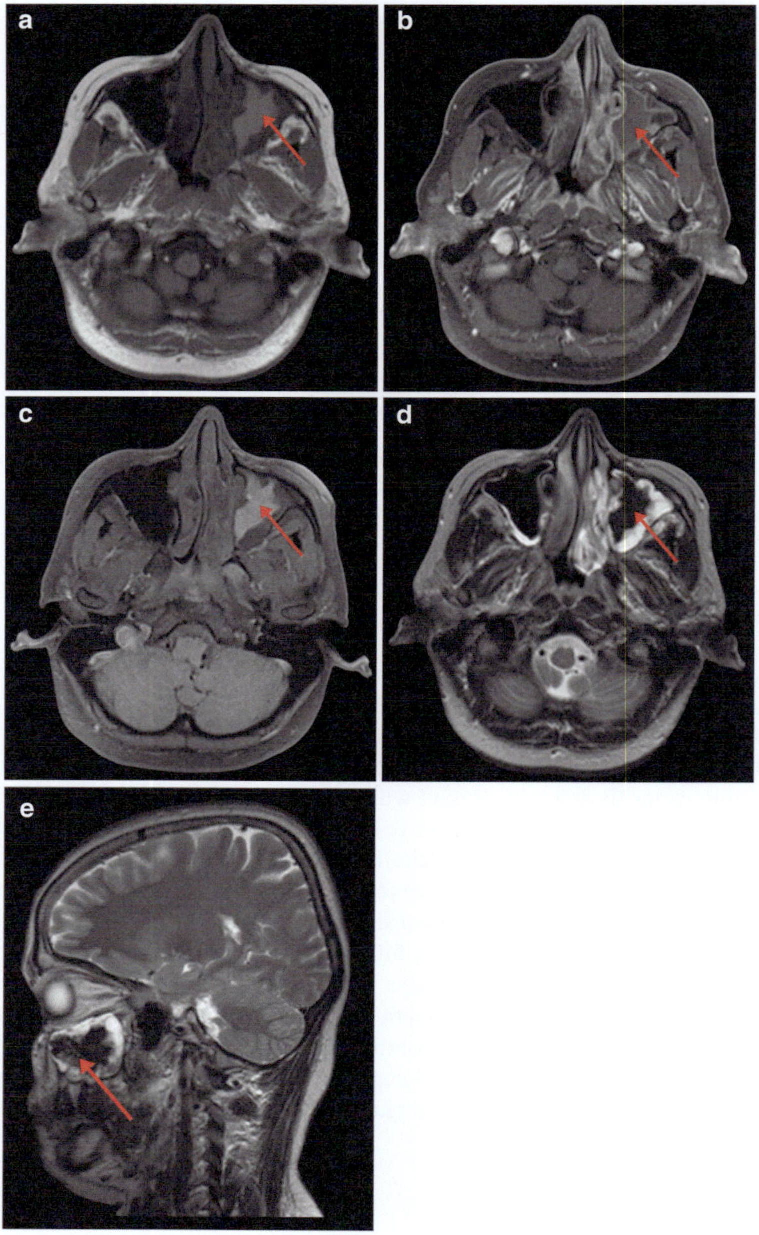

Fig. 6.7 Evidence of diffuse extensive enhanced mucosal thickening involving all paranasal sinuses, more marked at the left side along with sinus filling by non-enhancing materials (arrows), which are dark on T2WI and bright on T1WI, thus suggesting fungal elements or high protein content. These are associated with left maxillary sinus boundary erosions, resulting in thickening and enhancement of the left orbital floor in the extra-conal compartment. There is an absence of focal mucosal enhancement at some of the sinuses concerning invasive infection. (**a**: Axial T1, **b**: Axial T1 with Fat Suppression and Contrast, **c**: Axial T1 with Fat Suppression, **d**: Axial T2, **e**: Sagittal T2)

Differential Diagnosis

Chronic invasive fungal rhinosinusitis may mimic many other disorders, including benign or malignant neoplasms, pituitary tumours, syphilis, tuberculosis, sarcoidosis, Wegener's granulomatosis, lymphoma, inflammatory pseudotumor, myospherulosis, mucopyocele, allergic fungal rhinosinusitis, and rhinoscleroma.

Distinguishing Between Invasive and Non-invasive Sinusitis

Invasive and non-invasive fungal sinusitis share many features. Both can occur in immunocompetent or immunocompromised individuals, may have an acute or chronic course, and may extend beyond the thin walls of the sinuses into the orbit, eye structures, and brain. Affected sinuses often contain purulent, pasty, and foul-smelling material, which may have few or many fungal elements that often fail to grow in culture. This fungal material is commonly associated with dense polyposis and calcification, resulting in areas of focal or diffuse radiodensity on computed tomography (CT) imaging of the sinuses and decreased signal intensities on T1- and T2-weighted magnetic resonance imaging (MRI). There have been no controlled trials of treatments for fungal sinusitis syndromes. *Aspergillus* is the most commonly reported cause of fungal sinusitis. Since non-invasive and invasive forms were historically considered a continuum, reports of "aspergillosis of the sinuses," including clinical management studies, often address both as a single entity (Zinreich et al. 1988). It is now clear that invasive fungal sinusitis can be distinguished from non-invasive disease using clinical criteria, radiologic diagnosis, and histopathological examination of sinus tissue. Radiologic findings associated with fungal sinusitis include those also seen with bacterial sinusitis, such as air-fluid levels or mucoperiosteal thickening greater than 8 mm, and those more specific for fungal sinusitis, such as calcifications and loss of bony sinus margins. Fungal cultures of nasal mucus are unreliable for diagnosing any form of fungal sinusitis. Stainable hyphae are not present in the mucosa of patients with chronic bacterial sinusitis; they are present only in mucopurulent material within the sinus in non-invasive disease. Hyphae penetrate the sinus mucosa, submucosa, blood vessels, or bone in invasive disease. To distinguish between these forms, adequate quantities of sinus contents and biopsy specimens of diseased and healthy mucosa and adjacent bone must be obtained for histopathological analysis. Since fungi do not stain well with routine stains (such as haematoxylin and eosin), silver-impregnation fungal stains and fungal cultures of surgical specimens are necessary whenever fungal sinusitis is suspected.

Are Granulomatous and Chronic FRS Separate Entities?

This remains an unresolved issue. In the granulomatous type, the histopathologic response is characterised by a granulomatous reaction with considerable fibrosis, typified by non-caseating granulomas with foreign body or Langhans-type giant cells, occasional vasculitis, vascular proliferation, and perivascular fibrosis. Hyphae are usually sparse, and *A. flavus* is consistently isolated. This form may be geographically or ethnically related, being most commonly seen in Sudan, India, Pakistan, and Saudi Arabia. In contrast, the chronic invasive type is characterised by a dense accumulation of hyphae, sometimes with vascular invasion, chronic or sparse inflammatory reaction, and isolation of *A. fumigatus* with direct destruction of adjacent tissues. It is unclear whether fibrosis is consistently present in the chronic invasive form. The clinicopathological distinction between these two types is not sharp. Both have a chronic course and often involve prominent orbital involvement. There is currently no apparent difference in prognosis or therapy based on this distinction. However, in a panel discussion, participants agreed that chronic invasive and granulomatous fungal rhinosinusitis (FRS) should be differentiated primarily on pathological grounds until more data are available (Chakrabarti et al. 2009a, b).

Treatment

The management of invasive chronic fungal rhinosinusitis (ICFR) has two main components: surgical debridement and antifungal therapy. A multidisciplinary approach is essential for successful management. Early involvement of appropriate medical specialists (e.g., endocrinology, haematology) and surgical specialists (ENT, maxillofacial, neurosurgery, ophthalmology), along with microbiology consultation, is fundamental (Watkinson and Clarke 2018).

Surgical intervention is crucial and typically involves endoscopic sinus surgery to establish an early diagnosis and obtain tissue samples. An example of endoscopic sinus surgery for an invasive fungal granuloma can be seen in Fig. 6.8. The primary goals are to debride necrotic tissue (including mucosa and bone, if necessary) and to clear the sinus. The debridement should continue until healthy bleeding tissue is encountered (Deutsch et al. 2019). This may include the removal of large amounts of nasal mucosa, turbinates, and extended sinonasal access procedures (e.g., medial maxillectomy, DRAF III) (Pagella et al. 2016). Often, repeat procedures are needed to address progressively developing necrotic tissue. Complete surgical debridement has been shown to improve survival. In advanced cases involving the orbit or intracranial complications, the need for more extensive and potentially disfiguring open surgery may arise. While evidence suggests that procedures such as orbital exenteration or radical maxillectomy do not significantly improve survival, these patients generally have very poor survival rates. Many authors agree that orbital exenteration should be reserved for cases involving a non-functioning eye (Zuniga and Turner 2014).

Early initiation of systemic antifungal therapy has been shown to improve survival. Appropriate fungal cultures are crucial to ensure the correct antifungal agents are used. The mainstay of antifungal therapy is Amphotericin B, effective against *Mucorales* and *Aspergillus*, though it has significant nephrotoxic side effects. The

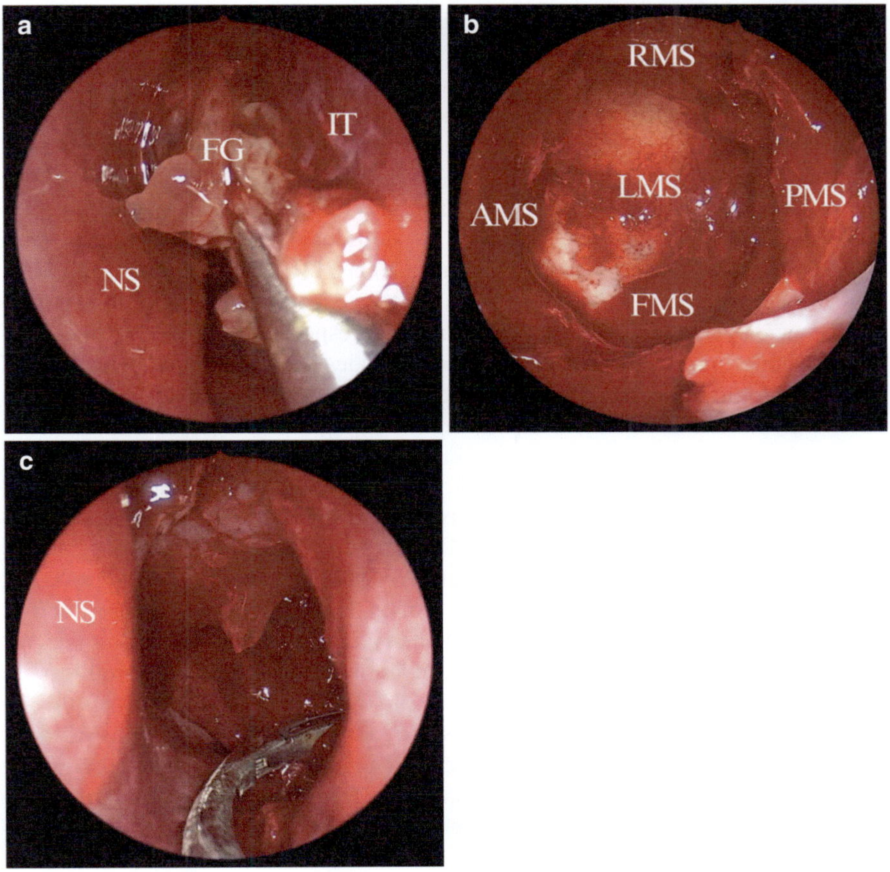

Fig. 6.8 This is an intraoperative video of a patient undergoing endoscopic sinus surgery (ESS) for a fungal granuloma. As can be seen in the thumbnails (right-side nasal cavity), (**a**) granulation tissue in the nasal cavity, which was later confirmed to be fungal granuloma by histopathology, (**b**) a 70° endoscopic picture of the maxillary sinus, and (**c**) a Heuwieser is used to remove the remnants of the granuloma. (*NS* nasal septum, *IT* inferior turbinate, *FG* fungal granuloma, *RMS* roof of maxillary sinus, *FMS* floor of maxillary sinus, *LMS* lateral wall of maxillary sinus, *PMS* posterior wall of maxillary sinus) (Audio 6.3 and Video 6.3)

development of liposomal Amphotericin has reduced nephrotoxicity to some degree. Once cultures are available, Voriconazole can be used for *Aspergillus* infections; it has a better side effect profile but is less effective against *Mucorales*. Other antifungals, such as Posaconazole and Isavuconazole, are reserved for second-line treatments and require further evidence; close collaboration with microbiologists is essential for appropriate management. Some evidence suggests that hyperbaric oxygen therapy, which releases oxygen-free radicals, may be beneficial as an adjunct to management, particularly in diabetic patients (Deutsch et al. 2019).

Granulomatous Invasive Rhinosinusitis

Fungal rhinosinusitis (FRS) is a rare disease associated with high morbidity and mortality rates, primarily reported in North Africa, the Middle East, and Asia, while it is rare in the Western world. It affects both immunocompromised and immunocompetent individuals. In recent decades, cases have notably increased due to both improved survival rates among at-risk individuals (e.g., diabetics and immunocompromised patients) and advancements in endoscopic and imaging diagnostics (endoscopy, CT, MRI) (Adelson and Marple 2005). FRS is an opportunistic infection caused by spores of the filamentous fungus *Aspergillus*. Aspergilli are saprophytes widespread in various environments, especially in the presence of decomposing organic material. The genus includes around one hundred species, grouped into fifteen categories based on cultural characteristics. Pathogenic strains for humans primarily belong to the *Aspergillus fumigatus* group (Pal et al. 2017).

Invasive infections are usually acquired through inhalation of spores or occasionally through direct invasion via broken skin. The spores germinate into hyphae, which invade blood vessels and, in invasive disease, can cause haemorrhagic necrosis and embolism. *Aspergillus* spp typically infect open spaces, such as lung cavities from previous diseases (e.g., bronchiectasis, tumours, tuberculosis), sinuses, or external ear canals. These infections are often locally invasive and destructive, though systemic spread can occur, particularly in immunocompromised patients with neutropenia or corticosteroid-induced immunosuppression. Aspergillosis is rare in HIV-infected individuals (Vergidis 2023). Focal infections can result in a fungal nodule (aspergilloma), characterised by tangled hyphae, fibrinous exudate, and few inflammatory cells, typically encapsulated by fibrous tissue. Occasionally, there is local invasion of tissue at the periphery of the cavity, but the fungus generally resides within the cavity with minimal local invasion.

Distinguishing Invasive and Non-invasive Fungal Rhinosinusitis

The most critical distinction is between invasive and non-invasive fungal rhinosinusitis. Invasive fungal rhinosinusitis includes acute necrotizing and chronic invasive forms (granulomatous and non-granulomatous), while non-invasive forms include saprophytic colonisation, fungus balls, and allergic fungal rhinosinusitis. Accurate classification is important for predicting prognosis and guiding therapy (Ferguson 2000). Both chronic invasive rhinosinusitis and chronic granulomatous rhinosinusitis describe locally invasive disease lasting at least 3 months, but they differ in pathology and clinical context (Chakrabarti et al. 2009a, b).

Chronic invasive fungal granuloma (CIFG) of the paranasal sinuses occurs in immunocompetent hosts, particularly in their second and third decades of life. It can be divided into two types: primary paranasal fungal granuloma and the form associated with chronic hypertrophic rhinosinusitis. In the secondary form, the sphenoid sinus is more frequently involved, and diabetes mellitus is a common concomitant disease (Han et al. 2007). Paranasal primary fungal granuloma is usually caused by

A. flavus and involves fungal invasion of the mucosa with a non-caseating granulomatous reaction. The form associated with chronic hypertrophic rhinosinusitis is challenging to diagnose and often discovered incidentally after surgery. Diagnosis is based on histological examination showing minimal fungal hyphae invasion reaching the submucosa, with an evident granulomatous reaction.

Symptoms

Chronic, slowly invasive granulomatous inflammation can present with fever, usually unilateral nasal obstruction, purulent rhinorrhoea, postnasal drip, facial pain, headache, and cough. Patients may also present with necrotizing skin lesions extending beyond the nose or paranasal sinuses, palatal or gingival ulcerations, signs of cavernous sinus thrombosis, or pulmonary or disseminated lesions. Often, the primary symptom is gradually progressive proptosis (Chavan et al. 2016).

Diagnosis of Aspergillosis

Diagnosing invasive fungal sinusitis is generally straightforward; however, when the infection presents as a granuloma, diagnosis can be challenging. CT and MRI are the preferred imaging modalities. CIFG typically shows homogeneous opacity (isodense or hyperdense relative to muscle tissue) on CT and an isointense or hypointense signal on T1- and T2-weighted MRI, respectively. It often involves only one or two sinuses, with homogeneous contrast enhancement, lack of sinus expansion, and localised bone erosion where the disease extends beyond the sinuses, with the extra-sinus component usually greater than the intra-sinus component (Reddy et al. 2010). MRI is generally superior to CT, and gadolinium-enhanced MRI can be used to differentiate granulomas from tumours of the rhinosinus tract (Lanzieri et al. 1991).

Routine haematoxylin-eosin staining may be inadequate, so special stains like GMS staining should be used in cases of suspected aspergillosis. A multidisciplinary approach is crucial for early diagnosis and timely intervention.

Culture and histopathology of tissue samples are usually necessary for confirmation. Histopathology helps distinguish between invasive infections and colonisations. Samples are typically obtained from the sinuses via anterior rhinoscopy. Since cultures take time and histopathology results can be falsely negative, treatment decisions often rely on strong clinical presumptive evidence.

Treatment of Aspergillosis

Invasive infections generally require aggressive treatment with Voriconazole or isavuconazole, which has similar efficacy but fewer adverse effects than Voriconazole. Amphotericin B (particularly lipid formulations) is effective but more toxic. Oral posaconazole or itraconazole (but not fluconazole) may be effective in some cases. Caspofungin can be used as rescue therapy. Combination therapy with Voriconazole and echinocandins may be effective for certain patients.

Aspergillomas do not require systemic antifungal therapy but may need surgical resection due to local effects. Traditional Caldwell-Luc surgery was previously used, but endonasal microsurgery has significantly improved the management of chronic fungal sinusitis, allowing for adequate removal of pathological tissue, even in advanced cases. The use of the microscope has been beneficial in some cases with extensive disease and skull base dehiscences.

Endonasal microsurgical techniques are now considered the appropriate approach for managing chronic fungal sinus disease, even in severe cases with radiological evidence of expansion or invasion of surrounding tissue. Further antifungal therapy is rarely indicated unless the fungal disease invades surrounding tissues or contralateral involvement is detected (Simmen et al. 1998). However, other studies suggest that pharmacological treatment combined with surgery can resolve chronic indolent invasive mycoses and prevent intracranial complications. Endoscopic surgery is indicated for all forms of paranasal sinus mycosis, although specific objectives may vary depending on the type. Timely surgical intervention can prevent intracranial complications and enable effective antifungal polychemotherapy (Castelnuovo et al. 2000).

References

Adelson RT, Marple BF (2005) Fungal rhinosinusitis: state-of-the-art diagnosis and treatment. J Otolaryngol 34:S18–S23

Alotaibi NH, Abu Omar O, Altahan M, Alsheikh H, Al Mana F, Mahasin Z, Othman E (2020) Chronic invasive fungal rhinosinusitis in immunocompetent patients: a retrospective chart review. Front Surg 7:608342. https://doi.org/10.3389/fsurg.2020.608342

Al-Radadi AM, Alnoury KI (2011) Optic chiasma involvement secondary to allergic fungal rhinosinusitis. J Pak Med Assoc 61(7):704–707

Anjum G, Ramesh DSV, Rukmangada T, Patil N (2020) Rhinocerebral maxillary mucormycosis: a palatal ulcer. Indian J Dent Res 31:652. https://doi.org/10.4103/ijdr.ijdr_234_18

Auluck A (2007) Maxillary necrosis by mucormycosis. A case report and literature review. Med Oral Patol Oral Cir Bucal 12(5):E360–E364

Bachert C, Pawankar R, Zhang L et al (2014) ICON: chronic rhinosinusitis. World Allergy Organ J 7:25. https://doi.org/10.1186/1939-4551-7-25

Ballenger JJ, Snow JB (2003) Ballenger's otorhinolaryngology. PMPH-USA

Bassichis BA, Marple BF, Mabry RL et al (2001) Use of immunotherapy in previously treated patients with allergic fungal sinusitis. Otolaryngol Head Neck Surg 125:487–490. https://doi.org/10.1067/mhn.2001.119585

Beck-Mannagetta J, Necek D (1986) Radiologic findings in aspergillosis of the maxillary sinus. Oral Surg Oral Med Oral Pathol 62:345–349. https://doi.org/10.1016/0030-4220(86)90019-8

Bhandari J, Thada PK, Nagalli S (2023) Rhinocerebral mucormycosis. StatPearls—NCBI Bookshelf. https://www.ncbi.nlm.nih.gov/books/NBK559288/

Bois E, Boucenna M, Sain-Oulhen C, Lecanu J-B (2017) Fungus ball of the middle ear: a case study. OTO Open 1:2473974X17746582. https://doi.org/10.1177/2473974x17746582

Bosi GR, De Braga GL, De Almeida TS, De Carli A (2012) Fungus ball of the paranasal sinuses: report of two cases and literature review. Int Arch Otorhinolaryngol 16:286–290. https://doi.org/10.7162/s1809-97772012000200020

Callejas CA, Douglas RG (2013) Fungal rhinosinusitis: what every allergist should know. Clin Exp Allergy 43:835–849. https://doi.org/10.1111/cea.12118

Castelnuovo P, Gera R, Di Giulio G, Staffieri A (2000) Paranasal sinus mycoses. Indian J Chest Dis Allied Sci 42(4):293–304

Chakrabarti A, Das A, Panda NK (2009a) Controversies surrounding the categorization of fungal sinusitis. Med Mycol 47:S299–S308. https://doi.org/10.1080/13693780802213357

Chakrabarti A, Denning DW, Ferguson BJ et al (2009b) Fungal rhinosinusitis. Laryngoscope 119:1809–1818. https://doi.org/10.1002/lary.20520

Chavan SS, Bhople KS, Deshmukh SD et al (2016) Chronic invasive fungal granuloma—a diagnostic dilemma in an immunocompetent host. Iran J Otorhinolaryngol 28(84):83–88

Chua AJ, Jafar A, Luong AU (2023) Update on allergic fungal rhinosinusitis. Ann Allergy Asthma Immunol 131:300–306. https://doi.org/10.1016/j.anai.2023.02.018

Clark DW, Wenaas A, Luong A et al (2012) Staphylococcus aureus prevalence in allergic fungal rhinosinusitis vs other subsets of chronic rhinosinusitis with nasal polyps. Int Forum Allergy Rhinol 3:89–93. https://doi.org/10.1002/alr.21090

Corvisier N, Gray F, Gherardi R et al (1987) Aspergillosis of ethmoid sinus and optic nerve, with arteritis and rupture of the internal carotid artery. Surg Neurol 28:311–315. https://doi.org/10.1016/0090-3019(87)90312-0

Crist H, Hennessy M, Hoeos J et al (2018) Acute invasive fungal rhinosinusitis: frozen section histomorphology and diagnosis with PAS stain. Head Neck Pathol 13:318–326. https://doi.org/10.1007/s12105-018-0965-8

D'Anza B, Stokken J, Greene JS et al (2016) Chronic invasive fungal sinusitis: characterization and shift in management of a rare disease. Int Forum Allergy Rhinol 6:1294–1300. https://doi.org/10.1002/alr.21828

Dave T, Sreshta K, Varma D et al (2021) Magnetic resonance imaging in rhino-orbital-cerebral mucormycosis. Indian J Ophthalmol 69:1915. https://doi.org/10.4103/ijo.ijo_1439_21

deShazo RD, Chapin K, Swain RE (1997) Fungal sinusitis. N Engl J Med 337:254–259. https://doi.org/10.1056/nejm199707243370407

Deutsch PG, Whittaker J, Prasad S (2019) Invasive and non-invasive fungal rhinosinusitis—a review and update of the evidence. Medicina 55:319. https://doi.org/10.3390/medicina55070319

Dufour X, Kauffmann-Lacroix C, Ferrie JC et al (2006) Paranasal sinus fungus ball: epidemiology, clinical features and diagnosis. A retrospective analysis of 173 cases from a single medical center in France, 1989–2002. Med Mycol 44:61–67. https://doi.org/10.1080/13693780500235728

Dutre T, Dousary SA, Zhang N, Bachert C (2013) Allergic fungal rhinosinusitis—more than a fungal disease? J Allergy Clin Immunol 132:487–489.e1. https://doi.org/10.1016/j.jaci.2013.02.040

Dykewicz MS, Rodrigues JM, Slavin RG (2018) Allergic fungal rhinosinusitis. J Allergy Clin Immunol 142:341–351. https://doi.org/10.1016/j.jaci.2018.06.023

Ferguson BJ (2000) Definitions of fungal rhinosinusitis. Otolaryngol Clin N Am 33:227–235. https://doi.org/10.1016/s0030-6665(00)80002-x

Flint PW, Haughey BH, Lund VJ et al (2020) Cummings otolaryngology. Elsevier

Fokkens WJ, Lund VJ, Mullol J et al (2012) EPOS 2012: European position paper on rhinosinusitis and nasal polyps 2012. A summary for otorhinolaryngologists. Rhinology 50:1–12. https://doi.org/10.4193/rhino12.000

Garcia-Rubio R, Alcazar-Fuoli L (2018) Diseases caused by Aspergillus fumigatus. Elsevier eBooks

Grant P, Skilbeck CJ (2014) Rhinocerebral mucormycosis: a devastating rhinological condition. Pract Diab 31:37–39. https://doi.org/10.1002/pdi.1826

Grosjean P, Weber R (2007) Fungus balls of the paranasal sinuses: a review. Eur Arch Otorhinolaryngol 264:461–470. https://doi.org/10.1007/s00405-007-0281-5

Han DH, An S-Y, Kim SW et al (2007) Primary and secondary fungal infections of the paranasal sinuses: clinical features and treatment outcomes. Acta Otolaryngol 127:78–82. https://doi.org/10.1080/03655230701624913

Hathiram B, Khattar V (2009) Fungus balls of the paranasal sinuses. Otolaryngol Clin North Am 1:33–36. https://doi.org/10.5005/jp-journals-10003-1004
Hernández JL, Buckley CJ (2023) Mucormycosis. StatPearls—NCBI Bookshelf. https://www.ncbi.nlm.nih.gov/books/NBK544364/
Holbrook JF, Eastwood JD, Kilani RK (2011) Intracranial abscess as a complication of allergic fungal sinusitis. J Neuroimaging 24:95–98. https://doi.org/10.1111/j.1552-6569.2011.00670.x
Hora JF (1965) Primary aspergillosis of the paranasal sinuses and associated areas. Laryngoscope 75:768–773. https://doi.org/10.1288/00005537-196505000-00004
Hoyt AEW, Borish L, Gurrola J, Payne S (2016) Allergic fungal rhinosinusitis. J Allergy Clin Immunol 4:599–604. https://doi.org/10.1016/j.jaip.2016.03.010
Ibrahim AS, Spellberg B, Walsh TJ, Kontoyiannis DP (2012) Pathogenesis of mucormycosis. Clin Infect Dis 54:S16–S22. https://doi.org/10.1093/cid/cir865
Illing EA, Dunlap Q, Woodworth BA (2015) Outcomes of pressure-induced cranial neuropathies from allergic fungal rhinosinusitis. Otolaryngol Head Neck Surg 152:541–545. https://doi.org/10.1177/0194599814567302
Kumar JA, Babu P, Prabu K, Kumar P (2013) Mucormycosis in maxilla: rehabilitation of facial defects using interim removable prostheses: a clinical case report. J Pharm Bioallied Sci 5:163. https://doi.org/10.4103/0975-7406.114322
Lanzieri CF, Shah M, Krauss D, Lavertu P (1991) Use of gadolinium-enhanced MR imaging for differentiating mucoceles from neoplasms in the paranasal sinuses. Radiology 178:425–428. https://doi.org/10.1148/radiology.178.2.1987603
Lee J-H, Lee B-D (2020) Characteristic features of fungus ball in the maxillary sinus and the location of intralesional calcifications on computed tomographic images: a report of 2 cases. Imaging Sci Dent 50:377. https://doi.org/10.5624/isd.2020.50.4.377
Lund VJ, Howard DJ, Wei WI (2013) Tumors of the nose, sinuses and nasopharynx. Thieme Medical Publishers
Mabry RL, Mabry CS (1997) Immunotherapy for allergic fungal sinusitis: the second year. Otolaryngol Head Neck Surg 117:367–371. https://doi.org/10.1016/s0194-5998(97)70128-1
Marple BF (2006) Allergic fungal rhinosinusitis: a review of clinical manifestations and current treatment strategies. Med Mycol 44:277–284. https://doi.org/10.1080/13693780600778650
Marple BF, Mabry RL (2000) Allergic fungal sinusitis: learning from our failures. Am J Rhinol 14:223–226. https://doi.org/10.2500/105065800779954482
Marple BF, Gibbs SR, Newcomer MT, Mabry RL (1999) Allergic fungal sinusitis-induced visual loss. Am J Rhinol 13:191–196. https://doi.org/10.2500/105065899781389740
Montone KT (2016) Pathology of fungal rhinosinusitis: a review. Head Neck Pathol 10:40–46. https://doi.org/10.1007/s12105-016-0690-0
Mousavi B, Hedayati MT, Hedayati N et al (2016) Aspergillus species in indoor environments and their possible occupational and public health hazards. Curr Med Mycol 2:36–42. https://doi.org/10.18869/acadpub.cmm.2.1.36
Mucormycosis (2023) Mucormycosis: conversation with Dr Deepak Haldipur and Dr Aditya Moorthy. In: ENT & Audiology News. https://www.entandaudiologynews.com/development/interviews/post/mucormycosis-in-conversation-with-dr-deepak-haldipur-and-dr-aditya-moorthy
Mycetoma (2024a) Data and statistics on mucormycosis. Mucormycosis. https://www.cdc.gov/mucormycosis/data-research/index.html
Mycetoma (2024b) Clinical overview of mycetoma. Mycetoma. https://www.cdc.gov/mycetoma/hcp/clinical-overview/index.html#:~:text=Mycetoma%20is%20a%20rare%20implantation,agrarian%20populations%20in%20tropical%20regions
Myers EN, Snyderman CH (2018) Operative Otolaryngology: Head and Neck Surgery. 3rd edn. Elsevier, Philadelphia
Nomura K, Asaka D, Nakayama T et al (2013) Sinus fungus ball in the Japanese population: clinical and imaging characteristics of 104 cases. Int J Otolaryngol 2013:1–4. https://doi.org/10.1155/2013/731640

Nussenbaum B, Marple BF, Schwade ND (2001) Characteristics of bony erosion in allergic fungal rhinosinusitis. Otolaryngol Head Neck Surg 124:150–154. https://doi.org/10.1067/mhn.2001.112573

Pagella F, De Bernardi F, Gasperina DD et al (2016) Invasive fungal rhinosinusitis in adult patients: our experience in diagnosis and management. J Craniomaxillofac Surg 44:512–520. https://doi.org/10.1016/j.jcms.2015.12.016

Pai V, Sansi R, Kharche R et al (2021) Rhino-orbito-cerebral mucormycosis: pictorial review. Insights Imaging 12:167. https://doi.org/10.1186/s13244-021-01109-z

Pal M, Tsegaye M, Girzaw F et al (2017) An overview on biological weapons and bioterrorism. Am J Biomed Res 5:24–34. https://doi.org/10.12691/ajbr-5-2-2

Pasquini E (2016) XL Convegno Nazionale di Aggiornamento: evoluzione ed innovazione nella gestione della patologia rinosinusale. In: Atti del XL Convegno Nazionale AOOI, Bologna, Italy

Petrikkos G, Skiada A, Lortholary O et al (2012) Epidemiology and clinical manifestations of mucormycosis. Clin Infect Dis 54:S23–S34. https://doi.org/10.1093/cid/cir866

Prakash H, Chakrabarti A (2019) Global epidemiology of mucormycosis. J Fungi 5:26. https://doi.org/10.3390/jof5010026

Reddy CEE, Gupta AK, Singh P, Mann SBS (2010) Imaging of granulomatous and chronic invasive fungal sinusitis: comparison with allergic fungal sinusitis. Otolaryngol Head Neck Surg 143:294–300. https://doi.org/10.1016/j.otohns.2010.02.027

Roden MM, Zaoutis TE, Buchanan WL et al (2005) Epidemiology and outcome of zygomycosis: a review of 929 reported cases. Clin Infect Dis 41:634–653. https://doi.org/10.1086/432579

Sataloff RT (2015) Sataloff's comprehensive textbook of otolaryngology: head & neck surgery. JP Medical Ltd

Schubert MS, Hutcheson PS, Graff RJ et al (2004) HLA-DQB1-03 in allergic fungal sinusitis and other chronic hypertrophic rhinosinusitis disorders. J Allergy Clin Immunol 114:1376–1383. https://doi.org/10.1016/j.jaci.2004.08.029

Simmen D, Briner HR, Schär G, Schuknecht B (1998) Chronische Mykosen der Nasennebenhöhlen—Stellenwert der endonasalen Nasennebenhöhlenchirurgie. Laryngorhinootologie 77:444–453. https://doi.org/10.1055/s-2007-997005

Stone N, Gupta N, Schwartz I (2021) Mucormycosis: time to address this deadly fungal infection. Lancet Microbe 2:e343–e344. https://doi.org/10.1016/s2666-5247(21)00148-8

Stringer SP, Ryan MW (2000) Chronic invasive fungal rhinosinusitis. Otolaryngol Clin N Am 33:375–387. https://doi.org/10.1016/s0030-6665(00)80012-2

Tan BK, Peters AT, Schleimer RP, Hulse KE (2018) Pathogenic and protective roles of B cells and antibodies in patients with chronic rhinosinusitis. J Allergy Clin Immunol 141:1553–1560. https://doi.org/10.1016/j.jaci.2018.03.002

Thurtell MJ, Chiu AL, Goold LA et al (2013) Neuro-ophthalmology of invasive fungal sinusitis: 14 consecutive patients and a review of the literature. Clin Experiment Ophthalmol 41:567–576. https://doi.org/10.1111/ceo.12055

Tieu DD, Kern RC, Schleimer RP (2009) Alterations in epithelial barrier function and host defense responses in chronic rhinosinusitis. J Allergy Clin Immunol 124:37–42. https://doi.org/10.1016/j.jaci.2009.04.045

Dhingra PL, Dhingra S (2013) Diseases of Ear, Nose and Throat. 6th edn. Elsevier, New Delhi.

Tyler MA, Luong AU (2018) Current understanding of allergic fungal rhinosinusitis. World J Otorhinolaryngol Head Neck Surg 4:179–185. https://doi.org/10.1016/j.wjorl.2018.08.003

Tyler MA, Lam K, Marino MJ et al (2021) Revisiting the controversy: the role of fungi in chronic rhinosinusitis. Int Forum Allergy Rhinol 11:1577–1587. https://doi.org/10.1002/alr.22826

Uri N, Ronen O, Marshak T et al (2013) Allergic fungal sinusitis and eosinophilic mucin rhinosinusitis: diagnostic criteria. J Laryngol Otol 127:867–871. https://doi.org/10.1017/s0022215113001680

Vergidis P (2023) Aspergillosi. Manuali MSD Edizione Professionisti. https://www.msdmanuals.com/it/professionale/malattie-infettive/funghi/aspergillosi

Wackym PA, Snow JB (2016) Ballenger's otorhinolaryngology. PMPH USA

Walther N, Wagner N, Kurzai N (2019) Updates on the taxonomy of Mucorales with an emphasis on clinically important taxa. J Fungi 5:106. https://doi.org/10.3390/jof5040106

Watkinson JC, Clarke RW (2018) Scott-Brown's otorhinolarnygology and head and neck surgery. CRC Press

Wiesner DL, Klein BS (2017) Lung epithelium: barrier immunity to inhaled fungi and driver of fungal-associated allergic asthma. Curr Opin Microbiol 40:8–13. https://doi.org/10.1016/j.mib.2017.10.007

Wu P-W, Lee T-J, Yang S-W et al (2021) Differences in clinical and imaging presentation of maxillary sinus fungus ball with and without intralesional hyperdensity. Sci Rep 11:23945. https://doi.org/10.1038/s41598-021-03507-1

Yoon YH, Xu J, Park SK et al (2017) A retrospective analysis of 538 sinonasal fungus ball cases treated at a single tertiary medical center in Korea (1996–2015). Int Forum Allergy Rhinol 7:1070–1075. https://doi.org/10.1002/alr.22007

Zinreich SJ, Kennedy DW, Malat J et al (1988) Fungal sinusitis: diagnosis with CT and MR imaging. Radiology 169:439–444. https://doi.org/10.1148/radiology.169.2.3174990

Zuniga MG, Turner JH (2014) Treatment outcomes in acute invasive fungal rhinosinusitis. Curr Opin Otolaryngol Head Neck Surg 22:242–248. https://doi.org/10.1097/moo.0000000000000048

Mabry RL, Marple BF, Folker RJ, Mabry CS (1998) Immunotherapy for allergic fungal sinusitis: three years' experience. Otolaryngol Head Neck Surg 119:648–651. https://doi.org/10.1016/s0194-5998(98)70027-0

Chang CC, Incaudo GA, Gershwin ME (eds) (2014) Diseases of the sinuses: a comprehensive textbook of diagnosis and treatment. 2nd edn. Springer, New York. https://doi.org/10.1007/978-1-4939-0265-1

Luong AU, Chua A, Alim BM, Olsson P, Javer A (2022) Allergic fungal rhinosinusitis: the role and expectations of biologics. J Allergy Clin Immunol Pract 10(12):3156–3162. https://doi.org/10.1016/j.jaip.2022.08.021

González-Alcaide G, Llorente P, Ramos-Rincón JM (2020) Systematic analysis of the scientific literature on population surveillance. Heliyon 6(10):e05141. https://doi.org/10.1016/j.heliyon.2020.e05141

Benign Lesions of Maxillary Sinus

7

Goran Latif Omer, Vivek Sasindran, Mithra Sara, Saman W. Boskani, Ahmed Maki Merza, Othman Hussein, Kosar Hama Noori, Sahand Soran Ali, Fabbri Ilenia, Silvani Lorenzo, Giulia Marzocchella, Riccardo Maurizi, Pier Giorgio Giacomini, and Aland Salih Abdullah

Antrochoanal Polyp

Introduction

Antrochoanal polyps (ACPs) are isolated polypoid lesions of the sinonasal mucosa that develop in the maxillary sinus (antrum). In the region of the choana, they penetrate and widen the sinus ostium and the posterior nasal cavity (El-Feky and Bhuta 2010). They enter via the sinuses native or accessory ostia, travel down the back of the nose to the choana, and then into the nasopharynx (Al-Balas et al. 2020).

Sphenochoanal polyps are similar to nasopharyngeal polyps but occur less frequently in the sphenoid sinus and expand into the nasopharynx. Polyps can also form in the nasochoana, frontochoana, or ethmochoana (Antrochoanal polyp 2018).

Supplementary Information The online version contains supplementary material available at https://doi.org/10.1007/978-3-031-83468-4_7.

G. L. Omer (✉) · S. S. Ali · A. S. Abdullah
Department of Clinical Sciences, College of Medicine, University of Sulaimani, Sulaymaniyah, KRI, Iraq

V. Sasindran · M. Sara
KM Cherian Institute of Medical Sciences, Chengannur, Kerala, India

S. W. Boskani · A. M. Merza · O. Hussein · K. H. Noori
Royal Hospital, Sulaymaniyah, KRI, Iraq

F. Ilenia · S. Lorenzo · G. Marzocchella · R. Maurizi · P. G. Giacomini
Department of Otorhinolaryngology, University of Rome Tor Vergata, Rome, Italy

© The Author(s), under exclusive license to Springer Nature Switzerland AG 2025

G. L. Omer, S. Di Girolamo (eds.), *Maxillary Sinus: A Comprehensive Guide*, https://doi.org/10.1007/978-3-031-83468-4_7

History and Etymology

Palfijn was the first to report ACPs in 1753, but the German physician Gustav Killian was the first to characterize them in 1906 (Al-Balas et al. 2020). In his analysis of 22 cases, Killian concluded that these anomalies originated in the maxillary sinus and entered the nasal cavity via the accessory ostium. Killian's polyp, or an antrochoanal polyp (ACP), is a single, noncancerous lesion that has a high mucin content but is otherwise harmless (Antrochoanal polyp 2018).

Epidemiology

Although ACPs can affect anyone of any age, they are more common in those between the ages of 10 and 30. Approximately, 5% of sinonasal polyps are located in the antronasal region. They are more common in younger people (children and young adults) and in males (by a ratio of roughly 2:1) than in females. Cook et al. found a 70% male prevalence and a 30% female prevalence. Gender et al. and Kaushalt et al., on the other hand, found that the female-to-male ratio for ACPs was 1:1.5 (Al-Balas et al. 2020; El-Feky and Bhuta 2010; Meir et al. 2021).

Aetiology

Although its precise aetiology remains unknown, it is believed to exhibit fewer inflammatory reactions than the normal bilateral nasal polyps seen in cases of diffuse chronic rhinosinusitis (Meir et al. 2021). In fact, nasal allergies are not linked to this condition. An infectious aetiology has been linked to some of the proposed causes. Chronic rhinosinusitis has also been linked to Antrochoanal polyps. While approximately 25% of patients experience chronic sinusitis, a direct link between the two has not been demonstrated. Other hypotheses include the Bernoulli phenomenon, in which the polyp grows into the nasal cavity due to the negative pressure created by the respiratory airflow along the direction perpendicular to the ostium (Antrochoanal polyp 2018).

Clinical Presentation

Unilateral nasal obstruction and rhinitis are the initial signs of ACP. The presence of epistaxis, discomfort, and putrid discharges suggests an unusual cause. Larger masses have been known to prolapse far enough back from the nasopharynx that they are visible through the mouth.

It is unusual to find a bilateral form. Only 14 examples are known to exist, according to the published research. Nasal obstruction and anterior nasal discharge are the most typical symptoms of ACP, whereas epistaxis and discomfort may indicate a different aetiology and warrant further investigation to rule out more serious conditions, such as juvenile nasopharyngeal angiofibroma or sinonasal cancers. Antrochoanal polyps are rare in atopic patients and common in those who are not allergic to dust or pollen. Clinically, an ACP manifests as a greyish or pinkish mass that extends posteriorly to the choana via the middle meatus and nasal cavity (El-Feky and Bhuta 2010).

Pathogenesis

However, unlike the normal bilateral nasal polyps seen in cases of diffuse chronic rhinosinusitis, its specific aetiology is unknown, and it is expected to have fewer inflammatory reactions. Allergic persons, people with cystic fibrosis, those who are sensitive to aspirin, and people with specific infections are more likely to experience them. The obstruction of venous return from the polyp is what drives its expansion. This blockage exists at the ostium of the maxillary sinus. The swelling of the polypoid mucosa caused by venous stasis is depicted in Fig. 7.1 (Antrochoanal polyp 2018; Meir et al. 2021).

Antrochoanal polyps are pathologically similar to any other inflammatory polyp. In contrast to other types of polyps, maxillary polyps are characterized by a thin stalk that emerges from the maxillary sinus. However, the exact cause of chronic sinusitis, which affects about 25% of individuals, has not been determined. Neoplasia, inflammatory polyp, or cystic degeneration of the intramaxillary retention cyst may all contribute to its elusive pathogenesis. There is still debate in the scientific literature on whether or not ACP actually originates in the maxillary sinus. Although maxillary sinus polyps typically begin in the middle and back of the sinus, they can start almost anywhere (El-Feky and Bhuta 2010; Meir et al. 2021).

The polyp typically develops in the inferior and posterior regions of the nasopharynx because ACP leaves the maxillary sinus through the accessory ostium in at

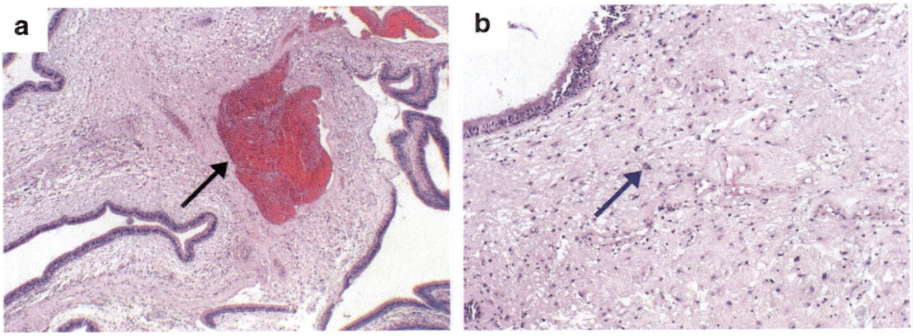

Fig. 7.1 This image (**a**: 4×, **b**: 10×) displays polypoid structures lined by respiratory-type epithelium without a thickened basement membrane. It is overlying a stroma containing stellate cells (Blue arrow) intermixed with mild chronic inflammatory cells. Moreover, dilated vessels filled with blood can be observed along with one vessel with thrombosis (Black arrow)

least 70% of instances. Recent research has shown that almost all ACPs reach past the accessory ostium. Choanal polyps can develop anywhere in the nasal cavity, including the sphenoid sinus, the nasal septum, and the choana (Meir et al. 2021).

Different types of ACPs exist based on where they adhere to the maxillary sinus wall. The inferolateral wall of the maxillary sinus was identified as the location of origin for all 15 cases of ACP examined by Berg et al. Deka; they discovered that the polyps came from the antero-inferior aspect of the antrum in 45% of his cases, the posterior medial wall of the antrum bordering the posterior fontanelle in 40% of his cases, and the site of origin could not be accurately determined in 15% of his cases (Al-Balas et al. 2020).

Various hypotheses have been proposed to explain the development of ACP, with some early research suggesting the condition develops from a type of cyst called antral mucous retention, which is found in a high percentage of the population (8–10%). Frosini et al. postulated that increased intra-sinus pressure brought on by partial occlusion of the natural ostium due to inflammatory changes and oedema explains why ACP occurs in only a subset of patients with retention cysts. This hypothesis may be supported by the histologic characteristics of ACP, which include a large number of inflammatory cells. The link between ACP and allergic reactions is debatable: although the specific cause of ACP remains uncertain, it has been linked to allergic rhinitis and ipsilateral maxillary sinusitis in children. Mantilla described a series of 27 cases of recurrent ACP in children, of which nearly half were considered to be passive smokers, indicating children who were exposed to cigarette smoke had an increased risk of recurrence after endoscopic surgery. Evidence like this may suggest a causal link between smoking and the onset of ACP, but this has not been established elsewhere, so more studies are warranted (Meir et al. 2021).

Differential Diagnoses (Antrochoanal Polyp 2018)

1. *Acute sinusitis* is characterized by prolapse of edematous mucosa from the maxillary antrum.
2. *Esthesioneuroblastoma*, which arises from the superior recess of the nasal cavity.
3. *Maxillary sinus mucocele*, revealing full opacification of the maxillary sinus alongside concomitant bony enlargement.
4. *Juvenile angiofibroma.*
5. *Nasal glioma.*
6. *Meningoencephalocele.*
7. *Inverted papilloma.*
8. *Mucocele.*
9. *Mucus retention cyst.*
10. *Tornwalt's cyst.*
11. *Grossly enlarged adenoids.*
12. *Lymphoma and nasopharyngeal malignancies.*

Diagnosing ACP, especially in younger children (aged 5–8), might be difficult. Adenoid hypertrophy is frequent in children and adolescents and can cause symptoms similar to atopic dermatitis, including nasal blockage, chronic rhinorrhoea, and snoring. Nasal endoscopy and/or lateral plain films of the neck are part of the preoperative treatment in these individuals, but ACP can still be missed in certain instances. The foreign body should also be eliminated as a cause of the child's unilateral nasal pathology because it typically presents with unilateral foul-smelling rhinorrhoea. Clinically, epistaxis is uncommon in patients with ACP. Neoplasia (inverted papilloma or malignant tumours) and vascular lesions (juvenile nasopharyngeal angiofibroma, hemangioma, or hemangiopericytoma) must be ruled out. Differentiating ACP from other illnesses relies on gathering extensive background information and doing a careful physical exam. Imaging can help diagnose when a physical exam is insufficient. Keep in mind that the diameter of the nasopharynx naturally narrows with age (particularly in children >8 years old), so the adenoid to nasopharynx ratio naturally decreases with age as well. Therefore, in order to rule out nasal polyps in children older than 8 years, a full nasal flexible endoscopy is required (Meir et al. 2021).

Histology/Histopathology

As shown in Fig. 7.1, Pearly white, edematous nasal mucosa that is pedunculated and prolapsed can be seen under the microscope. In most cases, the maxillary segment will be cystic, while the nasal and choanal ones will be solid. An ACP can be recognized by its "dumbbell" shape (Fig. 7.2), which is created by the cystic and solid components being connected by a thin stalk.

Cyst development, fibrosis, and squamous metaplasia are far more frequent microscopic findings in ACP than in scattered nasal polyps. In the antral (or intramaxillary) component of ACP, a cystic cavity is seen in the middle, surrounded by a homogenous edematous stroma with few cells. Occasionally, squamous metaplasia and reactive fibrosis can be seen in the choanal section of the polyp, while the intranasal portion is covered by respiratory epithelium that is identical to the normal mucosa of the sino-nasal tract (Fig. 7.3). ACP differs from allergic polyps by having more oedema and inflammatory cell infiltration but fewer eosinophils and submucosal glands. These results suggest that allergic reactions play a relatively modest role in the aetiology of ACP, but inflammatory alterations play a central role. The lack of submucosal glands also provides more evidence that ACP is caused by edematous hypertrophy of the respiratory epithelium rather than by distention of the glandular structure, as is the case with typical nasal polyps. The angiogenic markers vascular-endothelial growth factor (VEGF) and CD-34 are much less expressed in ACP than in nasal polyps caused by chronic rhinosinusitis. These results lend credence to the hypothesis that ACP results from a local inflammatory process and may shed light on the fact that, in contrast to other types of polyps, ACP is less likely to bleed as a presenting symptom or after endoscopic surgery. The presence of intramural cysts is a prominent feature of ACP. These cysts, which affect both the intramaxillary and

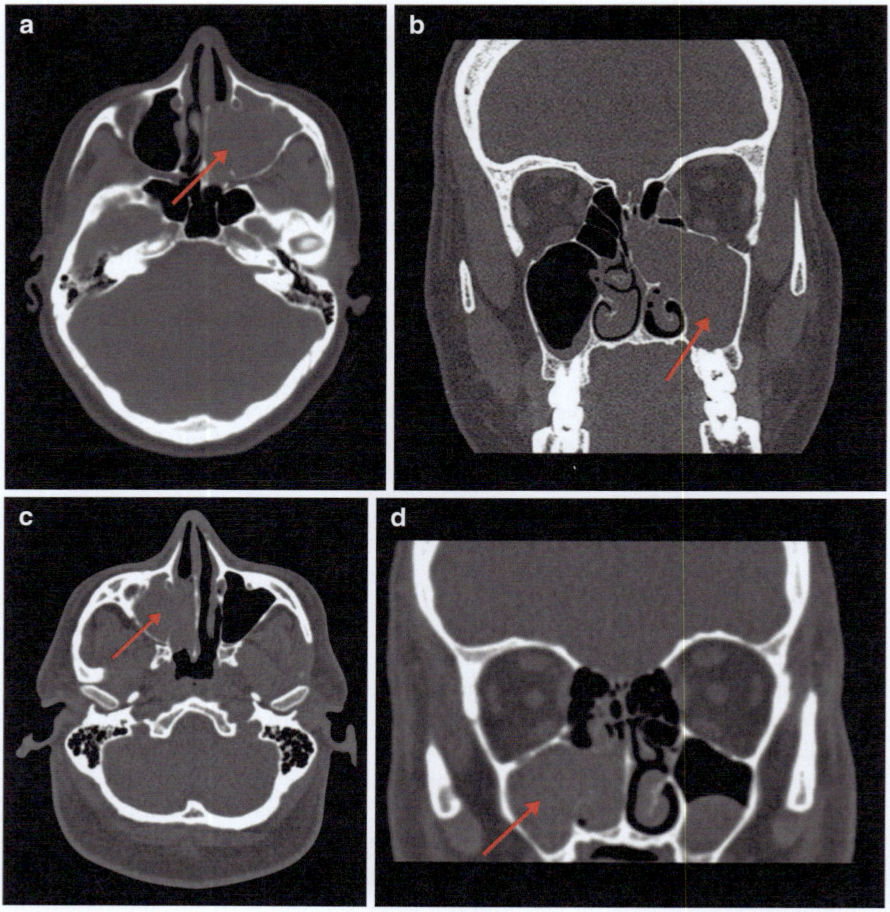

Fig. 7.2 (**a** and **b**) CT views of a female patient who has left maxillary sinus total soft tissue opacification, which is expanding and extending through the maxillary ostium into the left nasal cavity, reaching and obstructing the left posterior choana. (**c** and **d**) CT views of a male patient who has right maxillary sinus total soft tissue opacification, which is expanding and extending through the maxillary ostium into the right nasal cavity, reaching and obstructing the right posterior choana

intranasal regions of ACP, are thought to play a part in the disease's aetiology. The occurrence of intramural cysts also lends credence to Berg's hypothesis that chronic inflammation causes obstruction of the acinar glands or lymphatic ducts, which leads to the development of the polyps cystic portion. Significant oedema may be due to pressure created as the polyp expands through the ostium of the accessory sinus (Meir et al. 2021).

Cystic alterations are more common in ACP than in diffuse chronic rhinosinusitis with nasal polyps (d-CRS), which may be due to the distinct causes of the two conditions. Typical respiratory epithelium, with a thin lamina propria, cyst

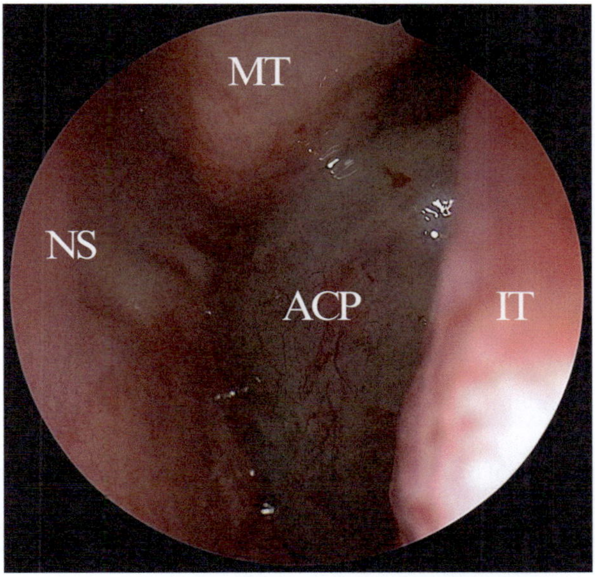

Fig. 7.3 This is an intraoperative video of a patient undergoing Endoscopic Sinus Surgery for an antrochoanal polyp. It can be seen in the thumbnail (left side nasal cavity); the polyp extends the maxillary sinus to the nasopharynx. (*ACP* antrochoanal polyp, *IT* inferior turbinate, *MT* middle turbinate, *NS* nasal septum) (Audio 7.1 and Video 7.1)

development, and fewer submucosal glands, is what gives rise to ACPs in the maxillary sinus. In contrast, the ethmoid sinus is a common starting point for nasal polyps in d-CRS due to its thick submucosal layer. The popular belief that ACP is more of a surgical issue than a medical one may be attributable to the lack of an inflammatory drive in the pathophysiology of ACP, which renders anti-inflammatory medication ineffective in this population (Al-Balas et al. 2020; Meir et al. 2021).

Diagnosis

Diagnosis is mainly clinical via endoscopic examination and supported by computed tomography (CT) imaging. The three components of the polyp may be detected on CT images: an intramaxillary portion, an intranasal portion, and a choanal component. Preoperative sinonasal CT scans are required for all patients because they are an important aspect of the diagnosis and give significant information about nasal and sinus bone landmarks prior to surgical intervention.

As shown in Fig. 7.2, a soft tissue mass occupying the maxillary sinus and extending through the accessory ostium into the middle meatus and the posterior choana can be seen on computed tomography (CT). ACP appears in CT as a hypoattenuating unilateral soft tissue mass that totally fills the maxillary sinus. It enters

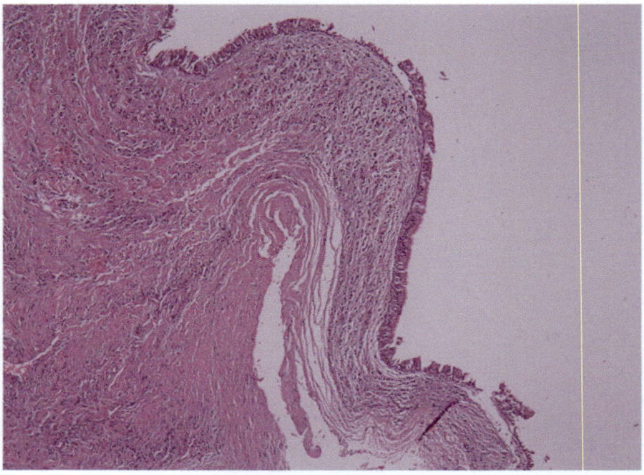

Fig. 7.4 Histopathological lamina of a mucous retention cyst within the maxillary sinus

the nasal cavity through the accessory maxillary ostium, medially to the inferior turbinate, and progresses to the nasopharynx (Fig. 7.4). In a few instances, the polyp extends anteriorly to the middle turbinate and anterior/inferior turbinate area. ACP generally doesn't lead to bony changes (bone erosion, breakdown, or sclerosis), but it can cause enlargement of the accessory maxillary ostium, which is mainly caused by an increasing cystic component of the polyp, resulting in the appearance of an expansile maxillary mass (Fig. 7.4). Other diseases, such as cancer, should be in mind in situations of suspected bone destruction on CT. Nevertheless, studies have revealed that weakening of alveolar bone in the maxillary sinus may develop as a result of ACP progression. Based on the radiological appearance of the lesion on CT, Lee classified ACP into three stages: Stage I (antronasal polyp without extension to the nasopharynx), Stage II (complete occlusion of the maxillary sinus ostium with nasopharyngeal extension), and Stage III (partial occlusion of the maxillary sinus ostium with nasopharyngeal extension). As previously stated, advanced CT stages (stages II and III) are more prevalent in children due to delayed diagnosis.

ACP is a grey-white-coloured mass with a smooth, round surface during nasal endoscopy. ACP is distinguishable from other allergic or inflammatory nasal polyps by its exclusive path from the maxillary sinus to the choana and bulging expansile behaviour (Al-Balas et al. 2020; Antrochoanal polyp 2018; Meir et al. 2021). A non-contrast CT scan is typically used to make a radiographic diagnosis. However, in a conventional X-ray of PNS, we can find a unilateral opacification of the maxillary sinus and nasopharyngeal mass. At times, we can observe a bilateral sinus involvement (23–42%). CT scans are often recommended because they provide precise information on the complete anatomy of the paranasal sinus as well as the extent of sinus involvement and anatomic variation.

The following features can be seen in a non-contrast PNS CT examination, which is best appreciated on true coronal or coronal reformatted scans:

(a) A homogeneous, well-defined mass emerging from the maxillary sinus, having mucin density.
(b) Generally expands the maxillary ostium and can protrude into the nasopharynx.
(c) Smooth enlargement of the maxillary sinus.
(d) There is no concomitant destruction of the bony structures around it. However, antrochoanal polyps may have a higher density if they have been present for a long period of time and/or have an accompanying fungal infection. A contrast-enhanced scan may demonstrate peripheral enhancement.

Magnetic resonance imaging (MRI) reveals hypointense T1 and enhanced T2 signals. The cystic component of the polyp is peripherally enhanced by gadolinium administration. Although CT is the ideal imaging modality for any nasal or sinus disease, including ACP, MRI may be used in children (due to the absence of radiation exposure) and in situations of complete unilateral nasal and sinus opacification in CT scans (to differentiate sinus secretions from the mass itself). Peripheral enhancement can be appreciated on post-contrast images. In T1 weighted sequences, impacted mucin/hemorrhagic content exhibits a high signal (Antrochoanal polyp 2018).

Plain Radiograph (El-Feky and Bhuta 2010)

Plain films are no longer regarded as sufficient for diagnosing sinus pathology. Nevertheless, they are still carried out in certain circumstances. The following findings were discovered:

- unilateral maxillary sinus opacification.
- a nasopharyngeal mass may be noticed on occasion. Bilateral sinus involvement is common (23–42%).

Treatment and Prognosis

Surgery is the gold standard of tCP treatment. Many surgical procedures for exposing the maxillary area have been developed since Killian's original description in 1906. As shown in Fig. 7.3, complete excision of the polyp's intramaxillary component is required for successful ACP resection. The optimal procedure should facilitate excellent access to all maxillary sinus walls while being as minimally invasive as feasible, particularly in infants. Endoscopic sinus surgery (ESS) involving polyp excision through either the inferior or middle meatus or a combination of both is now widely offered. Options such as ESS with adjuvant canine fossa puncture or ESS with "mini Caldwel-Luc " operation attempt to improve the visibility of the maxillary sinus's anterior and inferior walls (Meir et al. 2021). The classic treatment is intranasal snare polypectomy. However, if the stalk's base is not removed, the polyp could recur. Minimally invasive endoscopic surgery is done: the stalk attachment point is discovered and removed, along with a small cuff of nearby mucosa. Visualization of the stalk base can be achieved in many cases via a medial meatotomy, but it may require the creation of an additional window through the inferior meatus (El-Feky and Bhuta 2010). No studies on the efficacy of medical therapy for ACP have been reported, and the mainstay of treatment is still considered surgery, as already proposed by Stammberger in his "Polyposis Nasi" classification. In particular, the endoscopic technique has become the most widely accepted approach, even in children. To prevent a recurrence of the condition, it is critical to avoid simple polypectomy and to remove the underlying mucosa at the site of genesis of the ACP with little disruption of normal sinus physiology. However, due to the existence of coexisting sinonasal mucosal disease, it is not always feasible to define the site of attachment preoperatively and, as a result, to correctly plan the most appropriate surgical approach (Al-Balas et al. 2020).

In the past, the Caldwell-Luc procedure was used as the primary modality of treatment; however, the risk of damaging tooth development and the growth centres in children, together with frequent postoperative cheek swelling, affected its popularity. The endoscopic approach avoids swelling of the cheeks, decreases adverse effects on teeth and facial growth in children, and has a shorter hospitalization time compared with the Caldwell-Luc procedure. The introduction of angled optics and powered instrumentation, particularly angled micro-debrider blades that offer a good surgical field by shaving and excising soft tissue, allowing the intact mucosa to be saved during dissection around the point of attachment (Fig. 7.6), has improved the role of endoscopic sinus surgery (ESS). Nevertheless, it is not always possible to locate and reach the maxillary stalk of the ACP purely endoscopically, especially when it is on the anterior or inferior wall of the maxillary sinus. As a result, various surgical approaches have been advocated in conjunction with the endoscopic procedure in order to prevent recurrence owing to incomplete polyp removal by offering less morbidity and a lower rate of complications compared to a Caldwell-Luc procedure. Better visualization and access to the maxillary sinus can be obtained by combining ESS with a mini-Caldwell-Luc procedure, canine fossa puncture inferior meatal antrostomy, to a transnasal prelacrimal approach (recommended for revision surgery) or ESS with a large middle meatal antrostomy. If the stalk base is removed, the recurrence rate is modest (7%). Many surgical approaches for treating ACPs have been presented in order to reduce the frequency of postoperative recurrence with a minimum number of complications following the operation. All of these surgical approaches are based on the same fundamental principle: how to reach the point of its origin. Simple polypectomy (removing the polyp from the maxillary cavity using angled forceps without regard for the site of origin) is one of the surgical alternatives. However, ACP recurrence following this sort of procedure is reported to be 25%. Overall, many experts believe that the endoscopic technique for ACP removal is successful and safe. In research conducted by Franche et al., a recurrence incidence of 6.9% was recorded in 29 patients who had endoscopic transnasal surgery. Freitas et al. handled 16 cases of ACPs using the same approach and documented 12.5% recurrence, whereas Ozdek et al. recorded up to 22% of recurrences after middle meatal antrostomy alone. In a series of paediatric patients operated on in three ENT Italian Departments, Pagella et al. revealed a 22% recurrence rate in those who had undergone operation using the standard technique

(12/42 patients) and a 0% recurrence rate in four instances treated with a combined endoscopic and canine fossa approach.

Few writers removed the antral section of ACPs using merely inferior antrostomy. Gendeh et al. found that two of three patients who had an endoscopic intranasal polypectomy utilizing an inferior antrostomy route had a recurrence after a year of follow-up. Sato and Nakashima employed the same procedure to remove the antral section of ACPs; after a 10- to 46-month follow-up, none of the ten patients in this trial had a recurrence. Comoglu et al. have recently suggested a Transnasal prelacrimal recess approach in patients with recurrent antrochoanal polyps with an 83% success rate (10/12); according to the authors, this method of treatment ensured good exploration of the sinus and easy access to the origin of the polyp despite a higher risk of damaging the lacrimal pathway. The recurrence incidence of ACP following endoscopic surgical treatment does not differ substantially between children and adults. Galluzzi's meta-analysis revealed a 15% recurrence rate in children, with considerably higher rates in patients who received endoscopic surgical therapy alone vs a combination strategy (i.e. endoscopic and trans-canine sinusoscopy or mini-Caldwell-Luc) (Al-Balas et al. 2020; Antrochoanal polyp 2018; Cherrabi et al. 2021; Meir et al. 2021).

Special Consideration in ACP Resection; ESS in Children

As previously stated, ACP is more common among children and young people. Although there were no differences in pathophysiology or histology between children and adults, children are at a greater risk of recurrence. It is plausible to think that the physically small sinuses, unerupted teeth, and worry for maxillary development may influence the surgeon's surgical technique, resulting in a higher failure rate.

In his review of 200 patients with ACP, Forsini described recurrence in four patients (2%), all of which were children <7 years of age, in whom only polypectomy was performed. Eventually, in all cases of recurrence ESS was performed without evidence of recurrence (Meir et al. 2021).

Recurrence and Follow-Up

Recurrence rates range from 0%, recorded by Tsukidate, to 64%, as reported by Saito and associates, as seen in several published series. Recurrence rates vary depending on surgical approach, patient age, and other factors such as associated sinus diseases. This begs the question of how long we should follow-up with patients who have had ACP resection. Lee and Huang discovered that 65% of their paediatric ACP patients also had chronic sinusitis. Similarly, other writers have discovered a link between ACPs and allergic illness. Once there is persistent inflammation, the key idea is the difficulty of removing the completely diseased mucosa with the origin of the polyp. Natasha Choudhury reported 29 patients who had ACP treated with

(Endoscopic middle meatal antrostomy) EMMA surgery. They described no polyp recurrence, with a mean follow-up period of 14.7 months. Galluzzi examined 13 research studies and discovered that recurrence in children is greater than in adults, according to the previously mentioned factors. The research found that the combination approach had the lowest recurrence rate, with follow-up ranging from 6 to 120 months. The majority of recurrences occurred within 5 months to 3 years following the first operation. According to certain experts, various anatomic changes in the nasal cavity, such as septal deviation, conchal hypertrophy, and concha bullosa, may raise intramaxillary pressure, predisposing to the development of ACP. While these changes were found in up to 80% of ACP patients, none of them were associated with elevated recurrence rates. In most relevant studies, the time of recurrence was 1.2 ± 0.6 years. Therefore, it is advised to monitor ACP patients for at least 2 years after surgery in order to detect 95% of recurrent cases (Antrochoanal polyp 2018).

Retention Cyst

Introduction

Retention cyst is an epithelium-lined cyst containing mucous or serous fluid (yellowish or clear). It results from an obstruction of the ducts of mucosal serous and/or mucinous glands. Local infection and allergic reactions may cause obstruction of the duct and thus lead to the accumulation of fluid. The fluid accumulation within the obstructed duct can cause cystic dilatation of the gland. The cysts are usually found to develop under the mucous membrane of the sinus with a variation in their size and number. Rarely can these cysts enlarge to fill a maxillary sinus cavity, but they are usually small in size and are seen to have slow growth (Rastegar and Osmani 2022).

Without any therapeutic approach, the size remains constant in 60% of cases and decreases or disappears in another 30%, which leaves only 10% of cases that seem to have an increase in volume. This is the reason Wang et al. suggested that a "wait and see" approach was the best approach to be taken in the absence of clinical complications (Gonçales et al. 2015). Mucous retention cysts (MRC) may be unilateral in some cases but are more often found bilaterally (Rastegar and Osmani 2022). These cysts do possess an epithelial lining; however, there seems to be no epithelial wall (Rastegar and Osmani 2022). The cysts are mostly asymptomatic; however, nasal and postnasal discharge has been reported in certain cases with facial pain, headache and nasal congestion (Dağistan et al. 2021).

Mucous retention cysts are seen not only in dentate patients but also in edentulous patients, which gives rise to the suggestion that they have a non-odontogenic origin. If the mucous retention cyst is within the maxillary sinus, there is a possibility of radiological misdiagnoses since it can fill up the sinus, making the image blurry and giving the appearance of maxillary sinusitis (Gonçales et al. 2015). Even though the exact pathogenesis of the lesion is not agreed upon, it is known that local infection can possibly be a cause of obstruction (Rastegar and Osmani 2022).

Epidemiology

Mucous retention cysts (MRCs) are estimated to be present in about ten healthy adult populations. In a study done by M Bal et al., out of 510 patients who were reviewed for retention cysts, 29.4%(150 cases) of them were shown to have mucous retention cysts. The mean age of mucinous retention cysts was calculated to be 37.9 years (17–76) with a male-to-female ratio of 1.7:1. Majority of the cysts were found in the maxillary sinus either bilaterally or unilaterally with rare incidences of some ethmoid sinus retention cysts (Bal and Berkiten 2014). It is shown to affect patients of all races and both genders with a broad range of age groups. They are benign, self-limiting lesions that are most commonly found on the floor of maxillary sinuses, with the second most common sinus being the sphenoid sinuses. The pathogenesis of MRCs remains undefined, although it is strongly associated with allergies, inflammatory processes, infectious processes, trauma, relative humidity, and room temperature (Chang et al. 2014; Vieira et al. 2015; Rastegar and Osmani 2022).

Clinical Features

They are usually asymptomatic, while with MRCs, the most common complication is sinusitis. Sometimes, these lesions may cause headaches periorbital or facial pain, and they can even predispose to the development of recurrent rhinosinusitis and nasal obstruction (Caylakli et al. 2006). Retention cysts of the maxillary sinus are often incidental findings seen on radiographic images since they are asymptomatic (Gonçales et al. 2015); however, they can deviate the nasal septum and cause upper airway obstruction (Dağistan et al. 2021).

Histology

The pseudostratified columnar epithelium is seen with sparse occasional mucosal cells and minimal sign of inflammatory infiltrate; this can be seen in Fig. 7.4. The columnar epithelial lining of the cyst was observed to have cilia, and the surrounding connective tissue was fibro-elastic. The presence of the epithelium can help distinguish retention cysts from pseudocysts, which do not possess an epithelial lining (Mattos et al. 2019).

Diagnosis and Imaging

Physical examination, clinical history and radiological imaging are all part of the diagnosing process for mucinous retention cysts. Bone opacification and erosion can be seen in panoramic radiographs; however, computed tomography (CT) is still considered the gold standard for the diagnosis of mucous cysts. Retention cysts found within the maxillary sinus seem to have a homogenous, radiopaque, and sharply defined appearance. They are also seen to have a connection with the floor of the maxillary sinus (Mattos et al. 2019).

MRCs are a common incidental finding on CT and MRI of the sinuses. On radiographs, they are radiopaque, dome-shaped, rounded structures with a distinctly rounded edge on CT scan (Fig. 7.2) found along the floor of maxillary sinuses and sphenoid sinuses (Caylakli et al. 2006). Images are seen reflected with long T1 and long T2 features on MRI. These are, therefore, seen as low-signal intensity on T1W and as high-signal intensity on T2W MR images. Mucous retention types' cysts are seen to show slightly higher signal intensity on T1W images on MRI compared to the serous cyst type. The higher intensity of the mucous type is related to their elevated protein content. Retention cysts do not show contrast enhancement on enhanced CT and MRI scans (Chang et al. 2014).

Retention cysts found within the maxillary sinus are round-shaped masses with smooth surfaces and a radiopaque appearance on radiography. They are commonly seen to develop from the wall of the sinus and, more often, from the floor of the sinus. The biggest complication that arises due to these cysts is upper airway obstruction as a result of nasal septum deviation. Nasal septal deviation can narrow down the middle meatus, which subsequently leads to further sinus pathologies (Dağistan et al. 2021).

Treatment

Symptomatic cysts' treatment traditionally was by puncture and aspiration through the inferior meatus or excision through an intranasal antrostomy or by the Caldwell–Luc operation. With the development of the rigid nasal endoscope and the introduction of endoscopic intranasal sinus surgery, the management of sinus disease has changed. In the endoscopic approach, a rigid nasal endoscope is used, and most of the cyst is removed through the natural sinus ostium; this is also seen in Fig. 7.5. The endoscopic approach can be recommended as the surgical procedure and therapeutic approach of choice since it is associated with a very low rate of recurrence of 3% (Hadar et al. 2000). It is necessary to treat symptomatic cases of retention cysts in the maxillary sinus since it has been seen to lead to immediate improvement in the patient's breathing. Medical follow-up is usually not required unless the patient has a history of recent allergies.

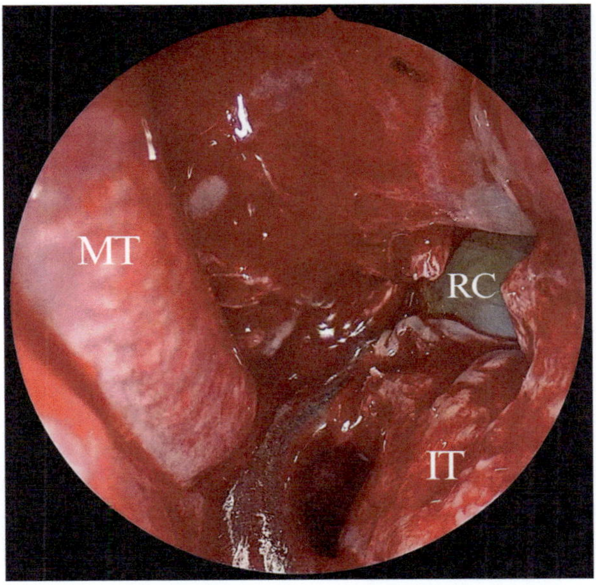

Fig. 7.5 This is an intraoperative video of a patient undergoing endoscopic sinus surgery for a retention cyst. As can be seen in the thumbnail (left side nasal cavity), maxillary sinusotomy type 1 is done, and the retention cyst can be visualized inside the sinus. (*RC* retention cyst, *IT* inferior turbinate, *MT* middle turbinate) (Audio 7.2 and Video 7.2)

Prognosis

About 6–23% of maxillary sinus cysts rupture spontaneously (Hadar et al. 2000). In the literature, spontaneous regression and disappearance rates of RCMs are reported between 17.6% and 38%, and RCMs are generally believed to be self-limiting (Dağistan et al. 2021). In most cases of sinus mucoceles, follow-up with panoramic radiographs is the only treatment required unless it is an extremely symptomatic case, and then an excision of the lesion is considered. This is mostly due to their stable size, which has been seen over the years. Cystic recurrence does happen, and it has been associated with difficulties in complete surgical removal of the lesion or other characteristics of the cyst at the cellular level (Mattos et al. 2019).

Differential Diagnosis (Choi et al. 2022; Hadar et al. 2000; Knipe and Claassen 2013)

(a) Sinus lining hyperplasia as a result as a result of odontogenic infection.
(b) Sinonasal Polyps: difficult to differentiate on CT and MRI, but retention cysts do not extend into the nasal cavity, unlike polyps.

(c) Paranasal sinus mucocele: the presence of air within the sinus does rule out mucocele.
(d) Antral pseudocyst: they form inflammatory exudate; however, unlike retention cysts, they do not have an epithelial lining.
(e) Neoplasia: it can be differentiated based on its association with systemic symptoms such as fatigue and weight loss tumour markers.

Dentigerous Cyst

Introduction

Dentigerous cysts are a form of odontogenic cysts that are generally present in young adults. The presence of a tooth that has failed to complete its eruption process is mandatory within the cyst. It is a slow-growing and benign cyst that is considered developmental in origin (Demiriz et al. 2015; Gaurkar et al. 2022). There have been reports of dentigerous cysts occurring because of a nonvital primary tooth impacted by periapical inflammation (Demiriz et al. 2015). It presents around the crown due to the fluid accumulation between the enamel organs. Facial deformities are common since the mass can undergo considerable expansion without causing any pain. This type of cyst does not commonly occur in the maxillary canine and is more frequent in the mandibular third molar teeth (Onay et al. 2019). Due to its slow growth and indolent growth, the lesion can remain asymptomatic for many years (Hamada et al. 2018). However, if it does evade the maxillary sinus, dentigerous cysts can present with epistaxis, purulent rhinorrhoea, facial pain and headache, obstruction, external nasal deformities, and swelling. In instances where it does occur in the maxillary sinus, the therapeutic approach necessary is surgery in conjunction with fenestration of the sinus (Hamada et al. 2018).

Epidemiology

A dentigerous cyst is the second most common odontogenic cyst (Onay et al. 2019). Among the developmental odontogenic cysts of the jaw, it is the most common (Kara et al. 2015). The average presenting age of the cyst is in patients aged between 20 and 40 years old and is very unlikely in children (Hamada et al. 2018). The frequency of the cyst in children ranges from 4% to 9% (Demiriz et al. 2015). The lesion is twice more likely to occur in males than in females. The majority of the cases are in the mandibular third molar, making odontogenic cysts of the maxillary sinus an infrequent phenomenon (Gaurkar et al. 2022).

Aetiology and Pathophysiology

Dentigerous odontogenic cysts have broadly been divided into inflammatory cysts and cysts that have a developmental origin. The latter is the most common type present around the crown of an erupted tooth. As mentioned before, in this type of cyst, the accumulation of fluid occurs between the layers of the enamel organs (Demiriz et al. 2015). It has been hypothesized that this fluid accumulation is due to a decrease in enamel epithelium (Shetty and Dixit 2010). The inflammatory type of cysts develops following periapical inflammation of a nonvital primary tooth. However, this form of dentigerous cyst is rare (Demiriz et al. 2015). Inflammatory dentigerous cysts could also occur from a spread of inflammation from an external source to the tooth (Shetty and Dixit 2010).

Clinical Presentation

The lesion can grow slowly for years without mediating any symptoms or discomfort in the patient. Symptoms typically arise when the cyst evades to involve the maxillary sinus (Hamada et al. 2018). The proliferation of epithelial cells, osmolality of fluid within the cyst and release of factors that result in bone resorption have all been hypothesized to be associated with the expansion and growth of the cyst. Therefore, although asymptomatic in the majority of patients, in cases with maxillary involvement, the cyst can manifest with rhinorrhoea, nasal defects, facial swelling, and excessive tearing (Tayşi et al. 2016). Swelling and pain are among the common presentations in patients diagnosed with symptomatic dentigerous cysts (Shetty and Dixit 2010).

Diagnostics and Imaging

The cysts are commonly found in routine radiographic examinations performed for evaluation of eruption failure in a tooth. Alternatively, the radiographic evaluation can also be conducted when there is a mal alignment, a missing tooth, or in cases of secondary inflammation presenting with pain and swelling (Gaurkar et al. 2022). On imaging, the cyst will appear as a unilocular radiolucency with a well-circumscribed border surrounding the tooth's crown. X-ray of the paranasal scan and orthopantomogram (OPG) are among the imaging tools since they're both easy to use and relatively cheap. A computed Tomography scan is used when precise dimensions and proximity to adjacent structures are required (Gaurkar et al. 2022). The lesion is generally anticipated when a follicular cyst exceeds 5 mm.

Histopathology

The soft tissue extracted from the tooth is stained with standard haematoxylin and eosin. On microscopy, the lesion will have a fibrous cyst wall that is lined with non-keratinized stratified squamous epithelium. The thickness of the epithelium varies (Austin and Nelson 2021).

Differential Diagnosis

Many differential diagnoses exist for odontogenic cysts, such as unicystic ameloblastoma, central giant cell granuloma, odontogenic keratocyst, and large radicular cysts. None of these lesions can be separated from an odontogenic cyst on the basis of radiography alone; therefore, histopathological evaluation may be required (Demiriz et al. 2015).

Treatment and Prognosis

The most common therapeutic approach for odontogenic cysts is surgery. Many different surgical approaches have been utilized, all tailored to the specificity of the case. Marsupialization, a technique that converts the cyst into a pouch, is among them. The procedure is carried out by making a surgical incision in the cyst capsule in order to minimize the intracystic pressure and evacuate its contents. Following this, the edges of the cyst are sutured to the healthy surface of the oral mucosa so that a large permanent opening is established. Maxillary cysts can be marsupialized into the maxillary sinus nasal cavity and can also be marsupialized into the oral cavity (Garip et al. 2015; Pogrel 2005). This procedure minimizes bone destruction; however, recurrence is one of its disadvantages (Kasat et al. 2012; Kara et al. 2015). An example of an endoscopic marsupialization of a maxillary cyst can be seen in Fig. 7.6. Alternatively, the cyst can undergo decompression to relieve the pressure. This is done by making a small opening in the cyst and keeping it open, which can be achieved by a drain or obturator. The obturator should be removed in this approach, and the cyst cavity should be soaked every day (Garip et al. 2015, Pogrel 2005). Regarding larger cysts, the approach of choice can be Waldron's procedure, a procedure that includes marsupialization followed by enucleation, which is performed when the size of the lesion has been reduced by marsupialization (Kara et al. 2015). The overall rate of success increases when the condition is diagnosed and treated early on. This is because the lesion has the potential to grow into more aggressive and painful forms (Pogrel 2005).

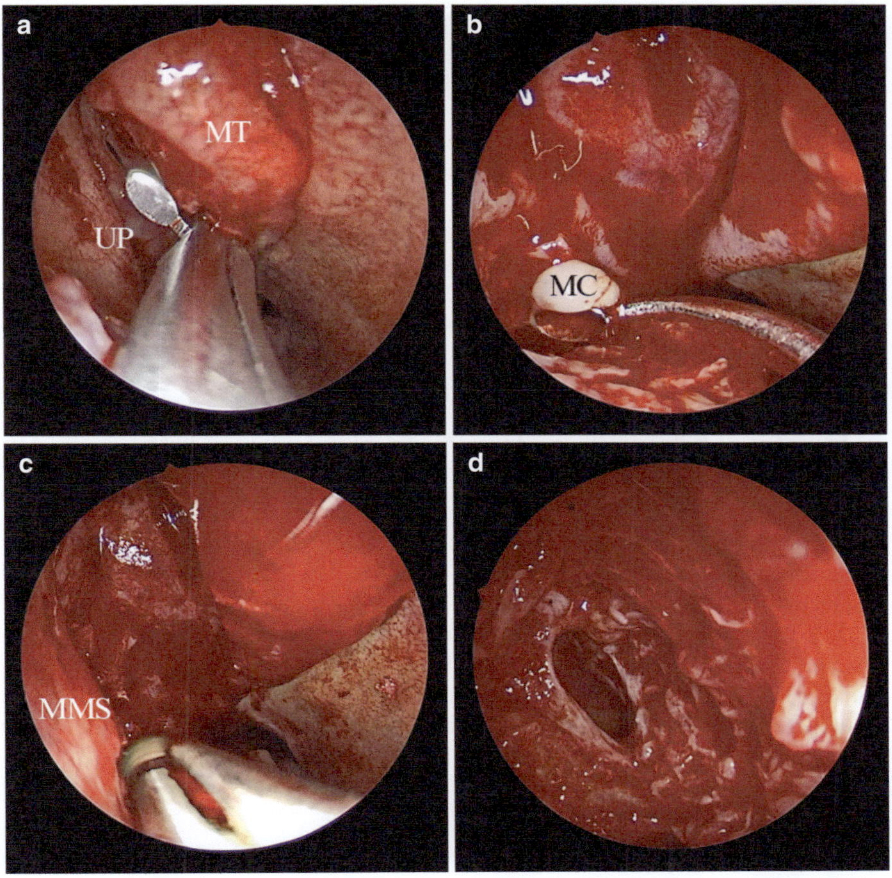

Fig. 7.6 This is an intraoperative video of a patient undergoing endoscopic sinus surgery for a maxillary cyst. As can be seen in the thumbnails (right side nasal cavity), (**a**) engaging the back-biter to the uncinate process to remove it, (**b**) opening of the maxillary sinus ostium by a J curette, (**c**) drilling of the inferior part of the medial maxillary wall to expose the area and therefore marsupialize the cyst, and (**d**) this is the maxillary cyst after marsupialization. (*UP* uncinate process, *MT* middle turbinate, *MC* maxillary cyst, *MMS* medial wall of the maxillary sinus) (Audio 7.3 and Video 7.3)

Maxillary Sinus Cholesterol Granuloma

Introduction

A cholesterol granuloma (CG) is granulation tissue that results from recurrent haemorrhage (Sataloff 2015). It is a chronic inflammatory lesion and is most often found in the petrous apex of the temporal bone. They resemble benign tumours, thus not easily diagnosed and have a cystic cavity filled with a fluid that is chocolate-brown in colour. The term "congenital epidermoid cysts" was once used to describe them, but they are now known as chocolate cysts because they are made of a fluid including cholesterol crystals, red blood cells and the breakdown products of those cells, multinucleated giant cells, and hemosiderin, all of which are encased in a fibrous capsule. This capsule consists of delicate blood vessels that are readily broken and prone to bleeding, which prevents the granuloma from healing (Ahmetgjekaj et al. 2022). Although CG is not found in the nasal cavity, the closed cavities of the paranasal sinuses, particularly the maxillary and the frontal sinuses, which are the most frequently affected sites, provide suitable conditions for their formation (Meirelles and Neves-Pinto 2006). In general, cholesterol granulomas in the maxillary sinus are uncommon and, both clinically and radiographically, resemble maxillary sinusitis (Alghulikah et al. 2021).

Epidemiology

The first report on cholesterol granuloma in the maxillary sinus was made in 1978 by Graham and Michaels (Meirelles and Neves-Pinto 2006). They are regarded as unusual in the maxillary sinus, and from 2005 to 2016, 12 of the approximately 50 instances that were published in English literature were described (De Freitas Filho et al. 2017). Additionally, they are most frequently observed in patients with cholesteatoma development and persistent otitis media (Mallon et al. 2014). The prevalence of CG is higher in middle-aged patients (mean age = 38 years old; age range from 27 to 56 years), with a male-to-female ratio of 3:1, thus a clear predilection for men (Da Motta Almada et al. 2008).

Pathophysiology

Haemorrhages inside these cavities, liberation from deteriorating tissue, or transudation appear to represent the pathogenesis of CG in the sinuses. The closed cavities of the paranasal sinuses have a long lymphatic drainage channel, which slows drainage. This would allow the cholesterol the time it needs to separate into crystals, precipitate, and then start the granulomatous transformation (Meirelles and Neves-Pinto 2006; Bütler and Grossenbacher 1989). Maxillary sinus CG may be caused by a variety of factors, including impaired sinus drainage, disrupted ventilation, and bleeding into the sinus with haemolysis. Cholesterol is thought to originate from the erythrocyte cell membrane that is damaged during bleeding. These crystals trigger a foreign body reaction, which was originally seen in animal experiments by Friedmann and Hiraide et al., which leads to leukocyte and macrophage migration and ultimately results in the development of giant foreign body cells. Cholesterol crystals can also be a result of connective tissue degeneration brought on by reduced ventilation caused by osteomeatal complex blockage due to injury and inflammatory substances. Maxillary sinus CG pathophysiology makes it common to link it to a history of rhinitis, sinusitis, trauma, and paranasal sinus surgery, especially as these conditions can result in localized bleeding foci (Bütler and Grossenbacher

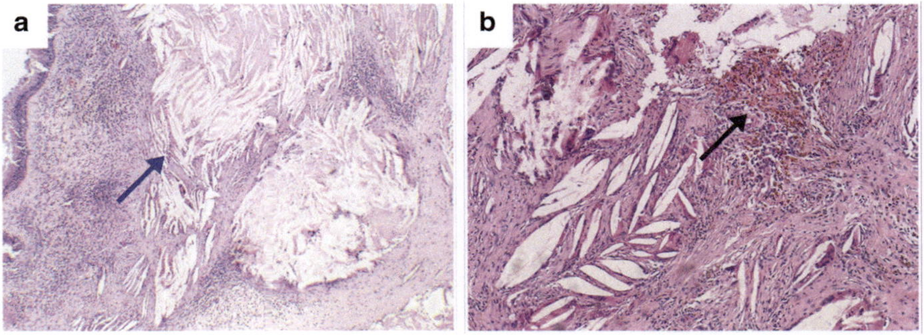

Fig. 7.7 This image (**a**: 4×, **b**: 10×) shows respiratory epithelium overlying multilobular aggregates of cholesterol clefts (Blue Arrow) that are surrounded by foreign body type multinucleated giant cells intermixed with lymphocytes, plasma cells and hemosiderin-laden macrophage (Black Arrow)

1989; Da Motta Almada et al. 2008). In summary, it has been proposed that three variables, including disrupted ventilation, poor drainage, and haemorrhage into a bone cavity with subsequent haemolysis and accumulation of cholesterol from red cell membranes, are responsible for the pathogenesis of paranasal cholesterol granuloma (Leon et al. 2002).

Histology

Due to the possibility that CG in the maxillary antrum could be confused for chronic sinusitis, histopathological investigation is crucial and needs to be performed on all specimens obtained following paranasal sinus surgery. As shown in Fig. 7.7, because of its distinctive morphology, CG does not easily resemble anything else (Meirelles and Neves-Pinto 2006). The cholesterol granuloma histopathology report states that thick masses of cholesterol crystals emerge as clefts that are surrounded by foreign body giant cells, plasma cells, foam cells, and lymphocytes. The areas that seem like intermixed clefts are evidence that cholesterol crystals have disintegrated as a result of the alcohol used in the staining method (Marina and Gendeh 2006).

Clinical Features

In the maxillary sinus, the clinical manifestations of CG are nonspecific and might be confused with those of other cystic or inflammatory disorders. It is frequently linked to a previous history of rhinitis, sinusitis, trauma, or paranasal sinus surgery, and it may be accompanied by symptoms such as facial pain, headache, otalgia, rhinorrhoea, and nasal obstruction. The most often reported symptoms were pain and blockage or congestion in the nasal cavity (Koo et al. 2016).

Diagnosis and Imaging

In order to establish a diagnosis of maxillary sinus CG, a microscopic examination of a foreign body reaction is required. This reaction is distinguished by foreign body giant cells and longitudinal cholesterol clefts, as well as granulocytes, foam cells, and macrophages packed with hemosiderin. In conclusion, it is feasible to witness fibrin deposition and local haemorrhage. These observations complete the picture (Koo et al. 2016). There are no specific X-ray findings that alert the surgeon to the diagnosis prior to operation; however, some patients may present with X-ray abnormalities that may suggest the diagnosis of CG (Meirelles and Neves-Pinto 2006).

On computed tomography (Fig. 7.8), CG lesions appear expansile and erosive, and they have well-defined margins; nonetheless, it might be challenging to differentiate them from other types of lesions, such as epidermoids and mucoceles, when utilizing this modality. Due to the fact that cholesterol granulomas exhibit high intensity in T1- and T2-weighted sequences, magnetic resonance imaging is able to provide improved specificity for the diagnosis of these lesions (Mallon et al. 2014). Opacification of the maxillary sinus, with a cystic arrangement or soft tissue density, usually well-defined by sclerotic cortical bone, although bone expansion and erosion can be noted, is one of the most common radiographic findings of maxillary sinus CG. Calcification foci are infrequent, and there is a possibility of bone erosion; however, it is not generally observed (Da Motta Almada et al. 2008).

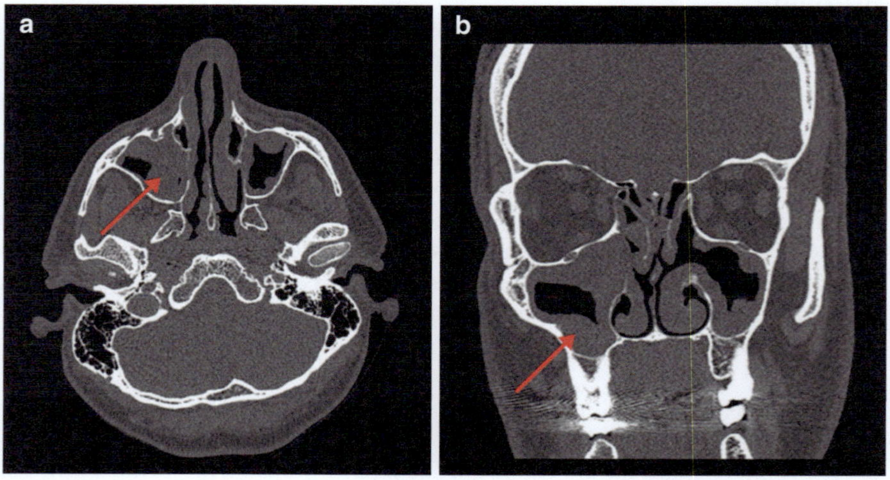

Fig. 7.8 Bilateral maxillary sinus mucosal thickening (**a**: Axial, **b**: Coronal), with the right cavity more than the left. The pathology in the right side maxillary sinus (arrow) was later proven to be a cholesterol granuloma

Treatment

The treatment of choice for maxillary sinus CG is surgical excision, either open or endoscopic (Da Motta Almada et al. 2008).

- The open techniques for surgical excision of the CG include:
  - *Caldwell-Luc Technique:* the tissue is removed via the canine fossa, and intranasal counter drainage is created through the inferior meatus (Matheny and Duncavage 2003).
  - *Weber Ferguson Incision:* it allows for the superior and inferior portions of the maxilla to be exposed and for its total en bloc excision from the upper alveolar ridge to the orbit (Gil et al. 2012).
  - *Modified Weber Ferguson Incision:*
  - *Midfacial Degloving Approach:* this approach leaves no visible external scars and provides great bilateral exposure of the maxilla, zygoma, paranasal areas, and infraorbital margins on both sides of the face (Zachariah and Neelakandan 2019).
  - *Maxillary Swing Technique*: wide access to the nasopharynx, pterygopalatine fossa, and pterygomaxillary fissure is provided by the technique. Also, soft palate function is maintained during the process (Vlantis et al. 2008).
  - Total Maxillectomy.
- The endoscopic techniques include (a case of endoscopic approach can be seen in Fig. 7.9):

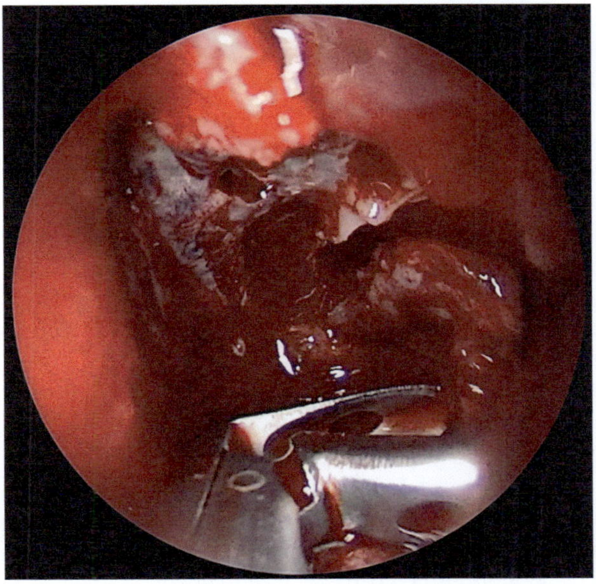

Fig. 7.9 This is an intraoperative video of a patient undergoing endoscopic sinus surgery for a cholesterol granuloma. As can be seen in the thumbnail (left side nasal cavity), a backward blacksley is used here to remove the granuloma from the maxillary sinus (Audio 7.4 and Video 7.4)

- Endoscopic Middle Meatal Antrostomy.
- Medial maxillectomy, with its modified types (I-IIb).
- Transseptal Approach.
- Prelacrimal Approach.

These approaches are further discussed in Chap. 11.

Differential Diagnosis

In these patients, the primary possibilities for a differential diagnosis were mucoceles of the maxillary antrum, cysts originating within the sinus, or cysts of dental origin. Malignant illness was also a possibility in the cases that showed extension or erosion of the maxillary sinus (Meirelles and Neves-Pinto 2006). Differential diagnosis of CG also includes allergic and inflammatory sinonasal diseases (Da Motta Almada et al. 2008).

Angiofibroma Involving the Maxillary Sinus

Introduction

Nasopharyngeal angiofibroma is a rare benign fibrovascular tumour (Stokes and Castle 2010). Although histologically benign, when it comes to its vascular entities, the tumour is considered aggressive. The majority of the cases are of the nasopharynx. In cases of extrapharyngeal angiofibroma, the tumour has a nonspecific clinical picture, mostly dependent on the location from which it arises. The exact cause for extrapharyngeal angiofibroma is yet to be found; however, there have been reports of ectopic tissue playing a role in pathogenesis (Cheah et al. 2023). The most common extrapharyngeal sites for angiofibroma include the nasal cavity, nasal septum, ethmoid and finally, the maxilla (Cheah et al. 2023). Juvenile nasopharyngeal angiofibroma originally arises from the sphenopalatine foramen. The tumour can then spread locally into the pterygopalatine fossa, nasal cavity, and paranasal sinuses (Acharya et al. 2017). Angiofibroma of the paranasal sinuses will likely present late; this is because the cavity has a large size, accommodating a large growth prior to symptom occurrence (Wan et al. 2022).

Epidemiology

Angiofibroma is an uncommon tumour, especially when outside of the nasopharynx. The tumour accounts for less than 1% of all head and neck neoplasms (Neel et al. 1973). Furthermore, it is mostly seen in males. Investigators have found testosterone, androgen, and dihydrotestosterone hormone receptors to have increased expression, whereas a decrease or even a lack of oestrogen and progesterone hormone receptors has been detected. Therefore, the diagnosis of angiofibroma in females should be done so after careful consideration and thorough evaluations (Neel et al. 1973). Regarding age, angiofibroma of the nasopharynx typically presents in younger individuals when compared to extrapharyngeal angiofibroma (Szymańska et al. 2012; Windfuhr and Remmert 2004). The average age of presentation in juvenile nasopharyngeal angiofibroma is 14 years (Acharya et al. 2017).

Aetiology

There are many hypotheses for the aetiology of angiofibroma; however, none have been proven (Tork and Simpson 2023). Among the many hypotheses, the majority revolve around a vascular origin, such as an arteriovenous malformation and/or an overexpression of the vascular-endothelial growth factor receptor (VEGFR). This hypothesis is very plausible, as it explains the highly vascular nature of angiofibroma (Tork and Simpson 2023). Furthermore, as previously mentioned, some others believe the tumour has an androgen overexpression and oestrogen downexpression origin (Alshaikh and Eleftheriadou 2015). This theory is reasonable as it accounts for the male gender predominance of angiofibroma and the fact that among women, the tumour is more common in older women with a lower oestrogen (Alshaikh and Eleftheriadou 2015). Regarding nasopharyngeal angiofibroma, there have been associations found with certain genetic anomalies, such as chromosome 17 deletions and their impact on TP53 tumour suppressor genes (Schick et al. 2005).

Clinical Presentation

The clinical picture of extrapharyngeal angiofibroma, unlike nasopharyngeal angiofibroma, which usually presents with nasal blockage and epistaxis, varies vastly and is mainly dependent on the tissue it arises from (Cheah et al. 2023). Angiofibroma of the sinuses generally presents late, and this is due to the large cavity size of the sinuses, permitting a great expansion before the tumour can cause compression and symptoms (Wan et al. 2022). Angiofibroma involving the maxillary sinus can present with long-term nasal discharge and gradual unilateral nasal blockage (Cheah et al. 2023). Patients with juvenile angiofibroma will present with a triad of a mass in the nasal cavity or nasopharynx, recurrent epistaxis, and progressive nasal obstruction (Acharya et al. 2017). According to a 26-patient review conducted by Wan et al., facial swelling, which presented in 14 patients, is the most common presentation of extrapharyngeal angiofibroma involving the maxillary sinus. Moreover, 11 out of the 26 patients also presented with obstruction and epistaxis (Wan et al. 2022). The mass can extend into the orbit, resulting in cranial nerve palsies and eventually leading to loss of vision (Alves et al. 2006).

Diagnosis and Imaging

To reach the diagnosis of nasopharyngeal angiofibroma, imaging modalities are required, along with consideration of the patient's clinical picture. Using nasal endoscopy, a reddish firm mass can be visualized within the nasal cavity. Even though radiographs can show the bulge or the inclination and the anterior displacement of the posterior wall maxillary sinus, computed tomography (CT) scan and magnetic resonance imaging (MRI) are still the gold standard imaging class (Tork and Simpson 2023). Since CT scan provides good hard tissue definition, it can highlight bone invasions such as that of the sphenoid's cancellous bone; however, since MRI provides better soft tissue definitions, it is preferred over CT scans for cases where soft tissue extensions are suspected. To determine the appropriate steps that need to be taken in surgery, it is better for the patient to undergo both MRI and CT scan (Acharya et al. 2017). On CT scans, an enhancing soft tissue mass will be visible within the posterior nasal cavity close to the sphenopalatine foramen. The tumour can be seen to extend into and beyond the nasopharynx, pterygopalatine fossa, and the nearby paranasal sinuses. No laboratory evaluation can aid in the diagnosis of juvenile nasopharyngeal angiofibroma (Tork and Simpson 2023).

Histology/Histopathology

Histologically, nasopharyngeal angiofibroma will appear as a well-circumscribed polypoid tumour. The mass will have both fibrous and vascular stromal tissue present in it, and it originates from myofibroblasts (Acharya et al. 2017; Tork and Simpson 2023). The spread of the tumour is usually submucosal. The vessels appearing within the stroma will have varying sizes and shapes. They could have a slit-like ectatic shape or a staghorn configuration (Tork and Simpson 2023). Interestingly, the blood vessels are often observed to be lined with endothelium alone and without the muscular coat needed for contraction. This lack of contractility in the vessels has been proposed as the reason for the continuous bleeding in the nasopharyngeal angiofibroma (Cheah et al. 2023). Furthermore, c-Kit/CD117 stains and androgen receptors are often positive (Oliveira et al. 2012). The mitotic activity is usually atypical, and cell types vary not only between different tumours but also within the same tumour (Tork and Simpson 2023).

Treatment and Prognosis

Surgery is still the mainstay treatment for juvenile nasopharyngeal angiofibroma. The type of surgery is mainly dependent on the size and the extent of the tumour (Acharya et al. 2017). There is a general consensus on endoscopic surgery as the most superior approach; however, this approach is best for juvenile nasopharyngeal angiofibroma confined to the cavity alone with little extension into the pterygopalatine fossa or the nearby sinuses (Dubey and Schick 2017). Due to its hypervascular nature, the tumour can first be embolized before the surgery to lower bleeding. It is necessary to perform the surgery within 24 h of embolization, as waiting any longer increases the risk of collateral circulation revascularizing the tumour (Dubey and Schick 2017). Although used in certain cases, embolization is expensive, and the procedure is not devoid of complications itself. The main aim in the endoscopic treatment of juvenile nasopharyngeal angiofibroma is to expose the tumour as much as possible but without traumatizing the surface to avoid extensive bleeding. The origin of juvenile angiofibroma is always the superior portion of the sphenopalatine foramen; however, the extension varies and based on the extension, different endoscopic approaches can be taken. Nonetheless, to expose the crucial area of the sphenopalatine foramen, at least ethmoidectomy, sphenoidotomy, and a large middle antrostomy extending posteriorly are required. For cases where the tumour has a large volume, it is rare for it to be resected in one bloc, and it is better to disassemble the juvenile angiofibroma first. This can be achieved by initially removing the nasal or nasopharyngeal portion of the tumour first before moving on to the deeper projections. The lateral extension of the tumour into the pterygopalatine fossa occurs frequently. From here on, the lesion can extend along many different pathways.

Juvenile nasopharyngeal angiofibroma can involve the maxillary sinus if the lesion from the pterygopalatine fossa extends anteriorly to displace the posterior wall of the maxillary sinus. Furthermore, the tumour can laterally extend into the infratemporal fossa through the pterygomaxillary fissure and into the hard palate through the descending palatine canal. To enhance the lateral exposure of the maxillary sinus's posterior wall, the opening of the metal wall is altered. To enlarge the medial maxillectomy anteriorly, either the lacrimal duct is sectioned at the inferior border of the lacrimal sac, or the Sturman-Canfield (or endonasal Denker) technique is used to remove medial portion of the maxillary sinus's anterior wall. It is essential to figure out the appropriate plane of dissection on the lesion after removal of the posterior wall of the maxillary sinus. Due to its close proximity, surgeons should be cautious not to damage the maxillary nerve. Due to the plane of dissection into the pterygopalatine fossa being posterior to the palatine nerves, the palatine nerves are not preserved except for lesions with little lateral extension. Regarding the maxillary artery, clipping it early on not only helps to lower intraoperative bleeding but also helps avoid damage during the operation.

In cases where the juvenile angiofibroma extends posteriorly, it goes from the pterygopalatine fossa into the cancellous bone and pterygoid root and grows along the floor of the sphenoid sinus. The tumour can erode the pterygoid process of the sphenoid bone to invade the pterygoid fossa and upper parapharyngeal space. To optimize exposure in these cases, the inferior turbinate and the medial wall of the maxillary sinus are resected to the floor of the nasal cavity. It is essential to work radically and extensively to drill the bony areas that are involved by the juvenile nasopharyngeal angiofibroma and continue past the infiltration margin indicated. This allows you to clear microscopic nesting of the tumours that are too small to be seen and prevent recurrence.

The tumour can extend from the pterygopalatine fossa into the cavernous sinus either by following the maxillary nerve or by going through the superior orbital fissure after going through the inferior orbital fissure and orbit. Wide exposure of the critical area is assured, and other portions of the tumour, such as the nasopharyngeal portion, are all resected before managing the cavernous portion of the tumour as the last step. Intraoperative navigation and Doppler are mandatory in this area to help correctly localize the artery and avoid life-threatening injuries. Furthermore, to avoid putting direct pressure on the artery, small cottonoids can be used when dissecting the juvenile angiofibroma. Due to difficulties in controlling the bleeding in instances of injury, the presence of an interventional radiologist is recommended to help quickly aid in haemostasis. Although the lesion can extend intracranially through the floor of the middle cranial fossa, infratemporal fossa and pterygomaxillary fissure into the inferior and superior orbital fissure or by direct erosion of the sphenoid sinus, among others, it is rare for actual dural invasion to occur. Thus, endoscopic approaches are sufficient to effectively remove the lesion. Due to difficulties in the visual field, two rubber catheters can be intranasally inserted following the resection of the tumour to anteriorly retract the palate and separate the posteroinferior nasopharyngeal attachment of the angiofibroma (Dubey and Schick 2017).

In cases where the angiofibroma is large and has extended into the adjacent sinuses and the infratemporal fossa, embolization becomes more necessary as bleeding is more likely. Furthermore, another way to endoscopically tackle large angiofibromas is the two-surgeon approach. This is when the second surgeon primarily provides high-volume suction to clear the operative area from bleeding. It is of utmost importance for the surgeon to preoperatively evaluate the case and have a thorough, detailed plan in mind, tailored to the presenting patient, on how to best approach the tumour based on its size, location and extension (Wormald 2008). Other approaches, such as lateral rhinotomy, midfacial degloving, and transpalatal surgery, can be used instead of the endoscopic approach for large juvenile nasopharyngeal fibroma that cannot be endoscopically dealt with. Radiotherapies are used for recurrent angiofibroma or for tumours that, either due to their size or their extension, are deemed unresectable (Tork and Simpson 2023).

Since the tumour is benign, the prognosis is considered good; however, disease recurrence can occur with advanced forms of the tumour. Furthermore, sometimes, in advanced diseases, it is not possible to completely resect the tumour. Although very rare, there have been cases reported of angiofibroma transforming into malignant tumours, possibly even undifferentiated sarcomas with a worse prognosis (Tork and Simpson 2023). For at least 3 years after surgical management, follow-up imaging should be performed every 6–8 months. A closer follow-up is necessary, possibly with contrast-enhanced MRI, for cases of persistent juvenile angiofibroma. A case of an endoscopic approach to an angiofibroma can be seen in Figs. 7.10 and 7.11.

Differential Diagnosis

The following are among the differential diagnoses of juvenile nasopharyngeal angiofibroma (Acharya et al. 2017; Fernandez et al. 2004; Tork and Simpson 2023):

Pyogenic Granuloma: small red bumps on the skin. It is a soft growth that bleeds easily and mostly occurs within the oral and nasal cavities.

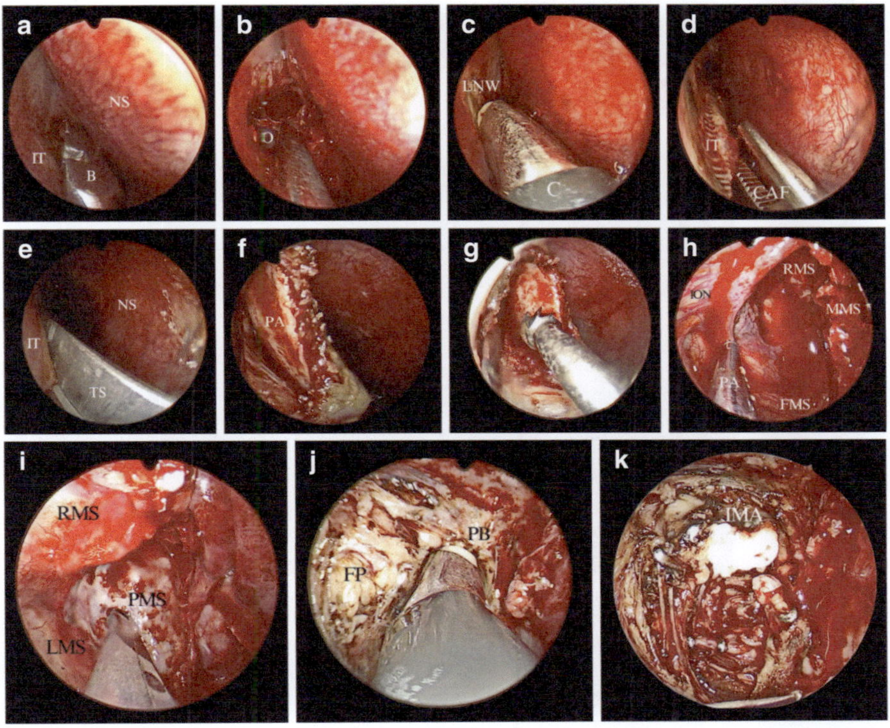

Fig. 7.10 This is an intraoperative video of a patient undergoing Endoscopic Sinus Surgery for an angiofibroma. As it can be seen in the thumbnails (left side nasal cavity), (**a**) uncinectomy is done by using a backbiter, (**b**) the maxillary sinusotomy is changed from type 1 to type 2, (**c**) the sinusotomy is changed to endoscopic medial wall maxillectomy type D (by Brescia classification) by using a coblator on the lateral nasal wall, (**d**) curved artery forceps are used to devascularize the inferior turbinate, (**e**) the devascularized inferior turbinate is cut with a turbinate scissor thus preparing the area for medial wall maxillectomy, (**f**) exposing the pyriform aperture, (**g**) drilling the pyriform aperture, (**h**) entering the maxillary sinus and exposing the posterior wall of the sinus, (**i**) removing the posterior wall of the maxillary sinus thus exposing the infratemporal fossa in order to reach the internal maxillary artery, (**j**) coblation of the infratemporal fossa fat pad, and (**k**) exposing the internal maxillary artery and ligating it using endoscopic clips. (*NS* nasal septum, *IT* inferior turbinate, *B* backbiter, *O* maxillary sinus ostium, *LNW* lateral nasal wall, *C* coblator, *CAF* curved artery forceps, *TS* turbinate scissor, *PA* pyriform aperture, *ION* infraorbital nerve, *RMS* roof of maxillary sinus, *MMS* medial wall of maxillary sinus, *FMS* floor of maxillary sinus, *LMS* lateral wall of maxillary sinus, *PMS* posterior wall of maxillary sinus, *FP* fat pad, *PB* pterygoid body, *IMA* internal maxillary artery) (Audio 7.5 and Video 7.5)

Sinonasal polyp: a polyp formed due to inflammation. Even Though it transforms into a hypervascular form following repeated injury, it is still much less vascular than juvenile angiofibroma.

Antrochoanal polyp: sinonasal polyps that arise from the mucosa of the maxillary sinus. This polyp can grow into the maxillary sinus and even reach the choana,

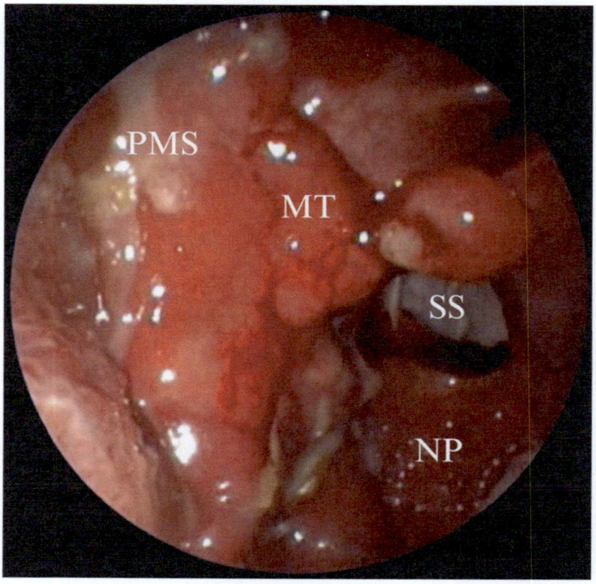

Fig. 7.11 This is a postoperative endoscopic video of a patient who underwent Endoscopic Sinus Surgery for angiofibroma. The posterior maxillary wall (PMS), middle turbinate (MT), sphenoid sinus (SS), and nasopharynx (NP) can be visualized in the thumbnail (Audio 7.6 and Video 7.6)

hence the name. Moreover, similar to juvenile angiofibroma, one of their most common symptoms is nasal obstruction.

Rhabdomyosarcoma: a sarcoma of striated muscle. Whenever present within the head and neck region, it mostly occurs in the orbit; however, it could also be observed in the paranasal sinuses, the nasopharynx and the pterygopalatine fossa, among others. It is a malignancy of young individuals.

Olfactory Neuroblastoma: nasal mass of the neuroepithelium with a clinical presentation and age of onset similar to juvenile nasopharyngeal angiofibroma; however, it is much more common in females.

Nasopharyngeal carcinoma: tumour of the mucosa arising from the superolateral nasopharynx. It has a peak incidence of 40–60 years, rarely occurring in paediatric and adolescent age groups, unlike juvenile nasopharyngeal angiofibroma.

Maxillary Sinus Inverted Papilloma

Introduction

Inverted papilloma is a benign epithelial growth that occurs in the underlying stroma of the nasal cavity and the paranasal sinuses. It is most well-known for its invasiveness, tendency to recur, and relationship with malignancy, which are the three characteristics that differentiate it vastly from other sinonasal tumours. IP is a benign epithelial growth (Lisan et al. 2016; Wackym and Snow 2016). It usually develops from the mucosal lining of the maxillary sinus and can have single or multifocal attachment sites (Wu et al. 2018). Ward was the first to report the presence of IP in the sinonasal cavity in 1854. Reingertz, on the other hand, histologically identified the tumour in 1935 and noticed its classic inverted nature in underlying connective tissue stroma. IP, inverting papilloma, epithelial papilloma, papillary sinusitis, Schneiderian papilloma, inverted Schneiderian papilloma, soft papilloma, transitional cell papilloma, cylindrical cell papilloma, polyp with inverting metaplasia, benign transitional cell growth are all names for this tumour (Wackym and Snow 2016). The World Health Organization has classified sinonasal Schneiderian papillomas into three subtypes: inverted, exophytic, and oncocytic lesions. While the overall rate of recurrence has decreased as a result of the widespread adoption of high-definition endoscopic optics and sophisticated surgical tools, there are still difficulties in managing tumours that are frequently recurrent or involve vital neurovascular structures (Eide et al. 2022).

Epidemiology

Out of the sinonasal Schneiderian papillomas, IPs are the most common subset and occur in 62% of cases. The tumour has an annual incidence of 0.2 to 1.5/100,000, and with a male-to-female ratio of 3.4:1, there is a male predominance. It is more likely to arise in older people in the fifth and sixth decades of life and has a mean age of diagnosis of 55 years (Eide et al. 2022; Wackym and Snow 2016; Wang and Noel 2017). IPs represent 0.5–4% of all sinonasal tumours (Wang and Noel 2017). As was indicated earlier, IPs can arise from either a single or many foci of origin, and the recurrence rate can range anywhere from 14% to 25% if the surgical resection is not performed in its entirety. This has important implications for clinical practice because IPs have been linked to a malignant transition rate of 5–15% to squamous cell carcinoma (Lisan et al. 2016). According to some studies, higher recurrence rates were associated with younger age (40 years), diabetes, advanced tumour stage, and HPV DNA. Pahler et al. also reported that patients who presented with recurrent papilloma infection were significantly younger at the time of initial diagnosis (48.7 years old on average) than those (60.2 years old on average) with non-recurrent tumours and multivariate logistic regression revealed that a younger age at initial diagnosis was the strongest risk factor for neoplasm recurrence (Makihara 2022).

Aetiology

The precise aetiology of IP is unknown. The embryologic origin of the sinonasal mucous membranes, the Schneiderian membrane, is at risk for developing this epithelial lesion; thus, the eponym has persisted. Due to the absence of an allergic history in many patients with IP, the function of allergy has been discounted. Chronic rhinosinusitis has also been suggested as a potential etiologic factor due to a temporal relationship and the increased incidence of sinusitis on the opposite side from the lesion; however, it has also been suggested that chronic sinusitis develops in these patients due to the obstructive nature of tumour itself. In addition, no association has been found between IP and environmental chemical exposure (Wackym and Snow 2016). Since the 1980s, it has been suspected that the human papillomavirus (HPV) may play a role in the aetiology of IP, although the precise cause of IP remains obscure. The HPV 16 and 18 serotypes have been discovered more frequently in tumours with dysplasia or malignant degeneration. Two recent meta-analyses found an association between HPV infection in IP tissue and progression to malignancy, predominately from high-risk HPV subtypes 16 and 18. Remarkably, more recent studies have discovered that epidermal growth factor receptor (EGFR) mutations are present in the majority of IPs and in a substantial proportion (30–88%) of IP-derived squamous cell carcinoma. When testing inverted and oncocytic papillomas for HPV DNA, only a small number of patients were positive (6.1% of IPs and 11.1% of oncocytic papillomas). Similarly, p16 expression, a proxy for HPV-driven oncogenesis, was not detected in the majority of samples (22.4% IP, 27.8% oncocytic papilloma). Thus, it has been hypothesized that both HPV and EGFR mutations can result in IP transformation into SCC and represent distinct tumorigenic pathways (Eide et al. 2022). Despite the abundance of evidence implicating HPV in the pathogenesis of IP, a number of studies provide contradictory evidence. Kraft et al. 15 detected HPV-11 in only one of thirty-nine IPs (3%) and none of the four IPs associated with SCC. Furthermore, a study of 66 patients with IP and five patients with IP-associated SCC did show HPV isolation in 20 (30.3%) patients with IPs and in three patients (60%) with IP-associated SCC; however, subsequent analysis revealed that the presence of HPV DNA was not a statistically significant predictor of the recurrence of IPs nor was it a statistically significant risk factor for IP-associated SCCs. These findings suggest that HPV infection may represent incidental colonization rather than a significant etiologic actor and that it is not necessarily a reliable predictor of malignancy or recurrence (Wang and Noel 2017). In addition to human papillomavirus, EBV genomes have been detected in IP tissues, and a few studies have postulated an association between EBV infection and IP (Nukpook et al. 2020). In contrast, it was documented in a previous review of sinonasal papilloma that EBV was no longer regarded as a significant factor in the development of IP. This claim was supported by a study of 73 Hong Kong patients with IP in which EBV DNA was not detected in any of the biopsies. In situ hybridization failed to detect EBV infection in a second review of 25 surgically resected IPs (Wang and Noel 2017).

Histology

As shown in Fig. 7.12, inverted papillomas have an endophytic or inverted growth pattern consisting of thickened squamous epithelial proliferation growing downward into the connective tissue stroma to form large clefts, ribbons, and islands. The epithelium is composed of squamous, transitional, and columnar cells (all three may

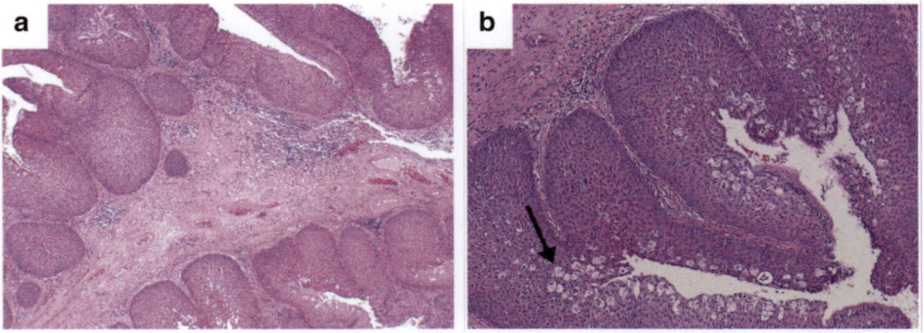

Fig. 7.12 This histopathological slide (**a**: 4×, **b**: 10×) shows a prominent downward endophytic growth of round to elongated interconnected squamous epithelial nests with smooth contours. Furthermore, it demonstrates focal mucosal ulceration transmigrating with neutrophils and neutrophilic microabscesses (Arrow)

be present in a particular lesion), with admixed mucocytes (goblet cells) and intraepithelial mucin microcysts. Typically, a heterogeneous chronic inflammatory cell infiltrate is observed in all layers of the surface epithelium. However, pleomorphism and cytoplasmic atypia may be present. Cells have a generally unremarkable appearance, with uniform nuclei and no accumulation. The epithelial component may exhibit numerous distinct cell characteristics indicating a high-glycogen content. In the basal and parabasal layers, mitotic figures may be observed, but atypical mitotic figures are not observed. Surface keratinization is possible. Components of the stroma range from myxoid to fibrous, with chronic inflammatory cells and variable vascularity. Intraepithelial mucocytes contain intracytoplasmic mucin that is Mucicarmine-positive, diastase-resistant, and PAS-positive (Upadhyaya et al. 2015).

Clinical Features

Unilateral nasal obstruction, discharge, and epistaxis are the most frequent clinical manifestations of inverted papilloma. Proptosis, diplopia, decreased vision, epiphora, and headache are uncommon symptoms that indicate intraorbital and intracranial extension. Inverted papilloma typically arises from the middle meatus region of the lateral nasal wall. Frontal and sphenoid sinuses are rarely affected, whereas maxillary sinuses and ethmoids are frequently affected (Sagar et al. 2019).

Diagnosis and Imaging

CT scan and magnetic resonance imaging (MRI) scan are the most common radiological investigations used to evaluate inverted papilloma. Bony alterations, such as the bowing of bones near the mass, are frequent CT findings (Fig. 7.13). On a CT scan, maxillary sinus tumours may cause the infundibulum to enlarge, making it

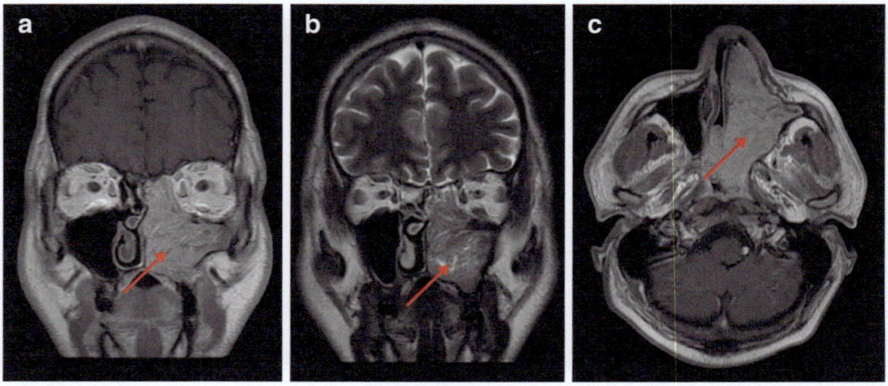

Fig. 7.13 Large enhancing soft tissue mass lesion obstructing the left nasal cavity, occupying the entire left maxillary sinus and ethmoidal air cells, focally extending to the frontal sinus, posteriorly obstructing the nasopharynx as well as focally bulging and obstructing the right posterior choana and posterior nasal cavity. The lesion has a convoluted cerebriform pattern on T2WI & contrast-enhanced T1WI, which is classical of inverted papilloma, associated with mucosal thickening and retained secretions in the left frontal and sphenoid sinuses. (**a**: Coronal T1 with Contrast, **b**: Coronal T2, **c**: Axial T1 with Contrast)

difficult to discern the uncinate process. "Bone-remodelling" may be an appropriate term to describe the changes that occur as a result of the constant pressure and mass effect of inverted papilloma on the surrounding bony structures, which are typically observed at the medial wall of the maxillary sinus and lamina papyracea. It is hypothesized that the bony skull base may have some response to pressure caused by an inverted papilloma, resulting in erosive rather than remodelling changes. In addition, a CT scan with contrast may reveal modest enhancement and calcification. T1-weighted images with contrast and T2-weighted images can be used to distinguish tumour mass from postoperative secretions on an MRI scan. Occasionally, in the absence of bony degradation, neither Coronal MRI can aid in the qualitative diagnosis, but they can at least raise the suspicion of a tumour. After the excision of an inverted papilloma, MRI is the first imaging modality to be performed in the follow-up evaluation (Upadhyaya et al. 2015). There have been numerous IP classifications published. Krouse devised a classification based on radiologically determined tumour extension in 2000. Although this classification has not been shown to be superior to others in terms of prognosis or therapeutic decision-making, it has the advantage of being simple to implement and reproducible and is, therefore, the most widely used in the international literature, making it easier to compare the results of various studies (Wackym and Snow 2016).

Treatment/Management

IP treatment is surgical and attempts to alleviate symptoms and allow for a complete specimen to be examined pathologically, especially for the presence of malignancy. The gold standard for surgery up until the mid-1990s was an external technique,

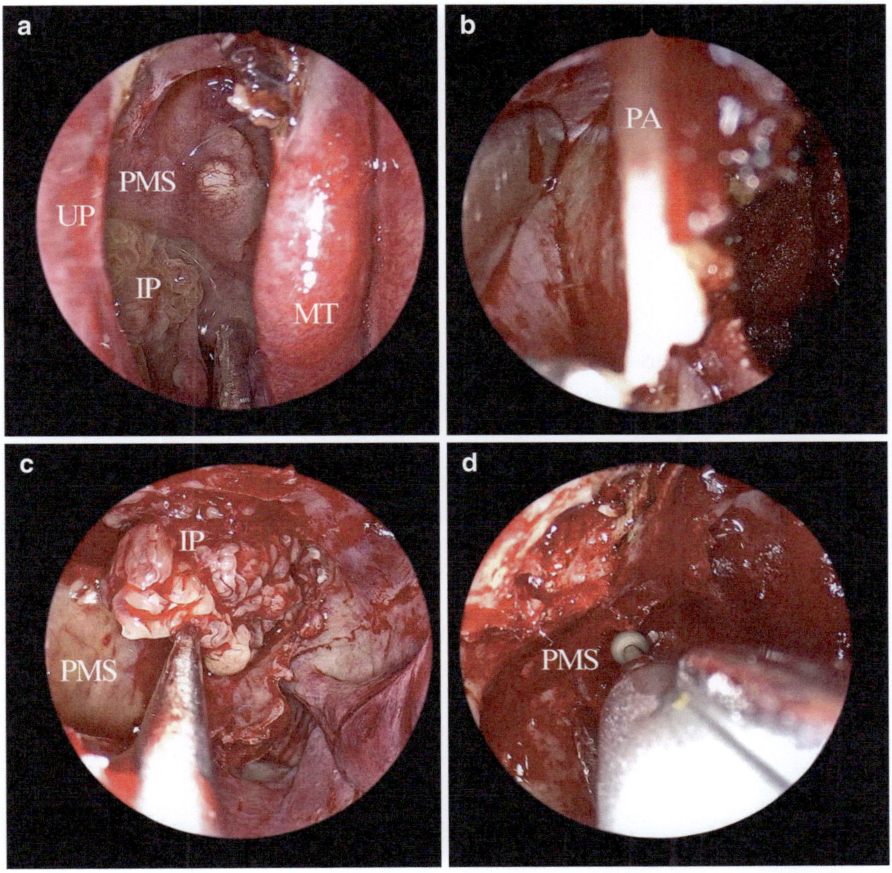

Fig. 7.14 This is an intraoperative video of a patient undergoing Endoscopic Sinus Surgery for a recurrent inverted papilloma. As can be seen in the thumbnails (left side nasal cavity), (**a**) the inverted papilloma can be seen on the posterior maxillary wall, (**b**) exposing the pyriform aperture and preparing the area for endoscopic medial wall maxillectomy type D (by Brescia group classification), (**c**) the lesion is being excised, and (**d**) the origin of the lesion is drilled. (*UP* remnants of the uncinate process, *PMS* posterior wall of maxillary Sinus, *IP* inverted papilloma, *MT* middle turbinate, *PA* pyriform aperture) (Audio 7.7 and Video 7.7)

namely a paralateronasal incision with a medial maxillectomy. Endoscopic treatment for IP, first described by Waitz and Wigand and Kamel in the same year, 1992, has since become the standard of care, according to numerous authors. Tumours with a restricted spread are the best candidates for endonasal endoscopic techniques; however, in some cases, an external or combination of external/endoscopic approaches is still necessary (Wackym and Snow 2016). Surgical procedures for IP excision are increasingly tailored to the pedicle of the inverted papilloma as part of a pedicle-oriented strategy. Some maxillary IP pedicle sites, particularly those in the lateral, anterior, and inferior sinus walls, have been reported to be inaccessible with the endoscopic technique alone. For total resection, some cases require external procedures like the Caldwell-Luc. However, with the development of endoscopic technology and techniques, maxillary sinus papillomas have been progressively treated with endoscopic methods only, as can be seen in Fig. 7.14. Although the pedicle position is crucial for surgical preparation, it is less certain if the number or location of IP attachment sites has any prognostic value (Wu et al. 2018).

Osteoblastoma

Introduction

A rare neoplasm characterized by osteoblast proliferation and formation of bone trabeculae within a vascular and fibrotic connective tissue stroma is referred to as osteoblastoma (Jones et al. 2006). This benign tumour generally arises in the posterior elements of the spine and the sacrum (Limaiem et al. 2023). To diagnose osteoblastoma, a clinical, radiological, and histopathological examination is necessary. This is not very straightforward as the radiological entities of osteoblastoma are highly variable, ranging from indolent features to very aggressive-appearing tumours (Sharma et al. 2009). Although the tumour generally occurs in the vertebrae and the long bones, it can rarely rise within the maxillary bone and, to a lesser extent, even in the maxillary sinus (Osguthorpe and Hungerford 1983). When in the maxillary sinus, the patients present with a painful facial swelling and like any other osteoblastoma that of the maxillary sinus requires histopathological examination to confirm the diagnosis (Osguthorpe and Hungerford 1983).

Epidemiology

Osteoblastoma is a rare benign bone-forming neoplasm that makes up 1% of all primary bone tumours (Jones et al. 2006). The primary site for this already rare tumour is the vertebrae, and the head and neck region only account for 18% of these benign lesions. Incidence of the lesion within the sinonasal tract is even more uncommon. Within the head and neck, this fibro-osseous tumour typically affects individuals of young age (Jaswal et al. 2007). Osteoblastoma has a 2:1 male gender predominance and is typically observed in the second decade of life (Vella et al. 2016).

Aetiology and Pathophysiology

Neither the aetiology nor the predisposing factors leading to osteoblastoma have been figured out (Jones et al. 2006). Similar to osteoid osteoma, new bone is formed in osteoblastoma; however, these new bones are also much more vascularized (Marcove and Alpert 1963). As previously mentioned, the degree of aggressiveness varies widely with these tumours. In the less aggressive and indolent form, the growth appears to be slow and well-demarcated with proper vascularity. This contrasts with the more aggressive types of osteoblastoma, which not only present with a higher recurrence rate but are also more difficult to differentiate from well-differentiated osteosarcomas due to their atypical histopathological characteristics (Toyodome et al. 2017; Woźniak et al. 2009). Although a benign tumour, osteoblastoma can have significant bone destruction properties and infiltrate the surrounding soft tissue. Very rarely, there have been reports of benign osteoblastomas undergoing malignant transformation and even metastasizing (Limaiem et al. 2023).

Clinical Presentation

The majority of osteoblastomas all over the body are slow-growing and asymptomatic. As a result, they are mostly found incidentally on imaging performed for other complaints (Limaiem et al. 2023). This is not the case for osteoblastomas of the head and neck region and, more specifically, those of the maxillary sinus since most patients present with painful facial swelling. This painful mass in patients with osteoblastoma of the paranasal sinus is typically not relieved by non-steroidal anti-inflammatory drugs. Moreover, the clinical signs and complaints are generally due to either obstruction or compression of the adjacent structures (Jaswal et al. 2007). Among the paranasal sinuses, the lesion is mostly of ethmoidal origin, and based on the structures they compress, patients can present with complaints of nasal obstruction, diplopia, and epiphora. For instance, when the tumour is large enough, the mass may be observed through the nostrils(Jaswal et al. 2007).

Diagnosis and Imaging

It is necessary to make an accurate diagnosis of osteoblastoma prior to initiating the tumour, and to do so, clinical, radiological, and histopathological approaches should all be considered (Sharma et al. 2009). Imaging modalities used to establish a diagnosis of osteoblastoma include a plain radiograph, a computed tomography (CT) scan and a magnetic resonance imaging (MRI) (Limaiem et al. 2023). A relatively well-circumscribed lesion can be seen on imaging without a lot of bone destruction (Bettinger and Loerz 2008). A mixture of fibrotic components with calcification combined with a dense sclerotic component is observed (Limaiem et al. 2023). The difficulty lies in distinguishing osteoblastoma from osteoid osteoma on imaging. This is because both lesions appear as round to oval, radiolucent lesions with well-demarcated margins and reactive sclerosis (Lucas et al. 1994). The appearance of the lesion tends to vary based on the age of the patient. A more radiolucent picture is observed among young individuals, whereas as patients grow older, the lesion tends to undergo sclerosis and ossifications. The radiological basis for a diagnosis of osteoblastoma is usually plain film radiography, with CT scans only serving a complementary role but with further detailed characterizations (Limaiem et al. 2023). No matter the imaging modality used, the confirmation of the diagnosis requires histopathological examination (Vella et al. 2016).

Histology/Histopathology

Similar to their radiographic features, the gross macroscopic appearance of osteoblastoma is similar to that of osteoid osteoma. The gross appearance of osteoblastoma is a red-brown vascular tumour with a sandpaper consistency. On average, the gross size of the tumour is 3–3.5 cm, but it can go up to a maximum of 15 cm (Lucas 2010). Histological appearance is not devoid of the similarities between osteoid osteoma and osteoblastoma since they both have osteoid deposition and immature bone trabeculae formation as their key feature. What differentiates the two lesions is that osteoblastoma deposits more osteoid than osteoma. Furthermore, the vascularity of an osteoblastoma is more than that of an osteoid osteoma, whereas the nidus appears to be a more organized osteoid osteoma. Although the mitotic rate is elevated, no atypical mitosis is observed. Moreover, osteoblastomas are differentiated from osteosarcomas since they do not infiltrate the preexisting normal lamellar bone but are rather separated from it by a thin area of fibrous tissue and no bone (Limaiem et al. 2023). An alternative method to differentiate between osteoblastomas and osteosarcomas is through immunohistochemical staining, in particular, staining for beta-catenin. The presence of nuclear beta-catenin is more indicative of an osteoblastoma, whereas, for osteosarcomas, cytoplasmic or membranous beta-catenin is more suggestive (Wan et al. 2014).

Treatment

Benign osteoblastomas of the sinonasal tract undergo complete surgical excision as treatment. There is a lot of controversy revolving around the role of irradiation for osteoblastoma; however, it could be used as a measure to prevent recurrence when the tumour is not completely excised (Jaswal et al. 2007). According to Woźniak et al., both adjuvant radiotherapy and adjuvant chemotherapy can be beneficial in patients with aggressive forms of osteoblastoma (Woźniak et al. 2009).

Based on the size and the extension of the mass, different routes can be taken to access it. For cases where it is found in the nasal cavity extending towards the maxillary sinus and has resulted in complete erosion of the medial wall of the maxilla, a lateral rhinotomy approach can be used (Jaswal et al. 2007). There have been reports of complete excision of the tumour through a buccal vestibular incision going from the canine to the second molar (Bokhari et al. 2012). Caldwell-Luc procedure is another alternative that can be used for maxillary sinus osteoblastomas. This has been reported for tumours of the maxillary sinus with extension into the left ethmoid sinus and erosion of the medial wall of the left maxillary sinus as well as the floor of the left orbit (Tom et al. 1980). Whenever local excision is not preferred, curettage or even partial resection can be performed. Although very rare, there are reports of tumour regression following partial resection (Smith 1972).

Moreover, the lesion can also be excised endoscopically using the Denker approach. This approach is a technique where an endonasal anterior maxillectomy is created without a separate sublabial incision. This technique can be used as an alternative to the more conventional Caldwell-Luc approach since they provide the same entry port into the maxillary sinus. In this approach, following lidocaine injection, unipolar electrocautery is used to make the first incision along the inferior mucosa at the junction of the nasal floor and the lateral wall to carry the incision through the periosteum. Superiorly, a second mucosal incision is performed along the lateral nasal wall. This incision is continuing anteroinferiorly so that it can lie just in front of the inferior turbinate's anterior head. Moving on to the soft tissue dissection over the maxilla, a dissection is made in the subperiosteal layer with a suction Freer elevator. This dissection exposes the anterior maxilla, the infraorbital foramen, and the lateral nasal wall. Furthermore, either an osteotome or a high-speed drill is used to produce a bony window into the anterior maxilla. It is essential to stay under the infraorbital nerve. This window is then connected to the inferior bony cut of the medial maxillectomy using either an osteotome or a bur. This allows access to the anterior portion of the maxillary sinus. The osteoblastoma can then be dissected and freed from the surrounding tissue. Following the isolation of the tumour, burs, osteotome and endoscopic scissors are used, respectively, to finish the remaining bony and mucosal cuts. A cut is made superiorly at the maxillary sinus roof, another is performed inferiorly at the junction of the nasal floor with the medial maxillary wall, and lastly, a posterior cut is made along the posterior wall of the maxillary sinus. This then makes room for the en bloc resection of the tumour with its bony attachment (Lee and Chiu 2019). A case of endoscopic resection of osteoblastoma can be seen in Fig. 7.15.

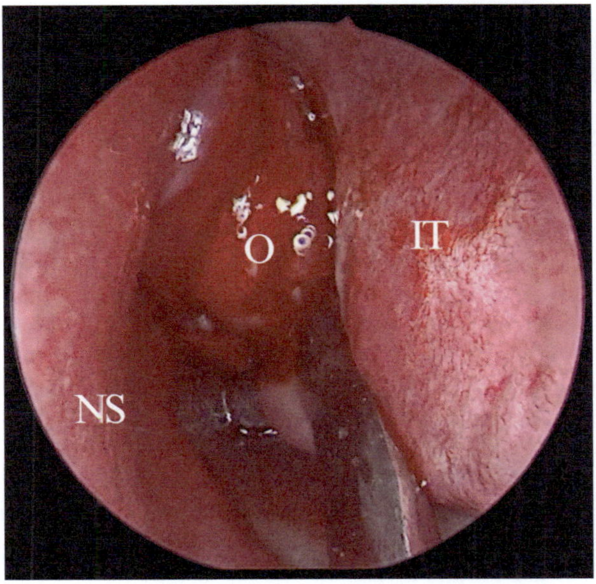

Fig. 7.15 This is an intraoperative video of a patient undergoing Endoscopic Sinus Surgery for osteoblastoma. As can be seen in the thumbnail (left side nasal cavity), the inferior turbinate is being outfractured to better visualize the mass. (*O* osteoblastoma, *IT* inferior turbinate, *NS* nasal septum) (Audio 7.8 and Video 7.8)

Differential Diagnosis

The list of differential diagnoses of osteoblastoma includes both histological and radiological differential diagnoses. Osteoid osteoma, osteosarcoma, metastasis, and aneurysmal bone cyst are all among the radiographical differential diagnoses. Regarding histology, the following are among the differential diagnosis (Lucas 2010):

Osteoid Osteoma

Although both osteoblastoma and osteoid osteoma can present with pain, it is still more common in osteoid osteoma. The pain in osteoblastoma is not relieved by salicylates. In some cases, unlike osteoblastoma, osteoid osteomas have been observed to regress spontaneously. Moreover, the key differentiating factor is that osteoblastomas generally tend to be larger than 2 cm, in contrast to osteoid osteomas, which are generally smaller. Furthermore, as mentioned above, the nidus in osteoid osteoma is more organized; however, the lesion is generally not as vascular as in osteoblastoma.

Osteoblastoma-Like Osteosarcoma

This is the case for certain borderline osteosarcomas that present with similarities to aggressive osteoblastomas. Whenever an osteoblastoma presents with cortical disruption, not-so-well-defined margins or involvement and extension of adjacent structures on imaging, a biopsy might be required to exclude osteosarcoma.

Fibrous Dysplasia

Introduction

The replaced fibro-osseous fibrous dysplasia (FD) is defined as a non-malignant bone disease with slow growth and a recurrent character in which the normal cancellous bone structure is replaced by a fibro-osseous tissue. This tissue subsequently leads to overgrowth and distortion of the affected part within the bone (Fusconi et al. 2013). The first author to describe Fibrous Dysplasia was Von Rechlinghausen in 1891 (Tinoco et al. 2009). McCune and Bruch were the first to suggest in 1937 that this lesion should be considered a specific entity and should be differentiated from other bone abnormalities (Kanazirska et al. 2010). Fibrous dysplasia typically shows an indolent course and grows slowly (Cruz-Ferreira 2019).

There are two categories of the disease: Monostotic FD, where only a single bone is involved and corresponds to (70%) of fibrous dysplasia cases, and Polyostotic fibrous dysplasia, in which several bones are involved and this corresponds to (30%) of fibrous dysplasias. Further division of the polyostotic form of FD gives both the McCune-Albright syndrome and the Jaffe-Litchenstein type (Sontakke et al. 2011). In the McCune-Albright subtype, there is an association found with multiple other endocrinopathies and involvement of the majority of the bones, although rare (Fusconi et al. 2013), while the Jaffe-Lichtenstein subtype is seen to have associations with 'cafe au lait' spots. The craniofacial bones are more frequently affected in the polyostotic form than in the monostotic form. The polyostotic form commonly involves not only the craniofacial bones but also the proximal femur and the rib. Maxillary lesions may extend to involve the maxillary sinus, zygoma, sphenoid bone and the floor of the orbit. Malignant transformation is rare, occurring only in 0.5% of monostotic and 4% of polyostotic forms. It is worth pointing out that there is no risk of conversion from the monostotic form transforming into the polyostotic form (Sontakke et al. 2011).

There are two categories of the disease: Monostotic FD, where only a single bone is involved and corresponds to (70%) of fibrous dysplasia cases, and polyostotic fibrous dysplasia, in which several bones are involved and this corresponds to (30%) of fibrous dysplasias. Further division of the polyostotic form of FD gives both the McCune-Albright syndrome and the Jaffe-Litchenstein type (Sontakke et al. 2011). In the McCune-Albright subtype, there is an association found with multiple other endocrinopathies and involvement of the majority of the bones (rare), while the Jaffe-Lichtenstein subtype is seen to have associations with "cafe au lait" spots (Fusconi et al. 2013). The craniofacial bones are more frequently affected in the polyostotic form than in the monostotic form. The polyostotic form commonly involves not only the craniofacial bones but also the proximal femur and the rib. Maxillary lesions may extend to involve the maxillary sinus, zygoma, sphenoid bone, and the floor of the orbit.

Malignant transformation is rare, occurring only in 0.5% of monostotic and 4% of polyostotic forms. The most common malignancies arising from FD are osteosarcoma, fibrosarcoma and chondrosarcoma. Previously, irradiation was reported as a possible risk factor; however, there have been cases of fibrous dysplasia in individuals never exposed to prior radiation therapy. There is no risk of the monostotic form transforming into the polyostotic form (Sontakke et al. 2011).

Epidemiology

The most frequent sites of origin are found in the Mandible and the Maxilla. It has a major preference for the white race, with males and females both being equally affected. FD represents about 2.5% of all benign osseous tumours and 7% of all bone tumours. The condition is a rare disorder with a reported incidence varying from 1:4000 to 1:10,000. The usual age of presentation is within the first to the second decade of life (Nilesh and Punde 2017; Tinoco et al. 2009).

Aetiology

The aetiology is not fully known and is somewhat controversial. However, there has been an association with a mutation of a gene within chromosome 20, which codes for a G-stimulatory protein (Kanazirska et al. 2010). The mutation results in somatic mosaicism since it occurs within the somatic cells (Fusconi et al. 2013). Other abnormalities were proposed by Lee e col. where disorders with the cAMP or intracellular regulation of kinase protein were suggested to have a role in the development of FD (Lee 1986).

The overproduction of cAMP is responsible for the majority of pathophysiology, as shown in the figure below. The abnormally elevated level of cAMP can lead to the overproduction of the tyrosinase enzyme, which can result in excessive production of melanin, resulting in dark skin lesions (Kushchayeva et al. 2018).

Clinical Features

The lesion is often found incidentally when imaging is done so for other clinical reasons since most patients with fibrous dysplasia are initially asymptomatic (Kushchayeva et al. 2018). Signs and symptoms of FD depend on the location of the lesion and the pressure effect it has on the adjacent structure as the tumour progresses slowly. It may cause either organic or aesthetic disorders such as facial asymmetry and deformity. These abnormalities will consequently also have a negative psychological impact on the patient. It may result in an expansion of the maxilla with loss of the nasomaxillary angle and generating a feline facial appearance. Expansion can also be seen to result in pathological fractures, obstruction of the paranasal sinuses, which cause recurrence of infections, cysts and mucoceles, anosmia, headache, visual disturbances due to compression of the optic nerve, alteration of the ocular movements, descent, exophthalmia, squint and conductive hearing loss (Tinoco et al. 2009; Park et al. 2023).

Histology

Histologically, a curvilinear trabeculae of woven bone is seen under a microscope. The spongy trabecular bone has no osteoblastic rimming, but it is seen to be entangled within a fibrous stroma; however, no cellular features of malignancy are observed. A biopsy of the tissue shows a characteristic pattern of Chinese letters. The macroscopic exam of fibrous dysplasia, on the other hand, shows an expansion of the osseous trabeculae into a thin cortical. An abrupt transition into healthy bone (Tinoco et al. 2009) occurs due to the lack of a definitive capsule, which aids in confirming the diagnosis of fibrous dysplasia (Eachempati et al. 2015).

There is great variation in the histological appearance between different cases of FD, even if they all meet the criteria for fibro-osseous disease (Davidova et al. 2019). Differences in the cellularity of the stroma were observed, ranging from sparse cellularity to very dense cellularity. Other differentiating factors, such as the presence or absence of calcified material mimicking cemento-osseous dysplasia and the presence or absence of osteoblastic rimming, were among the variations observed (Davidova et al. 2019).

Diagnosis and Imaging

The diagnosis is made through clinical examinations and histopathological and radiographic examinations. CT and MRI imaging of FD do not have pathognomonic radiological features and have been shown to result in a significant number of errors in diagnosis. According to Eversole et al., one feature that helps to differentiate the lesion from other fibro-osseous lesions is the presence of ill-defined margins (Eversole et al. 1972).

MRI aspects usually show an intermediate signal in both T1-weighted sequences and proton density, while heterogeneous hypointensity is the characteristic feature of images obtained with T2-weighted sequences. The CT aspect, on the other hand, mainly depends on the amount of bone and fibrous tissue and on the progressively increasing degree of mineralization (Fusconi et al. 2013). The appearance tends to vary based on the location since it can appear as a radiolucent ground glass matrix when in the axial skeleton, which usually appears smooth and homogenous, while craniofacial FD is usually seen as a dense and sclerotic lesion (Fig. 7.3) (Kushchayeva et al. 2018). The lesions in FD vary in size from a small focal abnormality and can go up as large as to involve most or all of a long bone (Kushchayeva et al. 2018).

The typical radiological exam shows a characteristic aspect of "opaque glass" or "ground glass" involving dense cortical tissue. The homogenous grey hazy density that gives rise to the ground glass appearance on imaging is due to the existence of both fibrous tissue and bone trabeculae simultaneously (Fusconi et al. 2013). CT is the test of choice for studying the lesion, evaluating its extension, and preparing it for surgery. Overall, there are three radiographic patterns in the fibrous dysplasia of the skull and facial bones, and they are described as pategoid, sclerotic and cystic patterns. Pategoid shows alternating radiodense and radiotransparent areas, sclerotic is homogeneously dense, and the cystic pattern is a spherical or ovoid radiolucent area surrounded by dense boundaries to give the appearance of a cyst (Domingues et al. 2018; Samieirad et al. 2021).

Treatment

The primary treatment for fibrous dysplasia depends on the size of the lesion. There are no uniformly accepted and set protocols for FD management; however, surgical treatment remains the main approach. Surgical management can be used to correct or prevent functional deficits as well as to help achieve normal aesthetics for the face (Eachempati et al. 2015); however, aggressive surgeries are still reserved for severe cases where dentition and vision are affected (Domingues et al. 2018). The delay in surgery, especially if the lesion is within the middle third of the face, which is difficult to access, is to prevent postoperative aesthetic and functional deficit (Domingues et al. 2018). Usually, a long-term follow-up is required due to the possibility of a flare-up of the continuous growth of the lesion (Eachempati et al. 2015).

Approaches such as trimming and surface contouring of the affected bone or curettage of bony cavities and packing with bone chips can be considered. Small lesions may need periodic follow-up. Surgical indications of FD are the presence of significant clinical symptoms and the control of large aesthetic or functional deformities. Because of the lesion's benign nature and its recurrence character, the surgery must be relatively conservative, with the main objective being the preservation of function. Important to note that surgery should be avoided until the patient reaches puberty since surgical intervention results in the loss or significant alteration of the normal anatomic features of the oral and facial structures, which creates significant cosmetic, physiological, and psychological deficiencies in the patient, to various degrees (Eachempati et al. 2015; Nilesh and Punde 2017).

Differential Diagnosis

Differential diagnosis of fibrous dysplasia is very broad and can include the following (Domingues et al. 2018; Rock and Singh 2008):

(a) Neurofibromatosis 1: osseous lesions are present, but the vertebra is the primary target.
(b) Metastatic osteoblastic lesions benign lesions.
(c) Osteofibrous dysplasia is usually seen in children younger than 10 years old and is exclusively found in the tibia.
(d) Paget's disease: mosaic pattern on histology with a similar radiographic appearance; however, the difference in demographics can aid in diagnosis.
(e) Osteochondroma: usually found within the metaphysis of long bone, while FD is found in the skull and femur (Rutkowski and Niewinska 2021).
(f) Cystic fibrous osteitis: overproduction of parathyroid hormone is the cause of cystic fibrous osteitis.

Ossifying Fibroma

Ossifying fibroma is a benign, noncancerous tumour. The tumour is composed of bone tissue forming within connective tissue. These tumours most often affect bones in your face with emphasis on the jawbones, and they are also slow-growing (Ossifying Fibroma 2022).

Ossifying fibromas are a particular kind of fibro-osseous lesions (FOL) that impact the head or neck. Lesions such as ossifying fibromas develop when fibrous tissue containing a material similar to bone replaces healthy bone (Ossifying Fibroma 2022). Treatment is necessary even if these tumours do not always present with symptoms. In addition to causing dental issues, they can also cause destruction of healthy bones. Oral surgery is required to resect the tumour.

There are many classifications in the literature, but they all agree that ossifying fibroma is considered a part of a spectrum of lesions known as benign fibro-osseous lesions. The spectrum includes fibrous dysplasia (FD), florid osseous dysplasia (FOD), and focal osseous dysplasia (FocOD). Despite behavioural differences, those lesions share similar histopathological and radiological characteristics in which the normal bone architecture is replaced by fibroblasts and collagen fibres containing variable amounts of calcified material, whether that being lamellar bone cementum or both (Shanab 2021).

Historic Background (Shanab 2021)

In 1872, Menzel was the first to describe ossifying fibroma, referring to it as cemento-ossifying fibroma in that group. The cementum-producing lesions were divided into four distinct types by the World Health Organization (WHO) in 1971. This reduced the name of cemento-ossifying fibroma to ossifying fibroma and three other lesions, including fibrous dysplasia, cemento-ossifying fibroma and cementifying fibroma. Other names were also given to OF, such as osteofibrous dysplasia by Campanacci in 1976 to emphasize that there is still a similarity between OF and monostotic fibrous dysplasia with the different pathological entities. Histopathological entities, aggressiveness, and destructive behaviours were used by Kempson to isolate ossifying fibroma from fibrous dysplasia. WHO reclassified them again in 2005 as a variant of three: ossifying fibroma, osseous fibroma, and fibrous dysplasia. In 2017, the fourth edition of WHO reclassified the bone-producing fibrous neoplasms into two major well distinct types, as differentiation from the non-neoplastic fibro-osseous lesions comprises fibrous dysplasia, osseous dysplasias, central giant cell lesion/granuloma, Cherubism, aneurysmal bone cyst, and simple bone cyst.

Types of Ossifying Fibromas

Bone-producing fibrous neoplasms are:

- Cemento-ossifying fibroma as benign Odontogenic (ectomesenchyme) tumour: composed of both cementum and bone that are differentiated from one cell of origin and that is a pluripotent stem cell of the periodontal ligament. They come from tooth-bearing sites and, hence, are of odontogenic origin. Another reason justifying the label (tumour) is the likelihood (despite its low rate) of recurrence (Shanab 2021). The tumour forms within the cementum, which is the hardened layer of connective tissue covering the root of a tooth. This tissue attaches and holds the teeth to the lower jaw(mandible). A fibroma can cause facial swelling as well as tooth loss. This type most typically affects women and people assigned female at birth (AFAB) in their 30s or 40s (Cleveland Clinic 2022).

- Juvenile ossifying fibroma (Shanab 2021). This faster-growing, more aggressive tumour typically affects youths between the ages of 5 and 15. Any portion of a child's skull may be impacted (Cleveland Clinic 2022).
  (a) Trabecular juvenile ossifying fibroma (TrJOF).
  (b) Psammomatoid juvenile ossifying fibroma (PsJOF) (Shanab 2021).
  - TrJOF and PsJOF are less frequent forms since they primarily affect younger people. While TrJOF targets the gnathic bones, PsJOF targets the ethmoidal sinus.
- Peripheral ossifying fibroma: This tumour appears on the top between the upper jawbone (maxilla) and the upper teeth. Adolescents and young adults are often the main groups affected (Cleveland Clinic 2022).

Aetiology

The aetiology is really unclear; however, it can be odontogenic, developmental, or traumatic.

In the literature, some postulated hypotheses (Shanab 2021):

- Hamner et al. considered 1968 for ossifying fibromas to be arising from pluripotent mesenchymal cells, which originate from the periodontal ligament, and so most of the fibro-osseous lesions.
- Kemposh did a study using electron microscopy where he found out that ossifying.
- Fibroma is formed from fibrous tissue in an attempt to repair a bony defect.
- Marx et al. suggested that an induction error at the mesenchymal cellular level can be related to the development of OF.
- Weing was the one to suggest that trauma can stimulate the progenitor cells.
- Pimenta et al. recently revealed a link between a novel tumour suppressor gene mutation (HRPT2) and OF and hypothesized that these lesions may stem from the gene's haploinsufficiency.
- Alghonaim et al. have described a case of OF affecting the paranasal sinuses with a history of bone grafting in that area (right maxilla) taken from the mandible, which was pathology-free. He suggested that it might be traumatic, developmental, or odontogenic (Shanab 2021).

Generally, medical experts are not sure why some people develop ossifying fibromas. However, potential causes may include (Cleveland Clinic 2022):

- Dental plaque build-up.
- Irritation of gum.
- Trauma to the face or jaw.
- Dental procedures (Cleveland Clinic 2022).

Clinical Presentation

Most patients with ossifying fibromas don't have any symptoms, and they rarely hurt. An X-ray taken as part of a dental exam or imaging test to look for another issue is the usual way the tumour is found (Cleveland Clinic 2022).

- Cemento-ossifying fibromas: Facial swelling (oedema) and shifting of teeth.
- Juvenile ossifying fibroma: Bulging eyes and nasal congestion.
- Peripheral ossifying fibromas: A red bump (mouth ulcer) on the upper gum or swollen gums (Cleveland Clinic 2022).

OF can affect any part of the facial bones and skull, with 70% affecting the head and neck region, mainly the jaws. Ossifying fibroma affects mainly the mandible (molar and premolar region) in 70–90%, followed by the maxilla and few cases reported in sinonasal bones, skull base, and orbit. Lesions in the maxilla commonly affect the posterior region, but few reported cases in the anterior (sinus antrum) region (Shanab 2021). It rarely affects the calvarium, mostly the frontal bone associated with paranasal sinuses. Gnathic OF is reported more commonly in female patients in their second to fourth decade of life, while sinonasal tract OF occurs later in life. According to the reported case, geographical distribution is another differential factor. Ossifying fibroma is found to be more common in middle-aged African women and least common in Caucasians. Moreover, clinical behaviour is different. In Africans, it does not tend to grow as much as in Caucasians, based on a retrospective study (Shanab 2021). It starts as a painless swelling, slowly growing, and can be discovered during routine radiographs. "Giant Ossifying Fibroma" is a name given for a lesion exceeding 8 cm in diameter and has more fibrous than osseous tissue. Although large lesions are rare, massive lesions can reach up to 10 cm or more. Other clinical presentations include surface ulceration and perforation of cortical bone when reaching a considerable size. OF tend to grow as round-shaped masses by equal expansion in all directions due to their centrifugal growth pattern. Extension to the inferior border of the mandible may cause paraesthesia of the inferior alveolar nerve. Lesions in the maxilla can cause obliteration in the oral vestibule or facial swelling. It may extend to the nasal cavity and cause epistaxis or obstruction. Moreover, it may extend to the orbital cavity, causing epiphora or bulging of the eye.

Although OF usually comes as an isolated lesion in patients without any significant medical conditions. TSC is a major neurocutaneous syndrome that can be associated with gingival hyperplasia or fibromas, but still, OF is a very rare finding. OF is found as monostotic in 80% of cases, but it can be found as multiple lesions, although it's very rare. Only 11 cases have been reported in the literature from 1968 to 2011.

It is very common to see off as a solitary lesion affecting patients with no medical background. However, co-existence in patients with other medical conditions is not rare. Association of OF with many syndromes (mainly neurocutaneous disorder) have been reported in the literature. Syndromes like Sturge-Weber syndrome,

Gnathodiaphyseal dysplasia, Buschke–Ollen–Dorff syndrome, and Oculocerebrocutaneous syndrome, Encephalocraniocutaneous lipomatosis, and neurofibromatosis. Two reported cases in a patient with neurofibromatosis type-1 (an autosomal dominant multisystem disorder) in calvarial and maxillary bone. Suggestions about the incidence of OF in those types of disorders may be related to developmental background, as it arises from multipotent cells of a periodontal membrane that are considered a neural crest in origin. Sometimes, it is associated with hormonal disturbances like hypercalcemia secondary to hyperparathyroidism. Hyperparathyroidism- jaw tumour syndrome develops 30–40% of single or multiple OF cases. (HPT-JT) is an autosomal dominant disorder characterized by multiple fibro-osseous lesions in the maxilla and mandible. Twenty-four reported cases were found in the literature (Shanab 2021).

Diagnosis of HPT-JT is always paramount in the treatment and prognosis by testing the level of calcium, phosphate, and parathyroid hormone. Inactivation of the HRPT2 gene is considered the main aetiology for HPT-JT. The treatment of those lesions is surgical removal with possible recurrence (Shanab 2021).

Diagnosis

Your dentist may notice an ossifying fibroma on a dental X-ray. You may also choose to get more detailed imaging scans like a CT scan or an MRI. The only way to obtain a definitive diagnosis is to do a biopsy of the tumour. This biopsy typically occurs after surgery to remove the tumour (Cleveland Clinic 2022).

Radiographic Features

Depending on the age of the lesion, OF shows different radiographical pictures. It starts to appear well-defined, with unilocular radiolucency and a sclerotic rim. When the lesion starts to be calcified, a mixed picture of radiolucency with radiopaque foci is more common (Fig. 7.3). When it gets fully mineralized, it appears as radiopaque with a rim of radiolucency. It may displace the roots, rarely causing their resorption. Fibro-osseous lesions look similar and can be the first differential diagnosis. Fibrous dysplasia is the main lesion in the differential diagnosis of OF. Despite the differences between OF and FD both radiologically and histopathologically, distinguishing them is still challenging (Shanab 2021; Vura et al. 2015).

OF in its early radiolucent stage mimics cemento-osseous dysplasia. Among the osseous dysplasia is focal osseous dysplasia (FOD) in early, intermediate, and late stages, which is an important differential diagnosis for OF. In contrast to OF, FOD occurs more frequently in older patients and usually presents ill-defined radiographic borders. Moreover, FOD is smaller than in OF and affects the periapical region more frequently. Other than fibro-osseous lesions, other diseases can be included in the differential diagnosis of OF according to its radiographic appearance; in the early radiolucent stage, the differential diagnoses include odontogenic cysts, ameloblastoma, periapical granuloma, radicular cyst and central giant cell lesions. In mixed radiolucent and radio-opaque radiographic appearance, calcifying cystic Odontogenic tumours, adenomatoid odontogenic tumours, osteoblastoma, and calcifying epithelial odontogenic tumours may also include. For matured lesions, completely radio-opaque resembling retained root, complex odontoma, idiopathic osteosclerosis, condensing osteitis, or osteoblastoma (if it is associated with the roots) (Shanab 2021).

Histopathological Features

The histology of ossifying fibroma varies; however, it is mostly composed of fibrous stroma and bone components with varying degrees of maturity. The stroma of connective tissue is made up of growing fibroblasts and collagen. OF hard tissue is divided into four types: lamellar bone, braided bone (which is the most prevalent), ovoid deposits, and anastomosing curvilinear trabeculae. It differs from fibrous dysplasia by having a more homogeneous pattern of hard tissue development. Cementifying fibroma is characterized by compact basophilic nodules, whereas ossifying fibroma has trabeculae of osteoblasts and osteocyte cavities. Ossifying broma stains positive for cytokeratin (Shanab 2021).

The difference between an ossifying fibroma and a non-ossifying fibroma (Ossifying Fibroma 2022):

Both an ossifying fibroma and a non-ossifying fibroma are benign bone tumours that develop for no obvious reason. There are some significant differences:

- A non-ossifying fibroma will not become bone material (ossify). These tumours typically develop on the long bones of children's legs. They seldom create issues or necessitate treatment.
- A non-ossifying fibroma disappears after a child's bones cease developing, but an ossifying fibroma hardens (calcifies) into a bone or skeletal substance. An ossifying fibroma can occur at any age. These tumours typically damage the face bones, particularly the jawbones. They can develop to be quite enormous, causing teeth to move. They nearly usually necessitate medical attention.

Management and Treatment

The tumour should be sent for histopathological study for the diagnosis. If the tumour is large, you may need a bone graft to replace the missing bone (Cleveland Clinic 2022).

The treatment will vary according to the clinical behaviour and radiological findings in the following treatment options (Shanab 2021):

1. Enucleation with or without grafting, when the lesion is not very large in size and well-demarcated from the surrounding osseous structure. Usually, they shell out easily during surgical procedures, and it's easier to do in the mandible than in the maxilla.
2. Curettage is used when there is no well-defined line of demarcation between the lesion and the surrounding bone or when the lesion is large and difficult to reach.
3. Radical treatment, in cases with massive and aggressive lesions reaching inaccessible areas like the nasal cavity, to avoid recurrences. OF has the ability to infiltrate about 1–2 mm, and a 5 mm resection is more than enough. This usually requires bone grafting or reconstructive surgery. This results in increased functional and aesthetic limitations, as well as the high cost of therapy.

Complications of Ossifying Fibromas

Untreated ossifying fibroma can get larger and replace the healthy bone. This raises your chances of getting a facial fracture. Tumours in the jaw might cause reabsorption of your teeth's roots, causing your teeth to shift (Cleveland Clinic 2022).

Prevention

Ossifying fibromas are rare. Medical experts aren't sure why some people develop these tumours, but you can't prevent them (Cleveland Clinic 2022).

Prognosis

An ossifying fibroma can grow back months or years after surgical removal. Children are more likely to experience a tumour recurrence. Your healthcare provider will schedule regular follow-up appointments for up to 10 years after surgery to check for signs of tumour regrowth (Cleveland Clinic 2022). The sarcomatous transformation has not been documented. The recurrence rate is 0–28%; thus, some authors advocate surgical resection; however, others still prefer the conservative treatment and rather a long follow-up since the recurrence is infrequent (Shanab 2021).

Recurrence rates vary depending on the type (Cleveland Clinic 2022):

1. Cemento-ossifying fibromas: Almost 30% recurrence rate.
2. Juvenile ossifying fibroma: 30% to almost 60% recurrence rate.
3. Peripheral ossifying fibromas: Up to 20% recurrence rate.

Maxillary Mucocele

Introduction

Mucoceles are epithelial lined mucus-containing sacs located within one of the paranasal sinuses, leading to expansion of the involved sinus cavity and remodelling of the sinus walls. It is lined by either pseudostratified or low-columnar epithelium in contradistinction to a cyst that has a distinct, separate membrane. Wherever bone erosion occurs, the mucocele's epithelium frequently fuses with the dura or orbital periosteum (Watkinson and Clarke 2018). The sinuses commonly affected by a mucocele in the order of frequency are the frontal, ethmoidal, maxillary, and finally sphenoidal (Dhingra 2010).

Mucoceles seem to be benign, but they can cause significant pathological issues as a result of their pressure effects on surrounding vital structures, mainly in the periorbital region (Caylakli et al. 2006).

Aetiology

The aetiologies of primary and secondary mucocele seem to be different. There will be inflammatory obstruction of mucus drainage in the primary mucocele, which will cause not only secretory duct obstruction but also cystic enlargement of mucosal glands and cystic degeneration of polyps. Contrastingly, the predisposing aetiology for the secondary mucocele tends to be the sequestration of residual mucosa after surgery and long-term tissue fluid retention. In sinuses that have already undergone surgery, such as the Caldwell-Luc operation (CLOP), secondary mucocele is more likely to develop, and the maxillary sinus is the most common sinus for secondary mucocele development (Yeom et al. 2022).

Epidemiology

Maxillary sinus mucocele is uncommon, occurring in less than 10% of all paranasal mucocele cases reported in English-language literature. However, due to the choice of surgery related to maxillary sinus inflammation, secondary maxillary sinus mucocele has been commonly found in Korea and Japan. They have been reported as postoperative cheek cysts, postoperative maxillary mucoceles, and postoperative maxillary cysts (POMCs), typically occurring as long-term complications of CLOP (Yeom et al. 2022). Although mucoceles can develop at any age and without regard to sex, the third and fourth decades of life seem to have a higher occurrence of the condition (Zhang et al. 2020).

Pathophysiology

In order for a mucocele to form, two factors must be found: an obstruction of the sinus outflow tract and an inflammatory process within the sinus. Within the epithelial lining of mucoceles, there are Osteolytic cytokine-IL-1 and tumour necrosis factors. This is important since it has been proposed that these cytokines may be responsible for the bony erosion in expanding mucoceles (Watkinson and Clarke 2018).

Histology

On a microscopic level, the cystic cavity is surrounded by a thin membrane made of pseudostratified ciliated cylindrical epithelium (sinus mucosa), which has alternating areas of hyperplasia and is supported by fibrous connective tissue. There are also numerous capillaries, some of which are congestive and mixed inflammatory exudates. The content is amorphous and eosinophilic, with inflammatory cells (lymphocytes and plasma cells) scattered in mucous material, as seen in Demicheri and Kornecki (2016).

Clinical Features

Mucoceles produce symptoms that are related to their expansion and subsequent pressure on the surrounding adjacent anatomical structures (Fig. 7.2). Medial expansion of the wall of the maxillary sinus into the nasal cavity leads to displacement of the inferior turbinate and causes nasal obstruction, while superior expansion of the maxillary sinus into the inferior orbit can cause displacement of the orbital contents and visual disturbance. On the other hand, downward displacement into the area of the alveolus can even cause loosening of teeth (Caylakli et al. 2006).

As a result of the expansion of the mucocele into the orbit, orbital symptoms are relatively common. These complaints are usually caused by ethmoidal, sphenoidal, and frontal mucoceles since ophthalmologic manifestation is unusual from maxillary mucoceles. Oedema and periorbital pain are the most common orbital findings. The most dreaded complication is amaurosis, but fortunately, it occurs less commonly, and its occurrence within maxillary mucoceles is extremely rare (Simões et al. 2015).

Diagnosis and Imaging

The diagnosis of mucocele is usually made on the basis of symptoms, imaging, surgical exploration, and histological confirmation. The most informative radiologic evaluation is CT. The mucocele appears as a homogenous lesion on the CT scan, which is isodense with the brain without contrast enhancement unless infected. In the walls of the sinuses, there are smooth, clear-cut margins of bone erosions. In contrast, in malignancy, the mass appears to be irregular in shape, with erosion and destruction of the surrounding structures, particularly the sinus walls, infiltration into the surrounding soft tissues and irregular margins of bone absorption. Magnetic resonance imaging is the best modality of choice reserved for mucocele formed secondary to sinonasal tumours in which the lining membrane of the mucocele will enhance after intravenous contrast. When there is destruction to the surrounding structures and expansion, the differential diagnosis can include both benign and malignant lesions of the paranasal sinuses. Dermoid, epidermoid, neurofibroma, cementifying fibroma, angiofibroma, inverting papilloma, and cylindroma are examples of benign lesions, while malignant lesions include adenoid cystic carcinoma, plasmacytoma, embryonal rhabdomyosarcoma, lymphoma, schwannoma, and tumours of dental origin (Caylakli et al. 2006). Figure 7.16 shows the maxillary mucocele demonstrated by the CT scan.

Differential Diagnosis

Mucoceles must be differentiated from several conditions, especially when there is no bone erosion, such as retention cysts, chronic sinusitis, antrachoanal polyp, and polyposis of the paranasal cavities. Retention cysts are commonly seen in the maxillary sinus and may be found in approximately 9% of the population in imaging studies. Their predisposing aetiology for the formation of the retention cyst tends to be as a result of obstruction of the ducts of seromucous glands in the sinus lining, creating a mucous- or serous-fluid-filled cyst that is lined by epithelium. They grow beneath the nasal mucous membrane, which explains why their walls are thin. The cyst appears as a soft tissue mass with a rounded, dome-shaped appearance on radiological imaging. It is most frequently located on the floor of the maxillary sinus and commonly contains clear, yellowish fluid. Mucoceles grow beneath the periosteum and are associated with obstruction of the duct or the natural ostium of any of the paranasal sinuses. The periosteum assists in the formation of the cystic wall, resulting in a strong and thick mucocele wall. Mucoceles usually tend to grow under the periosteum, while retention cysts grow under the mucosa of the sinus. This explains why retention cysts are non-expanding, well-circumscribed and have mucosa-covered masses, whereas mucoceles have osteolytic ability and a tendency to expand along the path of least resistance.

Another differential diagnosis is an antrochoanal polyp, which is believed to be a herniation of hypertrophic maxillary sinus mucosa into the nasal cavity by a natural or accessory ostia. The most common presenting symptoms are nasal obstruction and imaging; it appears as an opacity of the involved sinus on radiographical imaging. They never cause bony erosion. Nasal polyps can be both single or multiple and may be located in the sinus cavity or the nasal vault. They can expand the nasal cavity without bony erosion (Caylakli et al. 2006).

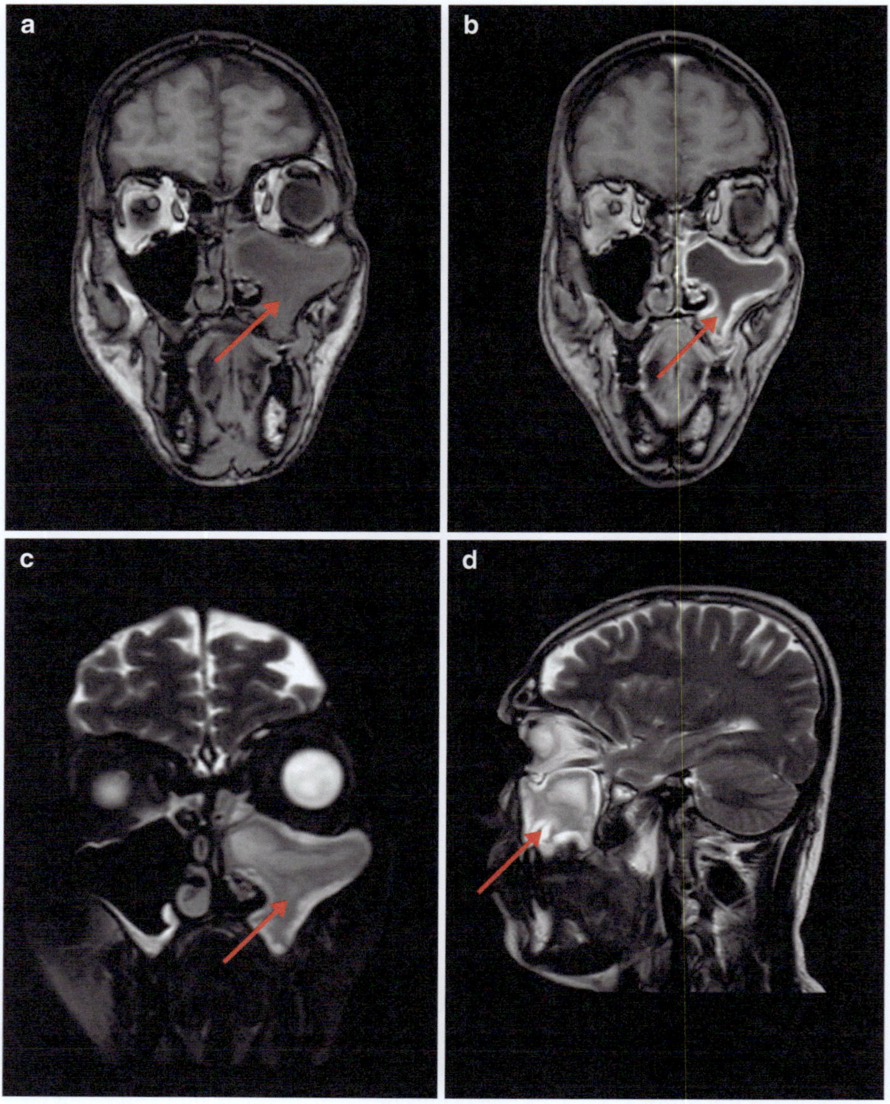

Fig. 7.16 Left maxillary expansion and complete filling by fluid signal intensity content (arrow) associated with smooth and thick enhanced mucosa, widening and obstruction of the ipsilateral osteomeatal complex, bulging into the middle meatus and obstructing the nasal cavity. The orbital floor is intact, and there is no intra-orbital extension or enhancing soft tissue component. (**a** Coronal T1, **b** Coronal T2 with contrast, **c** Coronal T2 with Fat Suppression, **d** Saggital T2)

Treatment/Management

Previously, Caldwell-Luc approach surgery with an inferior nasoantral window and excision of the mucocele lining were the mainstays of surgical therapy.

More recently, endoscopic evacuation via a wide maxillary antrostomy has been advocated.

An open approach may still be beneficial for large mucoceles, such as those with erosion of the anterior maxillary sinus wall, extension to the pterygomaxillary fossa, or multiloculated/complicated mucoceles as a result of prior trauma or surgery (Chang et al. 2014; Gür et al. 2016). A case of endoscopic treatment of mucoceles can be seen in Figs. 7.17 and 7.18.

Prognosis

After complete surgical excision, the prognosis is excellent. Complications include superimposed infection (pyocele), meningitis, and brain abscess. A correlation of clinical, radiographic, and pathologic findings is needed for the diagnosis of paranasal sinus mucocele (Wenig and Richardson 2009).

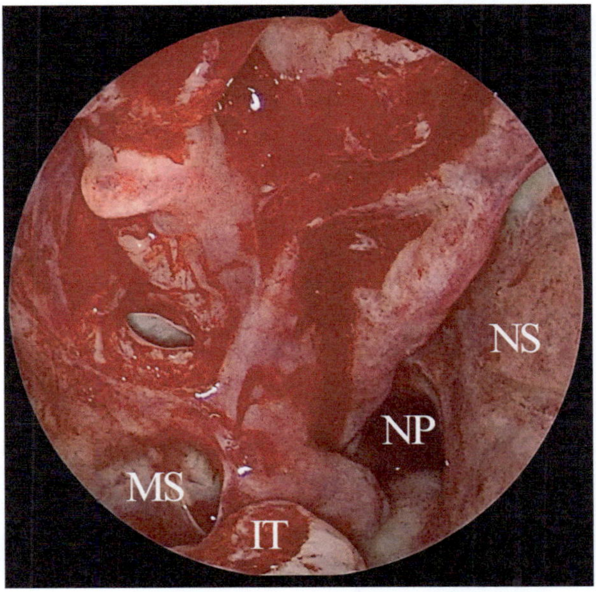

Fig. 7.17 This is an intraoperative video of a patient undergoing endoscopic sinus surgery for maxillary mucocele. As it can be seen in the thumbnail (right side nasal cavity), the mucocele is in the posterosuperior wall of the maxillary sinus, at the site of the Haller cells, with extension into the sinus cavity, and here, it has been marsupialised. (*MS* maxillary sinus, *IT* inferior turbinate, *NP* nasopharynx, *NS* nasal septum) (Audio 7.9 and Video 7.9)

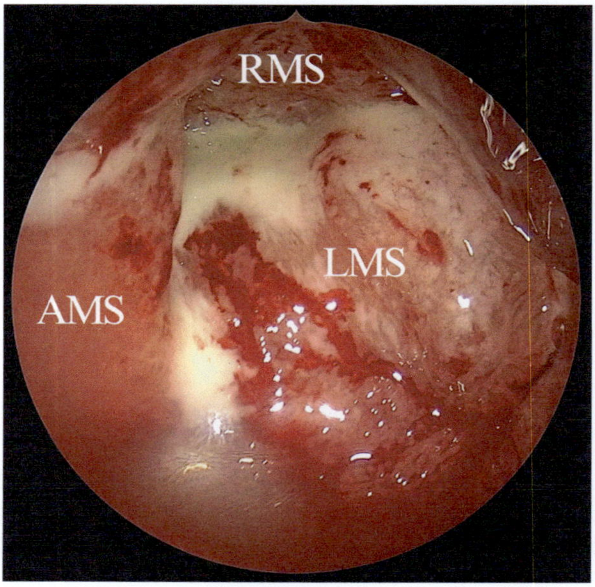

Fig. 7.18 This is an intraoperative video of a patient undergoing endoscopic sinus surgery (ESS) for an infected mucocele. As can be seen in the thumbnail (left maxillary sinus), the sinus is opened by a type 3 maxillary sinusotomy and pus is seen in its cavity. (*RMS* roof of the maxillary sinus, *LMS* lateral wall of the maxillary sinus, *AMS* anterior wall of the maxillary sinus) (Audio 7.10 and Video 7.10)

Schwannoma

Introduction

Schwannoma(SC), also known as neurilemmoma, is a benign tumour of nerve sheath origin arising from any nerve that is covered with a Schwann cell sheath. These include the cranial nerves (except for optic and olfactory), the spinal nerves, or nerves arising from autonomic nervous systems, especially the sympathetic system. Verocay was the first to describe them in 1910 and initially gave them the name "neurinoma". The term "neurilemmoma" was later on given by Stout in 1935. Reported cases of schwannoma (neurilemmoma) suggest that it is a slow-growing benign tumour that arises from the Schwann cells, which cover the nerve sheaths of all the peripheral nerves except those of optic and olfactory nerves since they do not possess Schwann cells and are enveloped by the meninges. It is rare for a Schwannoma to be reported to have arisen from the sinonasal tract (Alim et al. 2018; Verma et al. 2013).

Schwannomas are mainly composed of Schwann cells (SCs) found within a badly collagenised stroma. SCs are derived from neural crest cells and are subdivided into two types: myelinated and unmyelinated; both play a fundamental role in maintaining and regenerating axons of peripheral nervous system neurons;

however, they are also responsible for several demyelinating diseases and tumours such as schwannomas (Bueno et al. 2021).

The diagnosis is confirmed by the microscopic examination of the biopsy specimen. They can originate in any part of the body, but Schwannomas occurring in head and neck regions are quite frequent, with 25–45% of all reported schwannomas being found in this region. The neoplasm may develop at any age, and there is no sex predilection. When found within the nose and the paranasal sinuses, these tumours arise from intranasal nerves, ophthalmic and maxillary branches of the trigeminal nerve and branches of the autonomic nervous system (Khanna et al. 2003).

The soft tissue of the head and neck region is one of the most common sites for benign nerve sheath tumours, as well as the flexor surfaces of the extremities.

Although the head and neck region is the most common site for benign nerve sheath neoplasms, intra-oral lesions are unusual (only 1%). The most common site of occurrence is the tongue, and central jaw cases are rarer. In central jaw cases, the mandible is as common as the maxilla, which is very rare (Swami et al. 2019).

The maxilla is not a common region for the development of this tumour, and when it occurs, it is usually on the palate. In addition, it should be noted that the first case of schwannoma located in the mucosa of the alveolar ridge of the maxilla was described in a clinical case report. Polyp and mucocele are the commonest sinonasal tumours, and schwannoma is rarely found in the paranasal sinuses (Kandasamy et al. 2017).

Epidemiology

One of the most common sites for benign nerve sheath tumours is the soft tissue within the region of the head and neck, followed by the flexor surfaces of the extremities.

Although the head and neck region are the most common site for benign nerve sheath neoplasms, intra-oral lesions can also occur but are unusual (only 1%). The most common site of occurrence intraorally is the tongue, and the central jaw cases are less common. In central jaw cases, the mandible is more common than the maxilla, which is very rare. Wright and Jackson described 146 cases of soft tissue intraoral schwannomas, of which 52% occurred in the tongue. Intraosseous schwannomas are even more atypical, with the most common site being the posterior mandible, and are found in less than 0.2% of cases. The presence of a large inferior alveolar nerve could be the factor contributing to this. Chi et al. described 44 cases of intraosseous neurilemmoma, of which 39 were found involving the mandible and only five involved the maxilla (Knight et al. 2022).

According to Miranda et al. in 2017, the maxilla is not a common region for the development of this tumour, and when it occurs, it is usually on the palate. Winters and Simard were the first to describe a case of schwannoma located within the alveolar ridge's mucosa of the maxilla, and they did so in a clinical case report published in 1959. Therefore, in 2005, Sardinha et al. 16 said that approximately 146 cases of schwannomas were reported within the oral cavity. Salehinejad et al., on the other hand, published a systematic review in 2016 in which he reported 37 cases of oral schwannomas conducted between 2005 and 2015, and stated that among them, only three studies (2 from Iran and one from India) reported the origin of schwannoma to be from the mandibular gingival ridge. Hatziotia and Asprides did a study in which only 7 cases out of a total of 152 cases of oral schwannomas were reported. The purpose of reporting this clinical case is highly justified due to the rareness of the case, its difficult diagnosis and its unusual involvement. In addition to those, it also helps the scientific community with the approach and management of this type of tumour (Bueno et al. 2021).

Polyp and mucocele are the most common sinonasal tumours, and schwannoma is rarely found in the paranasal sinuses (Hegde et al. 2016).

Schwannoma of nasal and paranasal sinuses are also rare. About 25% and 45% of cases of schwannoma occur in the head and neck region, which makes them much more common than those in the nasal paranasal sinus since they only make up 4% of schwannomas. The rest of the exocranial tumours are distributed among the different sectors of the Neck. With regard to the nasal sinuses and cavities, the ethmoid sinus is the most common, followed by the maxillary sinus, nasal cavities, and sphenoidal sinus.

They are often encapsulated and attached to nerve tissue. Two different growth pattern presentations can be observed in a microscopic examination, which is referred to as Antoni A and Antoni B; however, both patterns show spindle-shaped cells that seem to be elongated with regular oval nuclei. Malignant transformation occurs in only 2% of the cases. Local recurrence is common in cases of incomplete tumour resection. Even though finding the exact nerve origin from which Nasosinusal schwannomas arise is hard to establish, it has been suggested that there is a probability they could arise from either the ophthalmic or the maxillary branches of the trigeminal nerve. Other nerves considered when it comes to the origin of Nasosinusal schwannoma are nerves from the autonomic fibres of the carotid sympathetic plexus or maybe even the sphenopalatine ganglion (Knight et al. 2022; Verma et al. 2013).

Aetiology

The aetiology is still unknown, and histogenesis remains a controversial argument. There are no known predisposing factors. J.Ch. Hatziotis et al. believe that trauma may be the cause, and this explains why neurilemmomas are more frequent in a recently traumatized area. There is an association between trauma and the development of the tumour (Verma et al. 2013).

Despite the lack of consensus in the literature about the aetiology of this tumour, however, Salehinejad et al., in a systematic review study composed of 26 articles in 2017, stated that schwannomas originate from the proliferation of vagus nerve and sympathetic fibres in the extracranial head and neck regions. Tumours with no known origin, on the other hand, make up 40%; however, another study states that the global incidence rate of this tumour is between 1 and 20 cases per 1,000,000 inhabitants. Abrahams et al. postulated in 2019 that its aetiology may be due to genetic predisposition or could follow chronic inflammation without a history of previous trauma. Young and middle-aged adults tend to be more affected, with women showing a slight predominance when it comes to the manifestation of the tumour as compared to men. It is worth pointing out that certain studies do not consider this difference a significant one, mainly because of the lack of corroborative epidemiological evidence, which may vary in size from a few millimetres to many centimetres (Bueno et al. 2021).

The aetiology is not fully known, but it is said that the lesion arises by the propagation of Schwann cells at one point within the perineurium. The growth of this lesion will cause the displacement of adjacent nerve tissue. Possible mechanisms through which schwannomas tend to involve a bone include either a tumour arising centrally inside the bone, a tumour arising in a nutrient canal, a soft tissue or a periosteal tumour causing secondary erosion and incursion into the bone (Swami et al. 2019).

Three different mechanisms of bone involvement by neurilemmomas include:

1. A tumour may arise centrally within a bone.
2. A tumour may arise within a nutrient canal.
3. Bone penetration and secondary erosion could be observed as a consequence of a soft tissue tumour or a periosteal one.

Most of these tumours are encapsulated and have a variation in size starting from 9.5 cm. They also have a mean diameter of 6.2 cm (Abdellatif et al. 2024).

Clinical Features

Schwannomas are slow-growing neoplasms and are usually asymptomatic till they attain a large size and become symptomatic. The symptoms depend upon the location/site of involvement and malignant transformation; it was found that epistaxis is usually associated with nose and ethmoid sinus neoplasms, while pain was more common with lesions of the maxillary sinus. Other symptoms include nasal blockage, rhinorrhoea, exophthalmos and facial swelling. Neuronal deficit has been noticed (Alim et al. 2018).

Schwannomas may develop at any age ranging from 2 to 72 years; however, there is a peak prevalence within the second and third decades of life as compared to other ages. Neurilemmomas involve males and females equally. The majority of the neurilemmomas are non-tender. With the expansion of the tumour, the nerve fibres become splayed over the outer aspect of the capsule rather than getting incorporated within the substance of the tumour. This explains the intact nerve function in all but very large neurilemmomas. The nerve from which the neurilemmoma arises may be seen as related to the capsule in 7% of cases (Verma et al. 2013).

It remains asymptomatic for quite a long period due to its slow growth. Nasal obstruction is the main symptom of this tumour, but other symptoms do arise in the later stages as the tumour enlarges, such as pain, bony dehiscence of the skull base and neural symptoms. It can also result in rhinosinusitis since clinical features are similar (Kandasamy et al. 2017).

In paranasal sinuses, these tumours arise from the fifth cranial nerve(trigeminal) and, more specifically, from the ophthalmic and maxillary divisions of it and not so much from the mandibular division (Hegde et al. 2016).

Schwannomas that are extracranial and within the head and neck are commonly seen in solitude, as well as demarcated lesions. The lesion presents as nasal obstruction, dysphasia, and hoarseness, depending on the site of the lesion. Schwannomas of the paranasal sinuses show varying clinical features, which are affected not only by the site but also by the nerve that is impacted and by the compression effect of the tumour on the adjacent neural structures. Epistaxis and pain may also be seen as a result of the involvement of ethmoidal sinus and maxillary sinus, respectively. Other clinical symptoms can also be observed and have been reported, such as anosmia, swelling, numbness, nasal obstruction, exophthalmos, and mucopurulent rhinorrhoea, although there tends to be a change in occurrence between cases (Swami et al. 2019).

Diagnosis and Radiology

This tumour does not possess a classical set of radiological signs; however, it does generally present as a unilocular radiolucency that tends to have a properly demarcated sclerotic border found on routine extraoral radiographs. The characteristic lesion on a CT scan is a well-demarcated mass that is seen to have resulted in thinning of the adjacent bone. CT scan is useful in evaluating the size, location, and erosion of bony surfaces (Swami et al. 2019).

CT scans of the nose and paranasal sinuses are the most useful investigation to this date, as they give complete reformation about the size and extent of the tumour and involvement or erosion of the adjacent bony structures. CT scan with contrast enhancement should be routinely used as some of the schwannomas are very vascular. Investigations like MRI and angiography are sometimes required to demonstrate any displacement of cerebral tissue and intracranial extension of the neoplasm (Alim et al. 2018).

The clinical course and radiographic appearance of this tumour are not unique. Hence, a preoperative diagnosis of schwannoma is rarely made. Usually, positive definite identification must await the results of histopathological analysis (Verma et al. 2013).

The diagnosis of neoplasms of nervous origin, such as schwannoma, is challenging due to the difficulty in defining the origin since they can affect several structures and are also easily confused clinically with other benign tumour lesions such as lipoma, mucocele, leiomyoma, granuloma, haemangioma, cyst, dermoid, epidermoid, salivary gland tumours, fibroma, neurofibroma, and traumatic neuroma (Bueno et al. 2021).

The imaging characteristics of neurilemmomas are important because, together with the symptoms, they allow a presumptive preoperative diagnosis and sometimes determine the nerve of origin. This allows for better surgery planning and the prediction of possible residual nerve deficits. On tomography, areas of central hypodensity are usually observed with peripheral enhancement due to greater vascularisation versus cystic and necrotic regions. In the MRI, they are isodense or hypodense on T1 and heterogeneously hyperintense on T2, and they tend to enhance a little with contrast (Villanueva et al. 1995). A high-resolution CT scan is considered the best imaging modality for such tumours as it provides details about the size and extent of the tumour and the presence of any bony erosions or dehiscence. MRI should be considered if there is a suspicion of intraorbital or intracranial extension on the CT scan.

Histopathology

The final confirmation of diagnosis can only be made after a histopathological examination, which is considered the gold standard for diagnosing any lesion.

Histopathological Examination

Incisional biopsy and anatomopathological evaluation are very crucial when it comes to the definitive diagnosis of schwannoma. Schwannoma has two patterns observed under microscopy, which tend to vary in quantity, present together or in isolation and can help define the diagnosis. Histopathological examination exhibits a typical biphasic pattern. It was classified by Antoni into two categories:

1. Antoni Type-A: Consists of spindle-shaped cells with long, slender fibres that form a parallel arrangement of nuclei, which is known as the palisading arrangement of the cells. Their cellularity is usually high, and their Schwann cells tend to form their palisade arrangement around a central eosinophilic area known as Verocay bodies, which are acellular (consists of reduplicated basement membrane and cytoplasmic processes).
2. Antoni Type-B: This type is not only less cellular but also has a pattern which is less organized and has oval spindle cells that are randomly arranged within a loose and myxomatous stroma. Within the stroma, microcystic degeneration and inflammatory cells can be found, and they are basically degenerative in nature, with myxoid changes seen in the connective tissue stroma. The cells and fibres run in a haphazard manner, and the entire tissue is loose in texture, which is present due to cystic degeneration (Hegde et al. 2016).

Out of all the types of schwannoma, the Plexiform schwannomas (PS) are the only tumour type that presents as a plexiform pattern (as the name suggests) of multiple nodules and intraneural growth.

Diagnostic immunohistochemistry is a valuable tool used daily in the assessment of soft tissue tumours through the identification and visualization of tissue antigens in clinical diagnostics and can characterize various biological processes or pathologies. Examples of these pathologies include immune responses, tissue rejection, and wound healing. It is an important diagnostic tool that, after careful evaluation of histopathology, can help separate differential diagnoses. Other than that, its highly specific antigen-antibody complex reactions can aid in locating key molecules associated with various processes within tissues that would be otherwise difficult to locate. These key molecules include tumour processes or markers, which allow for the identification of molecules and cell type markers present within a tumour, which can help in further analysis of cellular changes, especially phenotypic.

An important diagnostic tool for identifying and differentiating tumours is immunohistochemical staining. The S-100 protein (specific marker for neural tissue) is a marker that is routinely tested for, which is basically a neural crest marker antigen that gives rise to the intense diffuse immune staining, thereby giving a clear-cut diagnosis of schwannoma (Fig. 7.11b) (Hegde et al. 2016).

Histologically, five separate types can be separated: 1-Cellular 2- Ancient 3-Common 4-Epithelioid 5-Plexiform (Bueno et al. 2021; Hegde et al. 2016).

Malignant Transformation

Very rarely is a schwannoma seen with a malignant tendency. Signs of malignant transformation include the presence of tumour necrosis, cytological atypia, high mitotic activity ($\geq$3 mitotic figures per 10 high power fields), and a decreased expression of S100 protein (Knight et al. 2022).

Malignant tumours are an exception, as the majority of tumours are benign. Only 30–40 cases with malignancy of schwannoma have been described in the literature. A review was done for 430,000 cases of nonepithelial tumours of the nasal cavity, paranasal sinuses and nasopharynx, and the results showed that only four cases occurred (Villanueva et al. 1995).

The likelihood of malignant transformation of a schwannoma is very unusual.

There are only 12 reported cases of malignant schwannoma of the paranasal sinuses in literature (Swami et al. 2019).

Treatment

The treatment of choice in schwannoma of paranasal sinuses is complete surgical excision of the tumour. The surgical approach depends upon the site and extent of the neoplasm, with wide exposure and identification of adjacent structures.

For neoplasms of the nasal cavity and the ethmoid sinuses, lateral rhinotomy or external ethmoidectomy is preferred, but for sphenoid sinus lesions, a transantral approach or craniotomy is required for extensive intracranial lesions. The maxillary sinus is best approached by a Caldwell-Luc incision. For tumours of a limited extent, endoscopic resection is an approach that can be taken (Alim et al. 2018).

Although treatment always consists of surgical excision, small tumours of the maxillary sinus can be removed endoscopically. Radiation should not be employed as a form of therapy because schwannomas are highly radioresistant, and it will have no beneficial effect (Verma et al. 2013).

The therapeutic approach of choice regarding schwannoma is complete surgical excision the majority of times, as cases with recurrence are quite rare. Even though recurrence is not common, its likelihood increases when the surgical resection is not complete or in cases with either multiple nodules or intraosseous sites. Although schwannoma is a benign tumour with no malignant potential, it is suggested to perform a recurrent periodic follow-up of more or less than 2 years for early detection in cases of relapses if it occurs (Bueno et al. 2021).

Lately, sinonasal tumours are mostly managed with endoscopic surgery. A case of ethmoid schwannoma with intracranial extension was managed through nasal endoscopic surgery. Open surgery remains the standard option in cases with extensive disease, revision surgery, and endoscopy failure. Facial degloving, lateral rhinotomy, and Caldwell-Luc's approaches help remove large, extensive tumours. Complete excision is required for successful treatment; otherwise, relapse is inevitable (Kandasamy et al. 2017).

The selection of the approach depends on different factors such as size, location, extent of the tumour and involvement of the surrounding structures. For large tumours, the surgical approach of choice is controversial (Knight et al. 2022).

Different surgical approaches have been described for performing a complete excision of the tumour. Endoscopic excision is an appropriate technique due to its lower morbidity, excellent vision, and magnification of the surgical field, which is produced by high-definition endo cameras. Endoscopic surgeries are not only safer, but they also provide the possibility of reconstructions of the skull base with dissected flaps of the nasal cavity if deemed necessary. After treatment with complete surgical excision of the benign tumour, the next step is postoperative histopathological examination to establish and confirm the final diagnosis.

Endonasal surgery or the use of an external approach assisted with endoscopes are the most widely used techniques. These neoplasms are generally seen to have a poor vascular supply, and this is beneficial for endonasal resections, even if the tumour is large, as they are less likely to cause bleeding complications during operation. The intracapsular dissection techniques possess many uses, including the complete excision of the tumour, an extracapsular excision of the tumour, or even the collapse of the tumour.

In tumours involving the pterygomaxillary fossa, it is also possible to go for the endonasal approach with an endoscope.

It is unlikely to be able to identify the origin of the tumour and to maintain the function of the nerve when in either the nasal cavity or in the paranasal sinuses. There are studies that explain the intracapsular dissection technique of neck schwannomas. This is done especially for those schwannomas that tend to arise from the pneumogastric nerve, identifying and preserving some nerve fibres in order to keep some of the nerve's function. In a study of 52 patients with schwannomas of the nasal cavity and skull base, the frequency of operations done endo-nasally with an endoscopic approach was (18/52), while through a transmaxillary sublabial approach assisted with endoscopes (34/52), they reported a total resection rate of 80.8% (42 patients), subtotal of 15.38% (8/52), and partial of 3.84% (2/52). They had five cerebrospinal fluid fistulas that were repaired with fascia lata and a nasoseptal flap. During follow-up (6–134 months), there seemed to be 4 cases of relapse recorded. In another study, endoscopic surgery was chosen for ten patients who had schwannoma of the paranasal sinuses and of the nasal cavities. All were followed up for 2–120 months, and all of them were free of the disease and showed no sign of recurrence without the need for an external approach (Swami et al. 2019; Villanueva et al. 1995).

Differential Diagnosis

Differential diagnosis of schwannoma of the paranasal sinuses should include (Abdellatif et al. 2024; Swami et al. 2019):

(a) Leiomyosarcoma: Palisading and extensive degenerative changes are observed, but they are negative for S-100 and positive for SMA and desmin.
(b) Malignant Melanoma: Difficult to separate on biopsy; however, spindle cell and desmoplastic melanomas lose HMB45 expression.
(c) Neurofibroma: Usually has no capsule. It does have hypercellular mucoid areas but no hypocellular areas. Weaker S-100.
(d) Inflammatory polyps: Negative on immunostaining for S-100.
(e) Inverted papilloma: Negative on immunostaining for S-100.
(f) Spindle cell carcinoma of any type and any other mesenchymal tumours: Usually have weaker S-100.

Prognosis

It is very rare for recurrence to occur after successful en bloc removal of tumour (Alim et al. 2018).

Osteoma

Introduction

Osteoma is a benign and slow-growing osteogenic tumour that is made of either compact or cancellous bone. They are usually found in the cortical plate of long bones. Nonetheless, the paranasal sinuses are one of the most common sites for their occurrence in the head and neck region, and among them, osteomas usually form in the frontal sinus, followed by the maxillary sinus and ethmoid sinuses (Durão et al. 2012; Viswanatha 2012). Maxillary sinus osteomas are mostly asymptomatic and are regarded as a rare entity (Borumandi et al. 2013).

Aetiology

The aetiology of osteomas, in general, is obscure, especially solitary osteoma. However, the literature holds many theories regarding their development.

Gardner's syndrome, which is an autosomal dominant variant of familial adenomatous polyposis, has been proven to be a cause of multiple osteoma formations (Charifa et al. 2024). On the other hand, the theories regarding solitary osteoma, all of which are unproved, include traumatic, infectious, and developmental theories. The developmental/embryogenic theory states that osteomas form in the suture lines between endochondral and membranous ossification. Even so, this theory can explain ethmoid sinus osteomas only and does not explain maxillary sinus osteomas. According to the traumatic theory, a dysregulation of bone development and remodelling happens after trauma, especially during pubertal stages, while the infectious theory suggests that inflammation and infection in the area provide a secondary osteogenic stimulus (Janovic et al. 2013; Tiago et al. 2002).

Epidemiology

Generally, the incidence of osteomas in the facial region is up to 3%, with the frontal sinus accounting for 57% of the facial lesions. Additionally, males are 1.5–3 times more prone to the tumour compared to females (Lund et al. 2013).

Clinical Features

Osteomas are generally asymptomatic and are incidentally found. They usually become symptomatic through the pressure effect when sinus drainage is impaired or extraocular muscles are impinged (Flint et al. 2020).

Since the frontal sinus is the most common among the paranasal sinuses, most patients have headaches and nasal congestion (Cho et al. 2022; Kara 2022). However, according to the limited reports on maxillary sinus osteomas, patients mostly complain of facial deformity, rhinorrhoea, local pain, vision problems, and epiphora (Moretti et al. 2004; Saratziotis and Emanuelli 2014; Verma et al. 2012). Although osteomas grow slowly, by about 1.61 mm per year (Chang et al. 2014), they can extend to the neighbouring regions. For instance, the lesion can impinge the dura, which can lead to CSF leakage, meningitis, etc. With all that said, the malignant transformation of osteomas has never been described (Lund et al. 2013).

Subtypes

Osteomas have three types: ivory, trabeculated and mixed. Ivory osteomas have a wide base and consist of a haversian system; they are also slow-growing. On the other hand, trabeculated osteomas grow more rapidly and are more likely to be pedunculated (Arora et al. 2011). The most important clinical relevance of this histological differentiation is that when an ivory osteoma is being surgically removed, it requires more intense drilling since they are made of hard and dense bone with very few fibrous components (Chang et al. 2014).

Radiology

CT scans are generally accurate for diagnosing osteomas. On the CT scan, they appear homogeneous and well-circumscribed, with a high Hounsfield Unit showing their excessive density. Sometimes, finding the exact origin of the lesion can be difficult, as it can be lobulated and invaginated into the sinus contours; in these cases, MRI can be useful (Lund et al. 2013). The appearance on the MRI can be variable, depending on the amount of cortical and trabecular bone making up the lesion; nonetheless, there is no enhancement with contrast (Barajas et al. 2012).

Treatment

When osteomas are small, asymptomatic, and slow-growing, the literature suggests frequent follow-ups without surgery. However, in most other cases, where there is rapid growth, cosmetic disfigurement, and distressing symptoms, osteomas have to be surgically excised, either by open, endoscopic or mixed approaches. The open approaches include midfacial degloving, lateral rhinotomy, osteoplastic flap, and Caldwell-Luc procedure. On the other hand, endoscopic approaches include medial maxillectomy, either alone or combined with an anterior antrostomy (Lund et al. 2013; Viswanatha 2012).

Pyogenic Granuloma

Introduction

Pyogenic granuloma (PG) is an inflammatory hyperplasia that manifests as vascular growth on the skin or mucous membranes. Clinically, it is characterized by a soft mass with a smooth or lobulated appearance that can be sessile or pedunculated and does not contain purulent material. PG is a non-neoplastic tumour-like growth that frequently occurs in the oral cavity or on the skin. The term "inflammatory hyperplasia" encompasses a broad range of nodular growths on the oral mucosa, which represent inflamed fibrous and granulation tissues (Miller et al. 1999). PG may occasionally arise from the mucosa of the nasal cavity, with the anterior nasal septum, turbinates, and nasal vestibule being the most common locations. There are two types of PG: lobular capillary hemangioma (LCH) and non-LCH, which differ in their histological features (Martinez et al. 2023).

Aetiology and Epidemiology

Although PG can occur at any age (Al-Khateeb and Ababneh 2003; Lawoyin et al. 1997), it is more common in young adult females during their second decade of life, potentially due to the vascular effects of female hormones. Lesions are slightly more prevalent on the maxillary gingiva than on the mandibular gingiva. Clinically, PG appears as a smooth or lobulated exophytic lesion with small red erythematous papules on a pedunculated or sessile base, which is typically haemorrhagic and compressible (Eversole 2001; Neville et al. 2002; Regezi et al. 2003). It may develop as dumb-bell-shaped masses (Bouquot and Nikai 2001). However, in the literature, it is reported that the two types of PG are clinically different. They found that LCH PG occurred more frequently (66%) as a sessile lesion, whereas non-LCH PG mostly occurred as pedunculated (77%) (Epivatianos et al. 2005).

The size of the pyogenic granuloma can vary in diameter from a few millimetres to several centimetres (Neville et al. 2002; Regezi et al. 2003). However, it rarely exceeds 2.5 cm in size and typically reaches its full size within weeks or months, remaining indefinitely thereafter. The surface of the lesion is typically ulcerated and friable, covered by a fibrous membrane, and depending on the age of the lesion, the colour may range from red to purple. Interestingly, there is a correlation between pyogenic granuloma and pregnancy. Pyogenic granuloma is also known as a "pregnancy tumour" or "granuloma gravidarum" (Miller et al. 1999) because of the hormonal imbalance that coincides with pregnancy (Delbrouck et al. 2011). However, there is still no direct evidence to explain the mechanism by which steroid hormones modify the inflammatory response in pyogenic granuloma.

Histopathology

Histopathologically, pyogenic granuloma is a highly vascular proliferation that looks like granulation tissue. The blood vessels show a clustered or medullary pattern separated by less vascular fibrotic septa, leading some authorities to consider pyogenic granuloma as a polypoid form of capillary haemangioma (Figs. 7.19 and 7.20).

There are two different types of pyogenic granuloma. The first type is characterized by blood vessels organized in lobular aggregates. This type is called lobular capillary hemangioma (LCH). The second type consists of highly vascular proliferation that resembles granulation tissue (non-LCH). Probably, the presence of blood vessels with different luminal diameters in the lobular area of LCH pyogenic granuloma and in the central area of non-LCH pyogenic granuloma may be because different pathogenic factors influence their development (Bragado et al. 1999).

The expression of VEGF was analysed in histopathological examination from patients with pyogenic granuloma. The results disclosed the presence of a strong VEGF signal in pyogenic granulomas, which are constituted by a vast majority of cells of endothelial lineage (Al-Khateeb and Ababneh 2003).

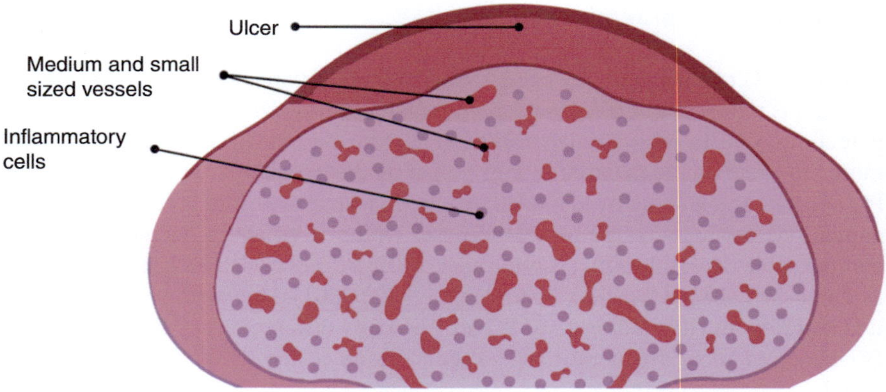

Fig. 7.19 Pyogenic granuloma

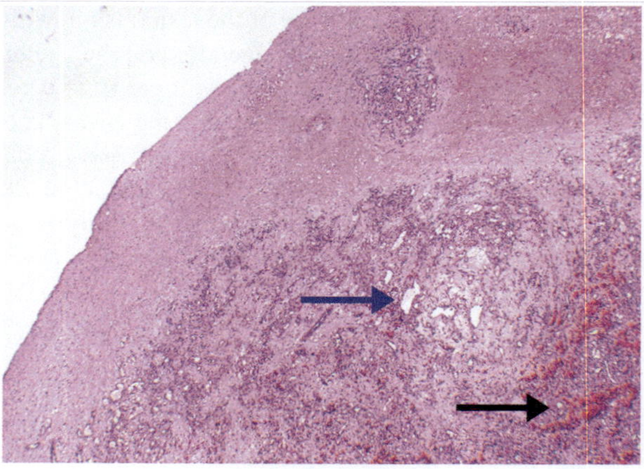

Fig. 7.20 Pyogenic Granuloma: This histopathological image (4×) shows a polypoid lesion with ulceration (Blue Arrow). There is also a focal lobular pattern of vascular proliferation with mild inflammation (Black Arrow)

Clinical Features

The clinical development of the lesion is slow, asymptomatic, and painless (Regezi et al. 2003), but it may also grow rapidly. The usual symptoms of the lesion include nasal obstruction and bleeding episodes, with intermittent epiphora and epistaxis, facial pain, or symptoms of cranial nerve deficits (Miller et al. 1999).

Diagnosis and Radiology

In terms of diagnosis and radiology, computerized tomography (CT) scans of the nose and paranasal sinuses are the most useful investigation to date. The characteristics of the imaging in the transverse section are that of a soft tissue lesion with a marked increase in contrast, hypoattenuated, not always uniform, occasionally with punctate/linear areas of hypoenhancement or central enhancement with hypoattenuated border with an average size of 1–2 cm (Anan 2021).

Magnetic resonance imaging (MRI) shows a gadolinium-enhancing mass of heterogeneous density arising from the right maxillary sinus that can extend to the nasal cavity through the ostiomeatal complex (Anan 2021). It presents as a mass of soft tissue that is homogeneously isointense in T1-weighted images and heterogeneously hyperintense with a hypointense border in T2-weighted images. Small cavities and intralesional foci of haemorrhage may also be observed (Neville et al. 2002). When the mass is found, it is important to formulate a differential diagnosis, as this would help further evaluation of the condition and management of the patient. Biopsy findings have an important role and are definitive in establishing the diagnosis.

Treatment

While many treatment techniques have been described for pyogenic granuloma, choosing an appropriate treatment can be difficult when the lesion is large or occurs in a surgically difficult area. The management of symptoms depends on their severity. If the lesion is small, painless, and free of bleeding, clinical observation and follow-up are advised (Martinez et al. 2023).

To avoid serious nasal bleeding, preoperative digital subtraction angiography and embolization of the sphenopalatine artery can be performed in selected cases. Following embolization, the lesion's size markedly decreases. The mass should be excised completely, under general anaesthesia, by an endonasal endoscopic approach (also seen in Fig. 7.21), which has become the most common method because it allows lower morbidity (Vukadinović et al. 2021).

After excision, recurrence occurs in up to 16% of the lesions, so in some cases, a new excision is necessary. Recurrence is believed to result from incomplete excision, failure to remove etiologic factors, or reinjury to the area (Martinez et al. 2023).

Differential Diagnosis

When a mass is found in the oral cavity, it is important to formulate a differential diagnosis as this would help further evaluation of the condition and management of the patient (Willies-Jacobo et al. 2000). Differential diagnosis of pyogenic granuloma includes peripheral giant cell granuloma, peripheral ossifying fibroma, SCC cancer (Eversole 2001; Regezi et al. 2003), haemangioma, pregnancy tumour, conventional granulation tissue, hyperplastic gingival inflammation, Kaposi's sarcoma, bacillary angiomatosis, angiosarcoma, and non-Hodgkin's lymphoma.

Peripheral giant cell granuloma (PGCG) is an exophytic lesion that is seen exclusively in the gingiva (Burket et al. 2003) and is clinically similar to pyogenic granuloma (PG). PGCG is often more bluish-purple compared to the bright red of a typical PG. Depending on its duration, PG can change in texture from soft to firm and can be suggestive of a fibroma (Eversole 2001, Regezi et al. 2003). Peripheral odontogenic or ossifying fibroma must be taken into consideration as a differential diagnosis, although these tend to be much lighter in colour (Regezi et al. 2003). Also, it is usually about 1.5 cm in diameter, although some have reached 6 cm in diameter. Like PG, it is commonly encountered among pregnant women, but unlike PG, this lesion is found exclusively on the gingiva and has a minimal vascular component.

One important differential diagnosis of PG is haemangioma, which is a developmental disorder, but small lesions may be clinically indistinguishable from PG. In comparison with PG, haemangioma is more meaty and shows histiocytoid and endothelial cell proliferation without an acute inflammatory cell infiltrate. Conventional granulation tissue is another differential diagnosis that should be considered. Despite the close relationship between PG and conventional granulation tissue, PG shows clinically different behaviour, such as rapid growth, multiple occurrences, and frequent recurrence, from those in granulation tissue.

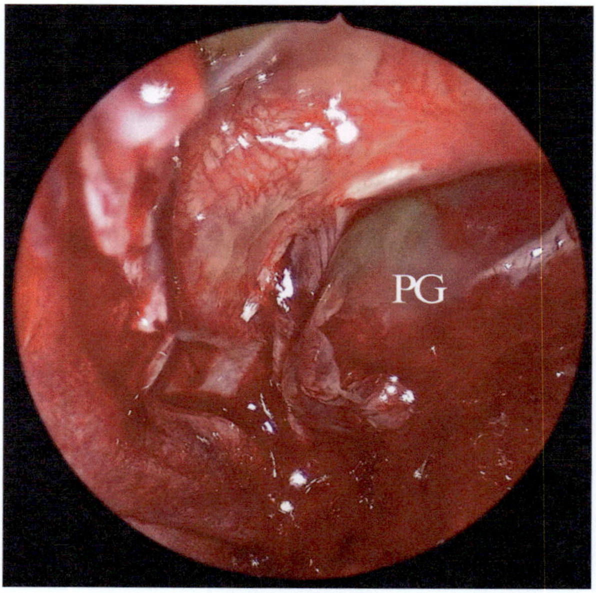

Fig. 7.21 This is an intraoperative video of a patient undergoing endoscopic sinus surgery (ESS) for pyogenic granuloma of the maxillary sinus. As can be seen in the thumbnail (left side nasal cavity), the pyogenic granuloma extends from the maxillary sinus to the nasal cavity. (*PG* pyogenic granuloma) (Audio 7.11 and Video 7.11)

References

Abdellatif E, Kamel D, Mantilla JG (2024) Schwannoma. PathologyOutlines.com. https://www.pathologyoutlines.com/topic/softtissueschwannoma.html. Accessed July 20th, 2024

Acharya S, Naik C, Panditray S, Dany SS (2017) Juvenile nasopharyngeal angiofibroma: a case report. J Clin Diagn Res 11(4):MD03–MD04. https://doi.org/10.7860/jcdr/2017/23729.9630

Ahmetgjekaj I, Harizi E, Rahman A et al (2022) Giant cholesterol granuloma of petrous apex. Radiol Case Rep 17:1220–1224. https://doi.org/10.1016/j.radcr.2021.12.046

Al-Balas HI, Farneti P, Bellusci A et al (2020) A comparison of two endoscopic techniques for the treatment of antrochoanal polyps. Acta Otorhinolaryngol Ital 40:290–296. https://doi.org/10.14639/0392-100x-n0259

Alghulikah A, Musallam N, Sumaily I et al (2021) Cholesterol granuloma of the maxillary sinus—a case report and literature review. Allergy Rhinol (Providence) 12:215265672098478. https://doi.org/10.1177/2152656720984785

Alim BM, Jomah M, Al-Thobaiti M (2018) Maxillary sinus schwannoma. BMJ Case Rep 2018:bcr-223946. https://doi.org/10.1136/bcr-2017-223946

Al-Khateeb T, Ababneh K (2003) Oral pyogenic granuloma in jordanians: a retrospective analysis of 108 cases. J Oral Maxillofac Surg 61:1285–1288. https://doi.org/10.1016/s0278-2391(03)00729-8

Alshaikh NA, Eleftheriadou A (2015) Juvenile nasopharyngeal angiofibroma staging: an overview. Ear Nose Throat J 94:E12–E22. https://doi.org/10.1177/014556131509400615

Alves FRA, Granato L, Maia MS, Lambert E (2006) Surgical approaches to juvenile nasopharyngeal angiofibroma—case report and literature review. Braz J Otorhinolaryngol 72(4):475–479

Anan R (2021) Lobular capillary hemangioma of the nasal cavity. Radiopaedia.org. https://doi.org/10.53347/rid-96158. Accessed 12 March 2023

Antrochoanal polyp (2018) J Cancer Prev Curr Res 9:00321. https://doi.org/10.15406/jcpcr.2018.09.00321

Arora A, Mukund A, Thapar S, Jain D (2011) Osteoma of the inner table of the skull. Indian J Otolaryngol Head Neck Surg 63(1):100–102

Austin RP, Nelson BL (2021) Sine qua non: dentigerous cyst. Head Neck Pathol 15:1261–1264. https://doi.org/10.1007/s12105-021-01327-3

Bal M, Berkiten G, Uyanık E (2014) Mucous retention cysts of the paranasal sinuses. Hippokratia 18(4):379

Barajas RF, Perry A, Sughrue M et al (2012) Intracranial subdural osteoma: a rare benign tumor that can be differentiated from other calcified intracranial lesions utilizing M.R. Imaging. J Neuroradiol 39:263–266. https://doi.org/10.1016/j.neurad.2011.11.003

Bettinger R, Loerz M (2008) Osteoblastom der Kieferhöhle: Eine seltene Knochenläsion. Laryngorhinootologie 70:275–277. https://doi.org/10.1055/s-2007-998037

Bokhari K, Hameed MS, Ajmal M, Togoo RA (2012) Benign osteoblastoma involving maxilla: a case report and review of the literature. Case Rep Dent 2012:1–4. https://doi.org/10.1155/2012/351241

Borumandi F, Lukas H, Yousefi B, Gaggl A (2013) Maxillary sinus osteoma: from incidental finding to surgical management. J Oral Maxillofac Pathol 17:318. https://doi.org/10.4103/0973-029x.119786

Bouquot and Nikai (2001)'s citation in the list was modified to: Bouquot JE, Nikai H (2001) Lesions of the oral cavity. In: Barnes L, Eveson JW, Reichart P, Sidransky D (eds) Diagnostic surgical pathology of the head and neck. Saunders, Philadelphia

Bragado R, Bello E, Requena L et al (1999) Increased expression of vascular endothelial growth factor in pyogenic granulomas. Acta Derm Venereol 79:422–425. https://doi.org/10.1080/000155599750009834

Bueno MV, Duarte ACC, Sinhorini PA et al (2021) Plexiform schwannoma in the maxillary alveolar ridge: a case report. J Oral Diagn 6. https://doi.org/10.5935/2525-5711.20210010

Burket LW, Greenberg MS, Glick M (2003) Burket's oral medicine. B.C. Decker

Bütler S, Grossenbacher R (1989) Cholesterol granuloma of the paranasal sinuses. J Laryngol Otol 103:776–779. https://doi.org/10.1017/s0022215100110059

Caylakli F, Yavuz H, Cagici AC, Ozluoglu LN (2006) Endoscopic sinus surgery for maxillary sinus mucoceles. Head Face Med 2:29. https://doi.org/10.1186/1746-160x-2-29

Chang CC, Incaudo GA, Gershwin ME (2014) Diseases of the sinuses. Springer

Charifa A, Jamil RT, Sathe NC, Zhang X (2024) Gardner syndrome. StatPearls—NCBI Bookshelf. https://www.ncbi.nlm.nih.gov/books/NBK482342/

Cheah SC, Lim EH, Japar R et al (2023) Angiofibroma of the maxillary sinus mimicking mucocele: a diagnostic challenge. Egypt J Otolaryngol 39:142. https://doi.org/10.1186/s43163-023-00504-1

Cherrabi K, Touihem N, Nakkabi I, Nadour K (2021) Bilateral antrochoanal polyps: a case report. Egypt J Otolaryngol 37. https://doi.org/10.1186/s43163-021-00090-0

Cho A, Jung Y, Park JH et al (2022) Clinical manifestations and surgical treatment outcomes of paranasal sinus osteoma. J Rhinol 29:19–25. https://doi.org/10.18787/jr.2021.00388

Choi MG, Hong CH, Choi EJ et al (2022) Sinus lifts in the presence of pseudoantral and mucous retention cysts. J Korean Assoc Oral Maxillofac Surg 48:101–110. https://doi.org/10.5125/jkaoms.2022.48.2.101

Cleveland Clinic (2022) Professional CCM ossifying fibroma. Cleveland Clinic. https://my.clevelandclinic.org/health/diseases/24275-ossifying-fibroma

Cruz-Ferreira AM (2019) Craniofacial polyostotic fibrous dysplasia initially diagnosed in a primary care unit. Korean J Family Med 40:58–60. https://doi.org/10.4082/kjfm.17.0129

Da Motta Almada CB, Fonseca DR, Vanzillotta RR, Pires FR (2008) Cholesterol granuloma of the maxillary sinus. Braz Dent J 19:171–174. https://doi.org/10.1590/s0103-64402008000200015

Dağistan H, CengİZ C, Can İH (2021) The relationship between maxillary sinus retention cysts and nasal septum. J Surg Med 5:687–690. https://doi.org/10.28982/josam.928949

Davidova LA, Bhattacharyya I, Islam MN et al (2019) An analysis of clinical and histopathologic features of fibrous dysplasia of the jaws: a series of 40 cases and review of literature. Head Neck Pathol 14:353–361. https://doi.org/10.1007/s12105-019-01039-9

De Freitas Filho SAJ, Esteves GG, Oliveira DT (2017) Cholesterol granuloma in the maxillary sinus: are endodontically treated teeth involved in its etiopathogenesis? Case Rep Pathol 2017:1–5. https://doi.org/10.1155/2017/5249161

Delbrouck C, Chamiec M, Hassid S, Ghanooni R (2011) Lobular capillary haemangioma of the nasal cavity during pregnancy. J Laryngol Otol 125:973–977. https://doi.org/10.1017/s0022215111001654

Demicheri G, Kornecki F, Bengoa J et al (2016) Maxillary sinus mucocele: review of case report. Int J Surg Case Rep 24:189–192

Demiriz L, Misir AF, Gorur DI (2015) Dentigerous cyst in a young child. European J Dent 9:599–602. https://doi.org/10.4103/1305-7456.172619

Dhingra PL (2010) Diseases of ear, nose throat. Elsevier India

Domingues PM, Gaffrée BG, Gomes SR et al (2018) Fibrous dysplasia in maxillary bone: case report. Int J Oral Dental Health 4:72. https://doi.org/10.23937/2469-5734/1510072

Dubey SP, Schick B (2017) Juvenile angiofibroma. Springer

Durão AR, Chilvarquer I, Hayek JE et al (2012) Osteoma of the zygomatic arch and mandible: report of two cases. Revista Portuguesa De Estomatologia, Medicina DentáRia E Cirurgia Maxilofacial 53:103–107. https://doi.org/10.1016/j.rpemd.2012.02.006

Eachempati P, Aggarwal H, Shenoy V, Baliga M (2015) Multidisciplinary approach for management of a patient with fibrous dysplasia of maxilla. BMJ Case Rep:bcr2015210330. https://doi.org/10.1136/bcr-2015-210330

Eide JG, Welch KC, Adappa ND et al (2022) Sinonasal inverted papilloma and squamous cell carcinoma: contemporary management and patient outcomes. Cancers 14:2195. https://doi.org/10.3390/cancers14092195

El-Feky M, Bhuta S (2010) Antrochoanal polyp. Radiopaedia.org. https://doi.org/10.53347/rid-9044

Epivatianos A, Antoniades D, Zaraboukas T et al (2005) Pyogenic granuloma of the oral cavity: comparative study of its clinicopathological and immunohistochemical features. Pathol Int 55:391–397. https://doi.org/10.1111/j.1440-1827.2005.01843.x

Eversole LR (2001) Clinical outline of Oral pathology. PMPH-USA

Eversole LR, Sabes WR, Rovin S (1972) Fibrous dysplasia: a nosologic problem in the diagnosis of fibro-osseous lesions of the jaws. J Oral Pathol Med 1:189–220. https://doi.org/10.1111/j.1600-0714.1972.tb01659.x

Fernandez MM, Martínez-Antón MA, Alobid I, Mullol J (2004) The antrochoanal polyp. Rhinology 42(4):178–182

Flint PW, Haughey BH, Lund VJ et al (2020) Cummings otolaryngology. Elsevier

Fusconi M, Conte M, Pagliarella M et al (2013) Fibrous dysplasia of the maxilla: diagnostic reliability of the study image. Literature review. J Neurol Surg B Skull Base 74:364–368. https://doi.org/10.1055/s-0033-1347374

Garip H, Aktop S, Gönül C, Göker K (2015) Treatment approaches for odontogenic cysts of the maxillary sinus. InTech eBooks

Gaurkar SS, Deshmukh PT, Singh CV, Khan FQ (2022) A rare presentation of dentigerous cyst. Cureus 14(6):e26098. https://doi.org/10.7759/cureus.26098

Gil Z, Margalit N, Fliss DM (2012) Open surgical approaches to the anterior skull base and paranasal sinuses. Head and Neck Cancer Clinics, pp 93–103

Gonçales ES, Gonçales AGB, da Silva Lima E, Rocha JF, Noleto JW, Hochuli-Vieira E (2015) Symptomatic mucous retention cysts of the maxillary sinus: case report. http://revodonto.bvsalud.org/scielo.php?script=sci_abstract&pid=S1984-56852015000200015&lng=pt&nrm=iso&tlng=en

Gür ÖE, Kaymakçi M, Yılmaz DNS (2016) Paranasal sinus mucoceles. J Craniofac Surg 27(5):e472–e475

Hadar T, Shvero J, Nageris BI, Yaniv E (2000) Mucus retention cyst of the maxillary sinus: the endoscopic approach. Br J Oral Maxillofac Surg 38:227–229. https://doi.org/10.1054/bjom.1999.0160

Hamada M, Takeshita A, Shimizu H et al (2018) Surgical simulation for dentigerous cyst in the maxillary sinus using full-color 3D salt modeling: report of a case. Oral Maxillofac Surg Cases 4:6–11. https://doi.org/10.1016/j.omsc.2018.01.001

Hegde O, Desai D, Bhandarkar GP, Paul T (2016) Benign schwannoma of the maxillary antrum. Eur J Dent 10:281–285. https://doi.org/10.4103/1305-7456.178307

Janovic A, Antic S, Rakocevic Z, Djuric M (2013) Paranasal sinus osteoma: is there any association with anatomical variations? Rhinology 51:54–60. https://doi.org/10.4193/rhino12.130

Jaswal A, Jana AK, Sikder B et al (2007) Benign osteoblastoma of maxillary sinus: a rare presentation. Indian J Otolaryngol Head Neck Surg 59:80–82. https://doi.org/10.1007/s12070-007-0026-1

Jones AC, Prihoda TJ, Kacher JE et al (2006) Osteoblastoma of the maxilla and mandible: a report of 24 cases, review of the literature, and discussion of its relationship to osteoid osteoma of the jaws. Oral Surg Oral Med Oral Pathol Oral Radiol Endod 102:639–650. https://doi.org/10.1016/j.tripleo.2005.09.004

Kanazirska P, Kanasirski N, Chenchev I, Cholakova RB (2010) Fibrous dysplasia in the maxillo-mandibular region—case report. Biotechnol Biotechnol Equip 24(Suppl 1):224–227

Kandasamy S, Rs N, John R (2017) Neurilemmoma of maxillary alveolus: a rare case report and review of literature. J Pharm Bioallied Sci 9:285. https://doi.org/10.4103/jpbs.jpbs_114_17

Kara İ (2022) Paranasal sinus osteomas: evaluation of surgical management with 13 cases. Eur Arch Otorhinolaryngol 279(11):5389–5394

Kara Mİ, Yanık S, Altan A et al (2015) Large dentigerous cyst in the maxillary sinus leading to diplopia and nasal obstruction: case report. J Istanb Univ Fac Dent 49:46. https://doi.org/10.17096/jiufd.10506

Kasat V, Karjodkar F, Laddha R (2012) Dentigerous cyst associated with an ectopic third molar in the maxillary sinus: a case report and review of literature. Contemp Clin Dent 3:373. https://doi.org/10.4103/0976-237x.103642

Khanna S, Gupta SC, Singh PA (2003) Schwannoma of maxillary sinus. Indian J Otolaryngol Head Neck Surg 55:132–135. https://doi.org/10.1007/bf02974623

Knight SWE, Knight TE, Santiago T et al (2022) Malignant peripheral nerve sheath Tumors—a comprehensive review of pathophysiology, diagnosis, and multidisciplinary management. Children 9:38. https://doi.org/10.3390/children9010038

Knipe H, Claassen B (2013) Paranasal sinuses retention cysts. Radiopaedia.org. https://doi.org/10.53347/rid-22374

Koo SK, Kim YJ, Jung SH, Son H (2016) Cholesterol granuloma of nasal septum. J Rhinol 22(1):44–46

Kushchayeva YS, Kushchayev SV, Glushko TY et al (2018) Fibrous dysplasia for radiologists: beyond ground glass bone matrix. Insights Imaging 9:1035–1056. https://doi.org/10.1007/s13244-018-0666-6

Lawoyin JO, Arotiba JT, Dosumu OO (1997) Oral pyogenic granuloma: a review of 38 cases from Ibadan, Nigeria. Br J Oral Maxillofac Surg 35:185–189. https://doi.org/10.1016/s0266-4356(97)90561-1

Lee PA (1986) McCune-Albright syndrome. JAMA 256:2980. https://doi.org/10.1001/jama.1986.03380210076028

Lee JT, Chiu AG (2019) Endoscopic Denker approach for anterior maxilla tumors. Elsevier eBooks, pp 183–190.e1

Leon ME, Chavez C, Fyfe B et al (2002) Cholesterol granuloma of the maxillary sinus. Arch Pathol Lab Med 126:217–219. https://doi.org/10.5858/2002-126-0217-cgotms

Limaiem F, Byerly DW, Mabrouk A, Singh R (2023) Osteoblastoma. StatPearls. https://www.ncbi.nlm.nih.gov/books/NBK536954/

Lisan Q, Laccourreye O, Bonfils P (2016) Sinonasal inverted papilloma: from diagnosis to treatment. Eur Ann Otorhinolaryngol Head Neck Dis 133:337–341. https://doi.org/10.1016/j.anorl.2016.03.006

Lucas DR (2010) Osteoblastoma. Arch Pathol Lab Med 134:1460–1466. https://doi.org/10.5858/2010-0201-cr.1

Lucas DR, Unni KK, McLeod RA et al (1994) Osteoblastoma: clinicopathologic study of 306 cases. Hum Pathol 25:117–134. https://doi.org/10.1016/0046-8177(94)90267-4

Lund VJ, Howard DJ, Wei WI (2013) Tumors of the nose, sinuses and nasopharynx. Thieme Medical Publishers

Makihara S (2022) Sinonasal inverted papilloma. Encyclopedia. https://encyclopedia.pub/entry/19696. Accessed 3 April 2023

Mallon A, Poletto E, Chennupati SK (2014) Large pediatric sphenoid sinus cholesterol granuloma: case report and review of the literature. Int J Pediatr Otorhinolaryngol Extra 9:103–107. https://doi.org/10.1016/j.pedex.2014.03.009

Marcove RC, Alpert M (1963) A pathologic study of benign osteoblastoma. Clin Orthop Relat Res 30:175–181

Marina MB, Gendeh BS (2006) Bilateral maxillary sinus cholesterol granuloma: a rare entity. Med J Malaysia 61(2):226–228

Martinez SML, Contreras NGC, Sandoval JRG et al (2023) Oral pyogenic granuloma: a narrative review. Int J Mol Sci 24:16885. https://doi.org/10.3390/ijms242316885

Matheny KE, Duncavage JA (2003) Contemporary indications for the Caldwell-Luc procedure. Curr Opin Otolaryngol Head Neck Surg 11:23–26. https://doi.org/10.1097/00020840-200302000-00005

Mattos RG, Egas LS, Oliveira P et al (2019) Mucous retention cyst in maxillary sinus with expansion of maxillary tuberosity: case report. J Oral Diagnosis 4

Meir W, Bourla R, Huszar M, Zloczower E (2021) Antrochoanal polyp: updated clinical approach, histology characteristics, diagnosis and treatment. IntechOpen eBooks

Meirelles RC, Neves-Pinto RM (2006) Granuloma de colesterol do seio maxilar. Rev Bras Otorrinolaringol 72(2):284–287

Miller FR, D'Agostino MA, Schlack K (1999) Lobular capillary Hemangioma of the nasal cavity. Otolaryngol Head Neck Surg 120:783–784. https://doi.org/10.1053/hn.1999.v120.a85324

Moretti A, Croce A, Leone O, D'Agostino L (2004) Osteoma of maxillary sinus: case report. Acta Otorhinolaryngol Ital 24(4):219–222

Neel HB, Whicker JH, Devine KD, Weiland LH (1973) Juvenile angiofibroma. Am J Surg 126:547–556. https://doi.org/10.1016/s0002-9610(73)80048-0

Neville BW, Damn DD, Allen CM, Bouquot JE (2002) Oral and maxillofacial pathology. W. B. Saunders, Philadelphia, pp 513–519. https://www.scirp.org/reference/referencespapers?referenceid=356419

Nilesh K, Punde P, Parkar M (2017) Craniofacial fibrous dysplasia of zygomaticomaxillary complex. World J Plast Surg 6(3):369–374

Nukpook T, Ekalaksananan T, Teeramatwanich W et al (2020) Prevalence and association of Epstein-Barr virus infection with sinonasal inverted papilloma and sinonasal squamous cell carcinoma in the northeastern Thai population. Infect Agent Cancer 15:43. https://doi.org/10.1186/s13027-020-00308-5

Oliveira JAA, Tavares MG Aguiar CV et al (2012) Comparison between endoscopic and open surgery in 37 patients with nasopharyngeal angiofibroma. Braz J Otorhinolaryngol 78:75–80. https://doi.org/10.1590/s1808-86942012000100012

Onay O, Suslu AE, Yilmaz T (2019) Huge dentigerous cyst in the maxillary sinus: a rare case in childhood. Turk Arch Otorhinolaryngol 57:54–56. https://doi.org/10.5152/tao.2019.1920

Osguthorpe JD, Hungerford GD (1983) Benign osteoblastoma of the maxillary sinus. Head Neck Surg 6:605–609. https://doi.org/10.1002/hed.2890060112

Park JK-H, Lee SY, Kim J-H, Kim B-K (2023) Long-term outcomes after core extirpation of fibrous dysplasia of the zygomaticomaxillary region. Arch Craniofac Surg 24:59–65. https://doi.org/10.7181/acfs.2023.00038

Pogrel MA (2005) Treatment of Keratocysts: the case for decompression and marsupialization. J Oral Maxillofac Surg 63:1667–1673. https://doi.org/10.1016/j.joms.2005.08.008

Rastegar H, Osmani F (2022) Evaluation of mucous retention cyst prevalence on digital panoramic radiographs in the local population of Iran. Radiolo Res Pract 2022:1–6. https://doi.org/10.1155/2022/8650027

Regezi J, Sciubba J, Jordan R (2003) Oral pathology clinical-pathologic correlations, 4th edn. WB Saunders, St. Louis, pp 376–380. https://www.scirp.org/reference/referencespapers?referenceid=1003721

Rock P, Singh G (2008) Fibrous dysplasia. Arch Pathol Lab Med 137(1):134–138. https://doi.org/10.53347/rid-4915

Rutkowski M, Niewinska K (2021) The epidemiology of benign proliferative processes of the skeletal system in children. Int J Environ Res Public Health 18:9338. https://doi.org/10.3390/ijerph18179338

Sagar P, Singh I, Rajpurohit P, Mandal S (2019) Inverted papilloma presenting as unilateral proptosis: a case report with review of literature. Saudi J Ophthalmol 33:413–416. https://doi.org/10.1016/j.sjopt.2019.01.008

Samieirad S, Momtaz MM, Mohtasham N et al (2021) Surgical treatment of fibrous dysplasia in the maxillary bone of a 12 year-old girl: a case report. World J Plast Surg 10:126–133. https://doi.org/10.29252/wjps.10.3.126

Saratziotis A, Emanuelli E (2014) Osteoma of the medial wall of the maxillary sinus: a primary cause of nasolacrimal duct obstruction and review of the literature. Case Rep Otolaryngol 2014:1–4. https://doi.org/10.1155/2014/348459

Sataloff RT (2015) Sataloff's comprehensive textbook of otolaryngology: head & neck surgery. J.P. Medical Ltd

Schick B, Veldung B, Wemmert S et al (2005) p53 and Her-2/neu in juvenile angiofibromas. Oncol Rep. https://doi.org/10.3892/or.13.3.453

Shanab HG (2021) Ossifying fibroma of maxilla: updated review of literature and a case report—ProQuest. https://www.proquest.com/openview/1d6b9c063509dd5fa9a6f1d5588a9ec5/1.pdf?pq-origsite=gscholar&cbl=2031963

Sharma V, Chew FS, Hoch B (2009) Periosteal osteoblastoma: multimodal imaging of a rare neoplasm. Radiol Case Rep 4:329. https://doi.org/10.2484/rcr.v4i4.329

Shetty RM, Dixit U (2010) Dentigerous cyst of inflammatory origin. Int J Clin Pediatr Dent 3:195–198. https://doi.org/10.5005/jp-journals-10005-1076i

Simões JC, Nogueira-Neto FB, Gregório LL et al (2015) Visual loss: a rare complication of maxillary sinus mucocele. Braz J Otorhinolaryngol 81:451–453. https://doi.org/10.1016/j.bjorl.2015.03.008

Smith WNH (1972) Benign osteoblastoma of the mandible: report of case. J Oral Surg 4:288–292

Sontakke SA, Karjodkar FR, Umarji HR (2011) Computed tomographic features of fibrous dysplasia of maxillofacial region. Imaging Sci Dent 41:23. https://doi.org/10.5624/isd.2011.41.1.23

Stokes SM, Castle JT (2010) Nasopharyngeal angiofibroma of the nasal cavity. Head Neck Pathol 4:210–213. https://doi.org/10.1007/s12105-010-0181-7

Swami P, Raval R, Kumawat V, Nyklesh V (2019) Maxillary schwannoma—a case report of a rare tumor. Natl J Maxillofac Surg 10:245. https://doi.org/10.4103/njms.njms_1_16

Szymańska A, Szymański M, Morshed K et al (2012) Extranasopharyngeal angiofibroma: clinical and radiological presentation. Eur Arch Otorhinolaryngol 270:655–660. https://doi.org/10.1007/s00405-012-2041-4

Tayşi M, Özden C, Çankaya AB et al (2016) Conservative approach to a large dentigerous cyst in an 11-year-old patient. J Istanb Univ Fac Dent 50:51–56. https://doi.org/10.17096/jiufd.85819

Tiago RSL, De Melo ECM, De Oliveira Fobé LP (2002) Osteomas fronto-etmoidais: aspectos clínicos e cirúrgicos. Rev Bras Otorrinolaringol 68:516–520. https://doi.org/10.1590/s0034-72992002000400010

Tinoco P, Pereira JCO, Filho RCL, Ruela KP (2009) Fibrous dysplasia of maxillary sinus. Arch Otorhinolaryngol 13(2):214–217

Tom LWC, Lowry LD, Quinn-Bogard A (1980) Benign osteoblastoma of the maxillary sinus. Otolaryngol Head Neck Surg 88:397–402. https://doi.org/10.1177/019459988008800414

Tork CA, Simpson DL (2023) Nasopharyngeal angiofibroma. StatPearls. https://www.ncbi.nlm.nih.gov/books/NBK545240/

Toyodome S, Nozoe E, Ishihata K et al (2017) A case of osteoblastoma arising in the mandible. Nihon Kyobu Geka Gakkai Zasshi 63:388–393. https://doi.org/10.5794/jjoms.63.388

Upadhyaya N, Khandekar S, Dive A, Mishra R (2015) Sinonasal inverted papilloma: a case report and mini review of histopathological features. J Oral Maxillofac Pathol 19:405. https://doi.org/10.4103/0973-029x.174644

Vella O, Cuny F, Robard L, Bazille C (2016) Osteoblastoma of the maxillary sinus in a child presenting with exophthalmos. Eur Ann Otorhinolaryngol Head Neck Dis 133:277–279. https://doi.org/10.1016/j.anorl.2016.01.007

Verma RK, Kalsotra G, Vaiphei K, Panda NK (2012) Large central osteoma of maxillary sinus: a case report. Egypt J Ear Nose Throat Allied Sci 13:65–69. https://doi.org/10.1016/j.ejenta.2012.02.001

Verma A, Banerjee K, Verma A et al (2013) Maxillary neurilemmoma—rarest of the rare tumour: report of 2 cases. Int J Surg Case Rep 4:1044–1047. https://doi.org/10.1016/j.ijscr.2013.09.006

Vieira EMM, De Morais S, De Musis CR et al (2015) Frequency of maxillary sinus mucous retention cysts in a central Brazilian population. J Dent (Shiraz) 16(3):169–174

Villanueva J, Gigoux C, Solé F (1995) Central neurilemmoma of maxilla. Oral Surg Oral Med Oral Pathol Oral Radiol Endod 79:41–43. https://doi.org/10.1016/s1079-2104(05)80071-x

Viswanatha B (2012) Maxillary sinus osteoma: two cases and review of the literature. Acta Otorhinolaryngol Ital 32(3):202–205

Vlantis AC, Yu BK, Kam MK et al (2008) Nasopharyngectomy: does the approach to the nasopharynx influence survival? Otolaryngol Head Neck Surg 139:40–46. https://doi.org/10.1016/j.otohns.2008.04.018

Vukadinović T, Labus M, Spasić S et al (2021) Maxillary sinus lobular capillary hemangioma in a 15-year-old boy. Ear Nose Throat J 102:117–120. https://doi.org/10.1177/0145561321993597

Vura NG, Gaddipati R, Ramisetti S et al (2015) Surgical management of ossifying fibroma in maxilla: report of two cases. J Int Oral Health 7(6):115–118

Wackym PA, Snow JB (2016) Ballenger's otorhinolaryngology. PMPH USA

Wan Y, Zhao W, Jiang Y et al (2014) β-Catenin is a valuable marker for differential diagnosis of osteoblastoma and osteosarcoma. Hum Pathol 45:1459–1465. https://doi.org/10.1016/j.humpath.2014.02.022

Wan MH, Govindaraju R, Narayanan P (2022) Maxillary extranasopharyngeal angiofibroma: a case report and a review of similar cases. Egypt J Ear Nose Throat Allied Sci 23:1–7. https://doi.org/10.21608/ejentas.2021.50903.1286

Wang M, Noel JE (2017) Etiology of sinonasal inverted papilloma: a narrative review. World J Otorhinolaryngol Head Neck Surg 3:54–58. https://doi.org/10.1016/j.wjorl.2016.11.004

Watkinson JC, Clarke RW (2018) Scott-Brown's otorhinolarnygology and head and neck surgery. CRC Press

Wenig BM, Richardson M (2009) Nasal cavity, paranasal sinuses, and nasopharynx. Icahn School of Medicine at Mount Sinai. https://doi.org/10.1016/B978-1-4160-3966-2/00009-6

Willies-Jacobo LJ, Isaacs H, Stein MT (2000) Pyogenic granuloma presenting as a congenital epulis. Arch Pediatr Adolesc Med 154:603. https://doi.org/10.1001/archpedi.154.6.603

Windfuhr JP, Remmert S (2004) Extranasopharyngeal angiofibroma: etiology, incidence and management. Acta Otolaryngol 124:880–889. https://doi.org/10.1080/00016480310015948

Wormald PJ (2008) Endoscopic sinus surgery. Thieme

Woźniak AW, Nowaczyk MT, Osmola K, Golusinski W (2009) Malignant transformation of an osteoblastoma of the mandible: case report and review of the literature. Eur Arch Otorhinolaryngol 267:845–849. https://doi.org/10.1007/s00405-009-1172-8

Wu V, Siu J, Yip J, Lee JM (2018) Endoscopic management of maxillary sinus inverted papilloma attachment sites to minimize disease recurrence. J Otolaryngol Head Neck Surg 47:24. https://doi.org/10.1186/s40463-018-0271-1

Yeom H-G, Lee W, Han S-I et al (2022) Mucocele in the maxillary sinus involving the orbit: a report of 2 cases. Imaging Sci Dent 52:327. https://doi.org/10.5624/isd.20210278

Zachariah T, Neelakandan RS (2019) Utility of the midface degloving approach for extended exposure in maxillary pathologies. J Maxillofac Oral Surg 19:217–224. https://doi.org/10.1007/s12663-019-01287-w

Zhang H, Hock LE, Robinson R, Simmons B, Walsh J, Shriver EM (2020) Maxillary sinus mucocele. EyeRounds.org. https://EyeRounds.org/cases/294-maxillary-sinus-mucocele.htm. Accessed 22 November 2023

Malignant Lesion of Maxillary Sinus

8

Goran Latif Omer, Vivek Sasindran, Mithra Sara, Pier Giorgio Giacomini, Sahand Soran Ali, Aland Salih Abdullah, Gianluca Velletrani, Beatrice Francavilla, and Riccardo Maurizi

Squamous Cell Carcinoma

Introduction

Following basal cell carcinoma, squamous cell carcinoma (SCC) is the second most common malignancy of the skin. The lesion commonly occurs in areas of the body exposed to sunlight and ultraviolet (UV) light (Howell et al. 2024). Although it generally follows an aggressive pattern, squamous cell carcinoma of the maxillary sinus is rare (Santos et al. 2014). The lesion accounts for approximately 3% of all malignancies in the head and neck region. Important risk factors include a history of chemical exposure or a viral infection along with Eastern country descendancy. Furthermore, middle-aged men are the most affected by the lesion. Symptoms include nasal obstruction, epistaxis, rhinorrhoea, pain, nasal stuffiness, and nasal fullness. The main therapeutic approach is surgical excision, which also aims to maintain and possibly even restore facial contours and function (Santos et al. 2014). Since the majority of the patients are diagnosed at an advanced stage, the malignancy tends to have a reduced survival rate and an unfavourable prognosis (Santos et al. 2014).

Supplementary Information The online version contains supplementary material available at https://doi.org/10.1007/978-3-031-83468-4_8.

G. L. Omer (✉) · S. S. Ali · A. S. Abdullah
Department of Clinical Sciences, College of Medicine, University of Sulaimani, Sulaymaniyah, KRI, Iraq

V. Sasindran · M. Sara
KM Cherian Institute of Medical Sciences, Chengannur, Kerala, India

P. G. Giacomini · G. Velletrani · B. Francavilla · R. Maurizi
Department of Otorhinolaryngology, University of Rome Tor Vergata, Rome, Italy

© The Author(s), under exclusive license to Springer Nature Switzerland AG 2025
G. L. Omer, S. Di Girolamo (eds.), *Maxillary Sinus: A Comprehensive Guide*, https://doi.org/10.1007/978-3-031-83468-4_8

Epidemiology

Malignant neoplasms of the nasal cavity and paranasal sinuses are rare, accounting for only 0.2–0.8% of all malignant neoplasms. As aforementioned, the malignancy makes up 3% of the total head and neck malignancies, with the majority (60–70%) of them occurring in the maxillary sinus, followed by the nasal cavity in 12–25% and the ethmoid with 10–15%. The average age of the lesion is in the mid-60s, with most patients presenting after the age of 50 (Dubal et al. 2015). Middle-aged men, mostly of white ethnicity, are the predominant patient population affected by this form of SCC (Santos et al. 2014).

Aetiology and Pathophysiology

Maxillary sinus SCC has a very broad range of risk factors. Exposure to chemical agents such as chlorophenol, nickel, and formaldehyde have all been previously reported. Furthermore, exposure to textile dust, wood, and cigarette smoking make up some of the other risk factors along with previous viral infections (Santos et al. 2014). Among the viral infections, human papillomavirus is the one particularly associated with squamous cell carcinoma. Another very important etiological factor is alcohol, especially when combined with cigarettes since they have been shown to pose a synergistic effect on the head and neck regions (Dubal et al. 2015). Although SCC generally has precancerous lesions, no precancerous lesion has been well established in the maxillary sinus, unlike other areas of the head and neck (Santos et al. 2014).

Clinical Features

The lesion remains either asymptomatic or presents with vague symptoms in the majority of the patients, at least till it reaches a more advanced stage (Dubal et al. 2015). By the time of diagnosis, most patients present with symptoms since the lesion has usually reached an advanced level by the time of presentation. There is a wide variation between patients regarding their symptoms. Swelling and pain are generally the most common symptoms. Other symptoms reported are rhinorrhoea, epistaxis, obstruction, nasal fullness, nasal stuffiness, paraesthesia to the tooth, diplopia, and lacrimation. The invasion of the lesion into the palate, nasal cavity, skin, mouth, orbit, skull, and other paranasal sinuses has a great impact on the patient's presentation (Santos et al. 2014). Furthermore, infraorbital nerve anaesthesia, serous otitis media and trismus can also be present (Stern et al. 1993). This variation in symptom presentation plays an important role in the delay of diagnosis.

Radiographic Features

SCC of the maxillary sinus generally arises from the alveolar ridge of the maxilla. As shown in Fig. 8.1, on imaging, a large mass is observed on the alveolar ridge, usually occupying the entirety of the maxillary sinus. Based on its aggressiveness,

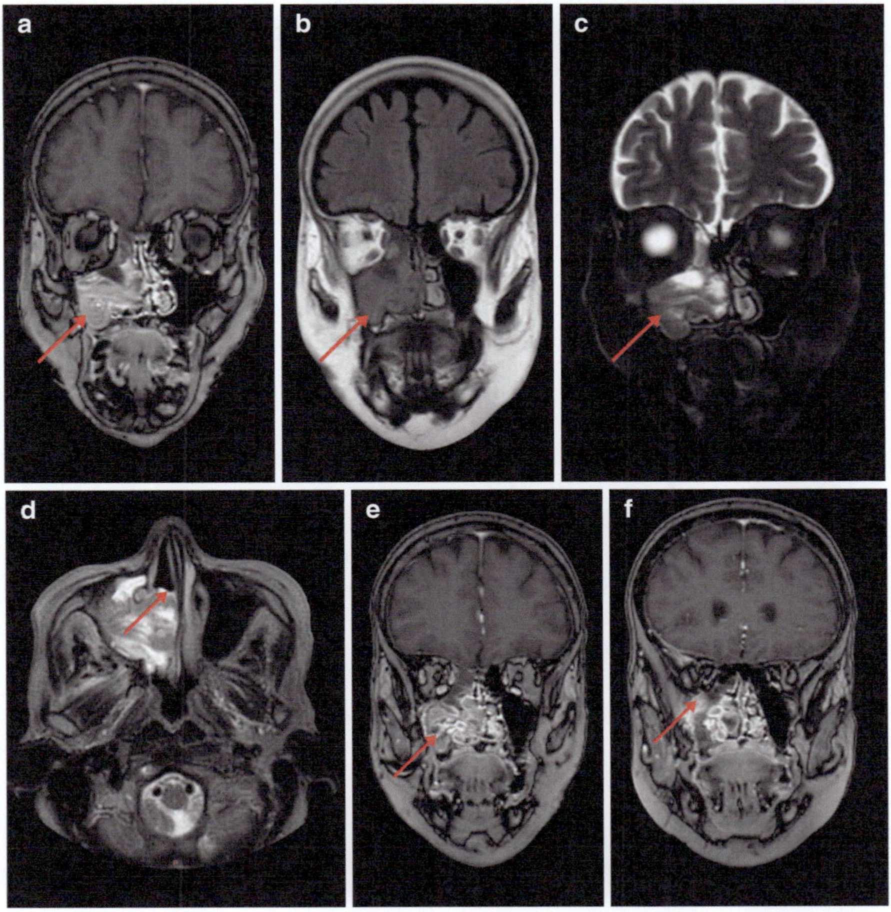

Fig. 8.1 A large lesion obstructs the right nasal cavity and posterior choana, extending through the osteo-meatal complex into and occupying the right maxillary sinus and focally extending to the right anterior ethmoidal air cells. The lesion has a convoluted cerebriform pattern on T2WI and contrast-enhanced T1WI, which is classical of inverted papilloma (it has transformed into SCC) which is: (1) Superiorly: Focally invading the bony floor of the right orbit at its posterior aspect, but there is no intra-orbital extension, and thus, a normal globe, ocular muscles and optic pathway are present. (2) Posteriorly: Infiltrating the sinus wall and focally invading the infra-temporal fossa and temporalis muscle, as well as abnormal signal intensity and enhancement at the origin of the lateral pterygoid muscle, suggesting infiltration during normal mandible and no invasion. (**a**: Coronal T1, **b**: Coronal T2 Flair, **c**: Coronal T2 Spair, **d**: Axial T2, **e** and **f**: Coronal T1 with Contrast)

the mass can evade and destroy the roof, anterior and lateral walls of the maxillary sinus, as well as its floor (Sheikh and Bickle 2017). Computed tomography (CT) scans can be of great help since they can help classify the tumour and determine its degree of resectability, as well as aid in the management plan (Kondo et al. 1986). Panoramic radiography can demonstrate the destruction of the walls of the maxillary sinus by the lesion, especially the inferior antral wall. Computed tomography (CT) scans and magnetic resonance imaging (MRI) are the imaging of choice for advanced lesions. This is primarily for their role in detecting the degree of invasion past the origin site (Vasudevan et al. 2012).

Histopathology

There are great similarities between the SCC of the maxillary sinus and those of the head and neck region in general. The degree of histological differentiation is not associated with the prognosis of the disease (Santos et al. 2014). Spindle and round epithelial cells can be observed on haematoxylin and eosin stains (Kondo et al. 1986). To further confirm the diagnosis, immunochemical staining can be performed for actin, desmin, cytokeratins, human epithelial membrane, HMB-45, and S-100. This can also be seen in Fig. 8.2.

Treatment

For tumours that have not metastasized and require local control, surgical excision is a good option, as it can also restore facial function and contour. However, no optimal management is available for advanced tumours since surgeries cannot provide appropriate loco-regional control. Furthermore, radiotherapy, even when combined with chemotherapy, does not provide promising results (Santos et al. 2014). The type of surgery is largely dependent on the stage of the tumour. For tumours of

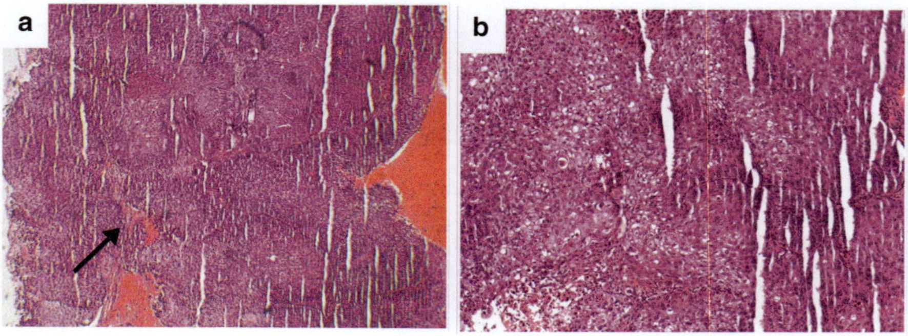

Fig. 8.2 Squamous cell carcinoma: This histopathological slide (**a**: 4×, **b**: 10×) demonstrates pieces of papillary growth (Arrow) that are lined by malignant squamous epithelial cells with large pleomorphic nuclei and prominent nucleoli

stages 1 and 2, the surgical approach is endoscopic medial wall maxillectomy type D, which can be seen in Fig. 8.3, whereas for tumours of stages 3 and 4, the Weber-Ferguson approach is preferred. Weber-Fergusson incision is used in total maxillectomy for tumours that are infiltrating the maxillary palate or lateral wall. It provides total exposure of the maxilla from the orbit to the upper alveolar ridge, permitting en bloc resection of maxillary tumours. The start of this facial incision is similar to that of a lateral rhinotomy, which then goes towards the philtrum in the middle and extends down towards the midline of the lip. This incision continues inferiorly along the gingivobuccal sulcus. From here, the incision extends laterally up towards the retromolar area. This is then followed by raising the cheek's soft tissue. For cases where the lateral and superior walls of the maxillary need to be approached, the infraorbital nerve and vessels should be transected. Lastly, an upper cheek flap is made that extends laterally and superiorly to reach both the inferior orbital rim and maxillary tuberosity, while inferiorly, it extends towards the pterygopalatine fossa (Fliss 2012).

Prognosis

Due to its aggressive nature and the fact that the lesion becomes advanced by the time the disease becomes symptomatic and is diagnosed, the survival rate decreases, and the prognosis is unfavourable (Santos et al. 2014). Lymph node metastasis is a

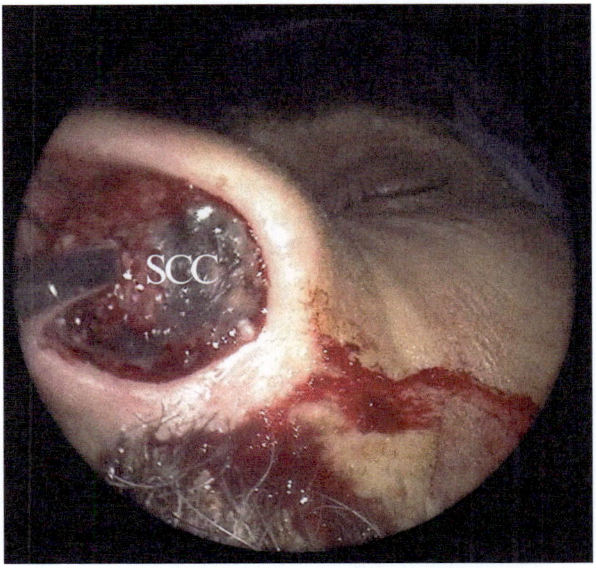

Fig. 8.3 This is an intraoperative video of a patient undergoing Endoscopic Sinus Surgery for squamous cell carcinoma (SCC). As can be seen in the thumbnail (right side nasal cavity), the mass has extended to the nostril (Audio 8.1)

great predictor of disease prognosis. Apart from their ominous prognosis, the rate of treatment failure is also high in these malignancies.

Differential Diagnosis

All primary sinonasal neoplasms within the maxillary sinus and other metastatic diseases need to be considered in the differential diagnosis. Examples of primary sinonasal neoplasms include undifferentiated sinonasal carcinoma, lymphoma, nasopharyngeal carcinoma, esthesioneuroblastoma, adenocarcinoma of minor salivary gland origin, and primary sinonasal melanoma (Vasudevan et al. 2012).

Adenocystic Carcinoma

Introduction

Adenocystic carcinoma is a slow-growing malignant tumour of the salivary gland. The tumour is uncommon, and it is characterized by features such as perineural spread, wide but local infiltration, and a tendency to recur following therapy (Chundru et al. 2013). It is rare for the tumour to occur in the maxillary sinus; however, it does have an inclination for distant metastasis when it does (Lahjaouj et al. 2021). It is thought that adenocystic carcinomas of the maxillary sinus arise from the mucosa of the paranasal sinus, more specifically, the seromucous glands (Li et al. 2021). Although the maxillary sinus carcinomas are described as slow-growing, they are still considered more aggressive than the adenocystic carcinomas of the minor and major salivary glands. This aggressive growth within the paranasal sinus is partly attributed to the fact the sinus is an air-spaced cavity in which the tumour can expand and the fact that the lesion can grow and spread in the submucosa of the sinus without showing any symptoms (Kim et al. 1999). Although rare, for patients complaining of pain, nasal obstruction, epistaxis, auditory symptoms, and a presenting nasal mass, the diagnosis of maxillary sinus adenocystic carcinoma should be considered (Gurung et al. 2022).

Epidemiology

The occurrence of this malignant lesion is uncommon, especially within the maxillary sinus. The lesion accounts for 20% of all salivary gland neoplasms (De Fátima et al. 2006). Adenocystic carcinoma of the maxillary sinus accounts for 0.3–1.0% of all sinonasal tumours (Rhee et al. 2006). The most common age group affected by the lesion are in the fifth to seventh decade. Although some studies implicate a female predominance, most do agree that both males and females are equally affected.

Aetiology and Pathophysiology

The exact aetiology and pathophysiology of this malignant tumour remains unknown to this day. Although adenocystic carcinoma is not considered hereditary, research does show that it can arise due to a genetic change that happens along the lifespan of an individual (De Fátima et al. 2006).

Clinical Features

Clinically, the tumour may appear as a small, indolent mass; however, this is deceptive since most of the early spread of the tumour is subclinical and does not cause any symptoms (Lahjaouj et al. 2021). This tumour can grow in an expansile form and invade minimum bone; however, it could also present with a destructive growth pattern and subsequently result in extensive bony defects (Andrade et al. 2014). Initially, this indolent growth could be mistaken for sinusitis or even allergic rhinitis since it presents with nasal obstruction, local pain, and epistaxis. As the tumour grows and extends further into the adjacent structure, the symptoms become more serious due to invasion of the orbit, pterygomaxillary fossa, meninges, and base of the cranium. With these advanced lesions, patients will often complain of ophthalmoplegia, ophthalmalgia, headache, and ocular proptosis, amongst others (Kato et al. 2013).

Radiographic Features

Multiple different modalities have been described to diagnose adenocystic carcinoma, ranging from imaging to Fine Needle Aspiration Examination (FNAC) and histopathological examination. The gold standard for diagnosis is computerized tomography (CT) scan and magnetic resonance imaging (MRI). CT scan is helpful as it can build a three-dimensional image to guide the surgeon in planning the surgical approach, whereas MRI can help showcase perineural invasion more (Gill and Frattali 2015). T2-weighted images can differentiate the cellularity of the tumours based on intensity, as hypointense tumours indicate a tumour with low cellularity, whereas a hyperintense tumour represents a tumour with high cellularity (Sigal et al. 1992). Imaging in general and CT scans specifically can show bony infiltration; however, it is difficult to distinguish benign and malignant lesions using imaging alone and make an appropriate diagnosis. It is for this reason that histopathological examinations are almost always ordered, as they help provide an ensuring diagnosis.

Histopathology

The tumour can be further subdivided histologically into a cribriform type, which is more differentiated (as seen in Fig. 8.4), and a solid form, which is less differentiated. The well-differentiated cribriform type will show darkly staining small islands

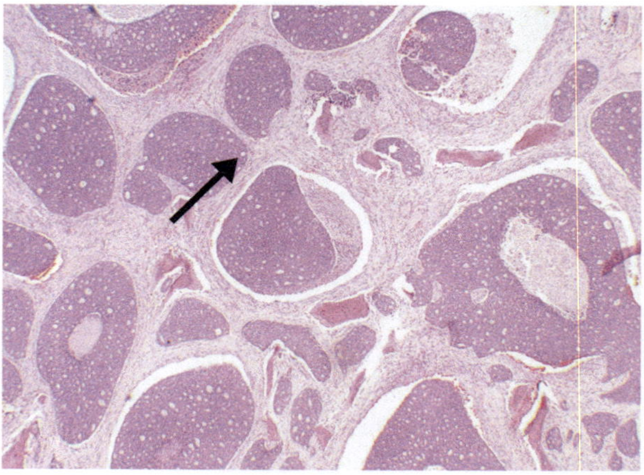

Fig. 8.4 Histopathological image of a glandular tumor composed of basaloid cells arranged in a cribriform pattern. H&E staining shows irregular nests and gland-like spaces. A black arrow indicates a cluster of tumor cells with characteristic architecture.

with minimal cytoplasm. This is in contrast to the hyperchromatic cells seen in the less differentiated solid form with indistinct borders and elevated mitotic activity (Lahjaouj et al. 2021). Based on histological appearance, the solid form is considered grade III. The cribriform grade II and grade I are reserved for a tubular subtype. All three subtypes do invade the perineural area; however, the grade III solid form has the worst prognosis, whereas the grade I has the best (Kato et al. 2013). Regarding adenocystic carcinomas of the maxillary sinus, the most common subtype is the grade II cribriform type, and the least common one is the grade III solid subtype (Rhee et al. 2006).

Treatment

Surgery, radiotherapy, chemotherapy, and combined therapy can all be considered as therapy for adenocystic carcinoma. Due to the broad subclinical expansion of the tumour that does not always appear on radiographic images, surgical excision is preferred with the widest possible margin (Chundru et al. 2013). In the setting of early presentation before much metastasis, endoscopic surgeries are preferred; however, this is not sufficient for advanced lesions as they require an open approach either a total or a partial maxillectomy. Apart from the extent of the tumour, other factors, such as the bone that has to be removed and the accessibility of the tumour, all dictate the surgical approach of choice. Endoscopic surgeries such as endoscopic sinus surgeries are the preferred approach for adenocystic carcinomas of the paranasal sinuses due to their minimal invasiveness (Li et al. 2021). It is difficult to aggressively approach the tumour and perform a complete excision with clean margins due to the complex anatomy surrounding the maxillary sinus. This is especially true since by the time the lesion generally presents, the dura, orbit, carotid arteries, brain, and cranial nerves are involved (Lahjaouj et al. 2021). With this being said, for surgeries to be successful, a tumour-free margin of at least 2 mm is required (Gill and Frattali 2015). The approach with the best overall survival and control of the tumour is surgery combined with radiotherapy (Michel et al. 2013).

Prognosis

Compared to other adenocystic carcinoma within the head and neck region, the long-term overall prognosis of maxillary sinus adenocystic carcinoma is worse. This is especially true for the grade III solid subtype. This worse prognosis of the lesion within the maxillary sinus could be attributed to its subclinical invasion and late detection. Furthermore, its surgical inaccessibility and lack of complete excision, along with its growth pattern, all contribute to this poor prognosis (Andrade et al. 2014). The overall 5-year survival for surgery with adjuvant therapy was 63%, whereas the overall disease-free 5-year was 43%.

Differential Diagnosis

Maxillary sinus adenocystic carcinoma should be considered with all sinonasal tumours whenever a patient presents with either a fleshy mass or a slow-growing swelling within or around the nose (Lahjaouj et al. 2021). Small cell neuroendocrine carcinoma, adenosquamous carcinoma, low-grade adenocarcinoma and basaloid squamous cell carcinoma are all among the differential diagnoses of adenocystic carcinoma (Rahmani et al. 2017).

Olfactory Neuroblastoma

Introduction

Olfactory neuroblastoma, also referred to as esthesioneuroblastoma, is a tumour arising from within the nasal cavity (National Cancer Institute). The neoplasm is rare, accounting for 3–6% of all sinonasal tumours (Tosoni et al. 2023). The lesion is known to arise from the neuroepithelium and to have neuroblastic differentiation. The common location for this tumour is the superior nasal cavity, including the superior nasal concha and the ethmoid bone, particularly the lamina cribrosa (Tosoni et al. 2023). Other locations for the neoplasm include the sphenopalatine ganglion, olfactory placode, the ganglion of loci, and autonomic ganglia of the nasal mucosa, among many others (Al-Osaimi et al. 2021). It is rare for the lesion to occur in areas such as the sphenoid sinus, sellar region, anterior ethmoid, pituitary gland, and maxillary sinus due to the lack of neuroepithelium (Holmes et al. 2016). A unilateral nasal obstruction followed by epistaxis is the most common presentation in patients (Al-Osaimi et al. 2021). The lesion has no gender predominance, and it occurs mostly in the sixth decade. Multidisciplinary care is required to properly manage olfactory neuroblastoma (Tosoni et al. 2023). This multi-discplinary approach will include surgery, chemotherapy, and radiotherapy, all combined.

Epidemiology

The tumour presents in 1 per 2.5 million persons each year, accounting for 3–6% of sinonasal tumours (National Cancer Institute 2024). There has been no report of any of the genders predominating. Regarding age, the neoplasm follows a bimodal age distribution, with the majority of the cases occurring within either the second or the sixth decade of life (Tosoni et al. 2023). The median age of the disease is 51.4 years. Ever since its first-ever report in 1924, there have been more than 1000 cases (Arnold et al. 2009). Interestingly, 85% of the patients present with advanced stages of olfactory neuroblastoma had low socioeconomic status. Patients with a lower socioeconomic status also suffered from more mortality (Sharma et al. 2022). These could be due to the lack of appropriate management and care in these patients, especially multidisciplinary care that is required in olfactory neuroblastoma.

Aetiology and Pathophysiology

The exact aetiology of olfactory neuroblastoma, like many other cancers, is not fully understood. Olfactory neuroblastoma does not run in families and is not hereditary; however, scientists have found genetic associations for the lesion. Certain parts of DNA on chromosomes 2, 5, 6, 7, and 20 might have an association with the development of the tumour (National Cancer Institute 2024).

Clinical Features

The neoplasm is locally aggressive and tends to metastasize in 20–48% of the patients. The cervical lymph nodes, accounting for 20–48% of the cases, are the typical site of metastasis. Other areas prone to metastasis are the bones and the lungs (Fiani et al. 2019). The tumour can extend to involve adjacent local structures such as the skull base and orbits. Olfactory neuroblastoma, when symptomatic, mainly presents with nasal obstruction and epistaxis. Other common symptoms, but all to a lesser extent, include anosmia, headache, pain, rhinorrhea, and excessive lacrimation. Furthermore, visual disturbances such as diplopia and proptosis could also occur (Dulguerov et al. 2001). Diagnosis can be delayed as symptoms are not always so obvious and can present similarly to inflammation (Holmes et al. 2016). It usually takes 6–12 months from the onset of symptoms to diagnosis (Tosoni et al. 2023). The growth pattern of the neoplasm has great variations. The tumour could have indolent growth and survival of up to 20 years and more but could also have an aggressive growth pattern with early metastatic spread, lowering the survival to months (Dulguerov et al. 2001). It is for this reason that apart from accurate diagnosis is necessary for olfactory blastoma, and it is essential to determine the stage and grade of the neoplasm (Holmes et al. 2016).

Radiographic Features

The most characteristic radiological finding of olfactory neuroblastoma is a "dumb-bell-shaped" mass observed across the cribriform plate. To evaluate the characteristics of the mass and possibly determine the stage, computed tomography (CT) scan and magnetic resonance imaging (MRI) are preferred. CT scan is better at indicating the bony Involvement of the mass, whereas MRI is preferred for assessing orbital and intracranial infiltration (Tosoni et al. 2023). Positron emission tomography (PET) scan can help better evaluate the tumour. For lesions within the maxillary sinus, a CT scan can demonstrate soft tissue thickening that will appear hypermetabolic on a PET scan (Holmes et al. 2016). The CT scan can also show the bony erosions within the maxillary sinus. Full-body CT and PET scans can be performed to show the extent of the spread of the disease (Bradley et al. 2003). No matter the findings on imaging, it is mandatory to perform a biopsy to confirm the diagnosis of olfactory neuroblastoma (Tosoni et al. 2023).

Histopathology

Without appropriate clinical knowledge, molecular techniques, and immunohistochemical markers, it is difficult to diagnose olfactory osteoblastoma by the pathologist. This is primarily due to the different histological types of the mass and the small amount of biopsy material available (Tosoni et al. 2023). Olfactory neuroblastoma will have cells with small round nuclei and sheets of punctate chromatin within a neurofibrillary stroma (Holmes et al. 2016). Other findings observed histologically in this lesion are Homer Wright and Flexner-Wintersteiner rosettes. Biomarkers such as CD-56, S-100, chromogranin, synaptophysin, and Neuron-Specific-Haemolysis (NSE) are all considered necessary and of great help in the diagnosis; however, they do not pose any prognostic determination (Tosoni et al. 2023).

Treatment

Due to the lack of randomized control trials, there is no standard treatment approach for olfactory neuroblastoma (Abdelmeguid 2018). However, less invasive Kadish A and B stages of the tumour are generally approached endoscopically (see Fig. 11.5), whereas open approaches are reserved for more advanced stages (Devaiah and Andreoli 2009). Kadish stage C can be approached endoscopically, but only if negative margins can be confident. For stage C Kadish tumours that have extended into the orbit or have spread laterally to reach the orbital axis, hard/soft palate or the midface, an open approach should be performed (Higgins et al. 2011). For cases of intracranial extension, due to the anatomical barriers present, both intracranial and extracranial approaches can be combined; however, due to the evolution in endoscopic procedures and their ability to showcase the suprasellar region, these open approaches have become less popular. Surgery, when combined with radiation therapy, whether neoadjuvant or adjuvant, has been shown to provide superior local control than when used alone. The local control with surgery alone was 17%, whereas when surgery was combined with radiotherapy, the rate increased to 86% (Faragalla and Weinreb 2009). Combination therapy becomes very crucial in cases where negative margins cannot be obtained (Meyer et al. 2017). Different chemotherapy approaches, such as induction chemotherapy, adjuvant chemotherapy or concomitant chemotherapy, can all be used. Induction chemotherapy mainly aims to reduce the risk of distant metastasis and preserve critical organs such as the eyes and the brain. Concomitant chemotherapy with radiotherapy is best utilized for cases where local recurrence poses an issue, whereas adjuvant chemotherapy is reserved for tumours with a high-grade stage (Meyer et al. 2017).

Prognosis

The overall survival rate of olfactory neuroblastoma is 55–90%; however, this varies based on many factors but primarily, the stage of the disease (National Cancer Institute), involvement of the nodes, which occurs in approximately 20% of all patients, is the greatest factor for predicting the prognosis (Tosoni et al. 2023). Compared to other sinonasal tumours, the overall prognosis is deemed high. The 5-year survival of the tumour is approximately 63%, and the progression-free survival is 57%.

Differential Diagnosis

Olfactory neuroblastoma needs to be considered, along with the extensive list of malignant tumours of the nasal cavity. The most common one is squamous cell carcinoma, accounting for 55% of all malignant tumours. This is followed by non-epithelial neoplasms and many other less frequently occurring malignancies. These include but are not limited to rhabdomyosarcoma, mucosa, mucosal melanoma, adenocarcinoma, sinonasal undifferentiated carcinoma, and extranodal NK/T-cell lymphoma (Faragalla and Weinreb 2009).

Maxillary Sinus Lymphoma

Introduction

Lymphoma is a cancer of abnormal proliferation of leukocytes originating from the lymphatic system. Broadly, lymphoma is classified into Hodgkin's and non-Hodgkin's lymphoma (Cancer Council 2024). Approximately, 40% of non-Hodgkin's lymphoma are extranodal; however, it is uncommon for primary non-Hodgkin's to arise from the paranasal sinuses (Usuda et al. 2021). The most common subtype of non-Hodgkin lymphoma is diffuse-large-B-cell lymphoma, which is a fast-growing malignancy. Although the aetiology is not fully understood, both immunosuppression and viruses have been hypothesized to play a role (Bhattacharya et al. 2013). A soft tissue mass can be identified within the nasal cavity. The mass will, to some degree, have bony Involvement; however, this is neither as aggressive nor as lytic as squamous cell carcinoma (DePeña et al. 1990). A quickly enlarging mass resulting in both local and systemic manifestations is the most common complaint of presenting patients. A combination of different chemotherapeutic drugs is the therapeutic approach used by the majority of patients. Unless the diagnosis is made in the early stages, the prognosis is not favourable, especially in older patients with stages 3 and 4 of the disease that have extranodal Involvement (Bhattacharya et al. 2013).

Epidemiology

Non-Hodgkin's lymphomas are the dominant type of lymphoma, accounting for roughly 90% of the cases. Among those, approximately 40% of non-Hodgkin's lymphoma are extranodal, and among those, the majority are in the stomach, liver, soft tissue and dura, among others (Usuda et al. 2021). It is uncommon for primary non-Hodgkin's lymphoma to occur in the paranasal sinuses as it accounts for 0.17% of all lymphomas and 8% of all paranasal malignancies (Usuda et al. 2021; Yasumoto et al. 2000). Among the paranasal sinuses, the maxillary sinus is the most frequently involved (Yasumoto et al. 2000). The nasal cavity is the most common primary site in patients from Asian/Pacific islands, whereas in Caucasian patients, the most common site becomes the maxillary sinus (Goel et al. 2016). The median age of patients affected by non-Hodgkin's lymphoma is 67 years.

Aetiology

No exact cause has been established for non-Hodgkin's lymphoma, but many in the literature emphasize viral and immunodeficiency aetiology. Among the infectious causes, Epstein–Barr virus, Human T-cell leukaemia virus, Hepatitis C virus, Human Herpesvirus 8, and Helicobacter pylori are all considered to contribute to the aetiology of non-Hodgkin's lymphoma. Apart from infections, other agents hypothesized to be involved are chemicals such as pesticides and phenoxy-herbicides and drugs such as phenytoin and TNF antagonists. Furthermore, any state of immunodeficiency is also considered a risk factor for the development of this lymphoma. This includes both congenital immunodeficiency disorders such as Wiskott-Aldrich syndrome and Severe Combined Immunodeficiency Disorder (SCID) and autoimmune disorders such as Sjögren syndrome and rheumatoid arthritis (Sapkota and Shaikh 2023).

Clinical Presentation

In cases of primary diffuse-large-B-cell-lymphoma originating from the maxillary sinus, the most common presenting complaint is a unilateral, slightly painful swelling of the maxilla. This could be accompanied by local symptoms such as nasal obstruction, nasal stuffiness, mucopurulent rhinorrhoea, recurrent epistaxis, diplopia, and the complaint of a rapidly enlarging mass. Moreover, the mass could also pose systemic symptoms such as weight loss, recurrent night sweats, and fever (Usuda et al. 2021). Although not common, the mass can present with no pain in certain patients and can even result in persistent toothache and palatal ulcer (Adouly et al. 2015; Yoon et al. 2001). The majority of these symptoms are non-specific and only indicate sinonasal obstruction; however, the unilateral presentation could possibly suggest malignancy (Adouly et al. 2015).

Diagnosis and Imaging

By the time of detection, a bulky mass occupying the maxillary sinus and its adjacent structure can be observed on CT scans (as seen in Fig. 8.5a). CT scans are excellent for detecting the bony changes associated with the tumour, whereas MRI scans (as shown in Fig. 8.5b) are considered the best for demonstrating the extent of spread due to their enhanced soft tissue definition (DePeña et al. 1990). According to a radiographic imaging review conducted by Peng et al., the most common imaging finding in DLBCL of the maxillary sinus is the presence of a discrete mass in 59% of the patients. This is followed by sinus opacification in 53% of the patients and bony erosions in 35% (Peng et al. 2014). Since MRI is more sensitive, it could detect focal haemorrhage in rare instances where it might be present (Yasumoto et al. 2000). Finally, the PET CT appearance of lymphomas is shown in Fig. 8.5c.

Histology/Histopathology

On hematoxylin and eosin stains, diffuse proliferation of large neoplastic B cells can be observed with large nuclei (Song 2016). Furthermore, immunochemical analysis can aid in the diagnosis and differentiate the tumour from other histologically similar tumours. It possesses high CD20 immunoreactivity in immunochemistry (Adouly et al. 2015). Other studies have stated that the masses are positive for vimentin, CD3, and CD45 (Song 2016).

Treatment and Prognosis

Radiotherapy and chemotherapy are the two main approaches of choice for non-Hodgkin's lymphoma of the maxillary sinus (Adouly et al. 2015). Radiotherapy is used for massive tumours, provided that the tumour is in its early stages. In the

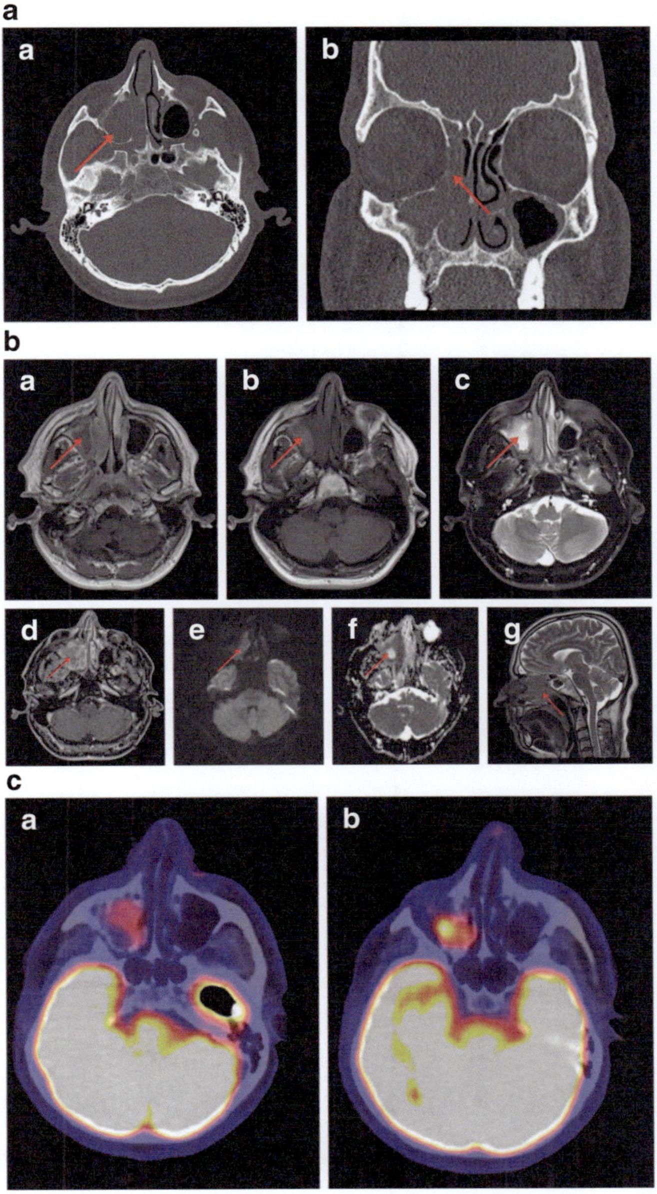

Fig. 8.5 (**a**–**c**) Evidence of an infiltrative soft tissue mass lesion centred at and obstructing the right nasal cavity (**a**), extending through the right osteo-meatal complex, infiltrating along the walls of the RT maxillary sinus as well as the ethmoidal air cells, which is hypointense on T2WI & T1WI (**b**: a: Axial T1 with contrast, b: Axial T1 without contrast, c: Axial T2, d: Axial T1 with Contrast and Fat Suppression, e: Axial DWI, f: Axial ADC, g: Sagittal T2), restricted on DWI and showed enhancement after contrast, PET (**c**: **a** and **b**) avid caused multifocal erosions of the right lamina papyracea and right orbital floor with extra-conal focal extension

majority of patients, initial chemotherapy is a combination. Regarding prognosis, unless the patient is older than 60 and the tumour is stage 3 or 4 with extranodal involvement, the prognosis is considered favourable. Therefore, the earlier the diagnosis is, the more likely it is for the patient to have a good prognosis (Bhattacharya et al. 2013). Following treatment, continuous close monitoring and follow-up is advisable. An endoscopic approach to maxillary sinus lymphoma can be seen in Fig. 8.6.

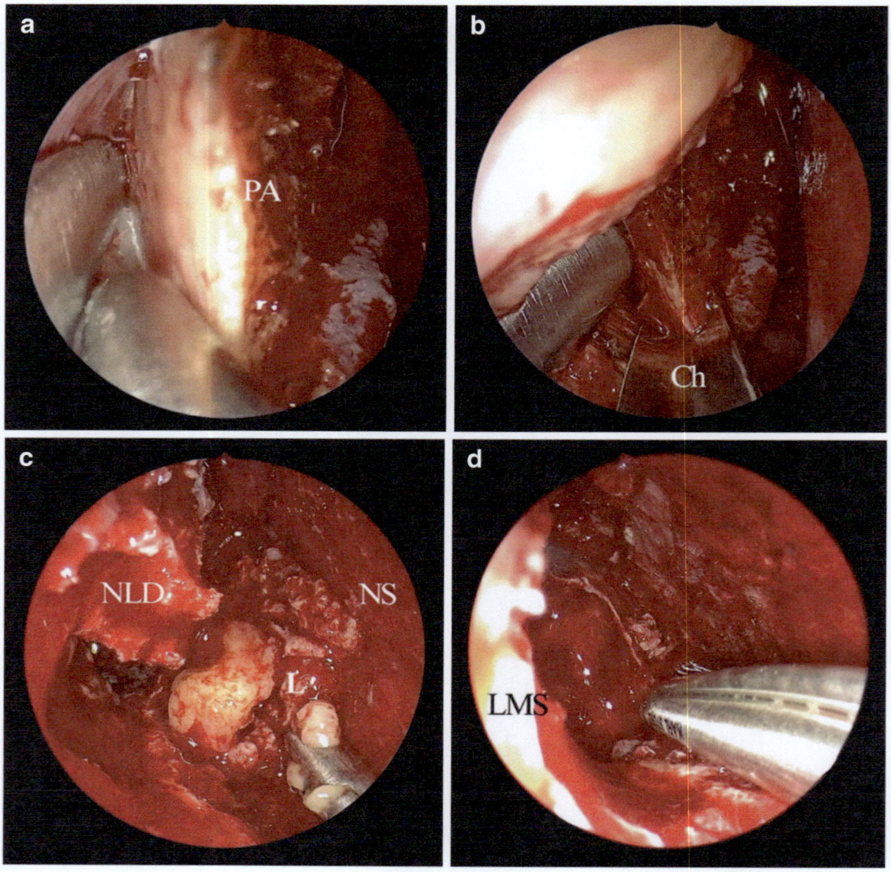

Fig. 8.6 This is an intraoperative video of a patient undergoing Endoscopic Sinus Surgery for a lymphoma. As can be seen in the thumbnails (left side nasal cavity), (**a**) exposing the pyriform aperture and preparing the area for endoscopic medial wall maxillectomy type D (by Brescia group classification), (**b**) removing the pyriform aperture by chisel and hammer, (**c**) removing the lymphoma from the maxillary sinus, and (**d**) inside of the maxillary sinus showing clearance of the tumour. (*PA* pyriform aperture, *Ch* chisel, *NLD* remnant of nasolacrimal duct, *L* lymphoma, *NS* nasal septum, *LMS* lateral wall of the maxillary sinus) (Audio 8.2 and Video 8.1)

Differential Diagnosis

Clinically, the tumour is similar to the common malignancies of the oral cavity. These include the likes of squamous cell carcinoma and minor salivary gland tumours. One feature that helps distinguish between squamous cell carcinoma and maxillary sinus lymphoma is the submucosal growth. Furthermore, squamous cell carcinoma has an ulcerative gross appearance (Bhattacharya et al. 2013). The clinical entity can also help differentiate inflammatory processes from neoplastic ones (Usuda et al. 2021). Despite being very rare, it is advisable for non-Hodgkin's lymphomas to be considered among the differential diagnoses of nasal cavity lesions (Adouly et al. 2015).

Rare Malignant Lesion of the Maxillary Sinus

Introduction

By the time malignant lesions of the maxillary sinus are present, they are usually advanced and have involved the surrounding structures. Due to the wide variety of malignant lesions that can present within the sinus, many different treatments exist. The therapeutic approach depends on the type of tumour, its extension and the areas involved (Dierks 1999). Apart from the lesions previously talked about in the previous chapters, there have been various reports of other lesions of the sinus. Among the many others are malignant epithelial tumours of the maxillary sinus, such as squamous cell carcinoma and adenocarcinoma. Furthermore, malignant soft tissue tumours such as rhabdomyosarcoma, fibrosarcoma, malignant fibrous histiocytoma, and leiomyosarcoma, although rare, have all been reported before (Bracigliano et al. 2021). The clinical signs and symptoms are shared largely by most malignant maxillary sinus tumours. According to Bashir et al., nasal obstruction, facial swelling, paraesthesia, and epistaxis are among the most frequently occurring early symptoms, whereas the presence of a palpable mass, lymphadenopathy, and diplopia are among the most common late clinical presentations of malignant maxillary sinus tumours (Bashir et al. 2023).

Adenocarcinoma

Arising from the glandular structures of epithelial tissue is a malignant tumour referred to as adenocarcinoma. Cancer can arise from many different parts of the body, and the aetiology of the cancer changes based on the site of the tumour. Although the etiologies vary, tobacco smoking seems to play a role in the majority of them. The breast, prostate, lung, and the gastrointestinal tract are among the common locations for the carcinoma. Regarding the sinonasal tract, adenocarcinoma, accounting for 10–15% of the cases, is the second most common malignancy after squamous cell carcinoma (Choi 2024). Within the maxillary sinus, adenocarcinoma is very rarely reported. According to Fukuda et al., who investigated the rareness of adenocarcinoma in the maxillary sinus relative to squamous cell carcinoma in the Japanese population, factors such as extensive use of softwood and high level of chronic rhinosinusitis play a role in this difference in prevalence (Fukuda et al. 1989). Both surgical means and radiotherapy are used in the treatment of adenocarcinoma of the nasal cavity and the paranasal sinuses (Canadian Cancer Society 2020).

Mucosal Melanoma

Melanoma is a form of cutaneous cancer that originates from melanocytes (Mayo Clinic 2023). A rare subtype of melanoma arising from the mucous membranes of the body, such as those lining the mouth, nose, and throat, among others, is referred to as mucosal melanoma (Cleveland Clinic 2024). Mucosal melanomas of the sinonasal tract account for 1% of all melanomas and 4% of all sinonasal tumours (Ascierto et al. 2017). The lesion has no gender predominance and most commonly occurs in the seventh decade of life. Unless there is pigmentation, it is difficult to diagnose mucosal melanomas of the maxillary sinus (Gautam et al. 2022). Furthermore, the maxillary sinus is the least frequent site for the tumour, in contrast to the nasal cavity, which is the most common (Bachar et al. 2008). The diagnosis can be confirmed with immunohistochemical and histopathological examination. Whether or not pigmentation is present, melanoma should be considered and examined whenever an intranasal mass with rapid progression exists. Due to its high vascularity, the cancer has an aggressive characteristic and can metastasize. The majority of patients present with epistaxis along with nasal congestion. The macroscopic image of the tumour is a dark mass with polypoidal growth. Imaging modalities such as computed tomography (CT) and magnetic resonance imaging (MRI) are used to investigate possible bony involvements; however, histopathological examination is required to help with the diagnosis (Gautam et al. 2022). In histology, the presence of melanin pigmentation can guide the diagnosis. Furthermore, positive immunohistochemical stains such as S100 and HMB-45 can aid in the diagnosis, especially since they are positive even in lesions without melanin pigmentation. The therapeutic approach used as first-line treatment is wide surgical resection until a negative margin is reached. However, despite aggressive therapeutic approaches, the malignancy has an undesirable prognosis with a 5-year survival rate of 12–30% (Gautam et al. 2022).

Rhabdomyosarcoma

It is a malignant tumour of striated muscle arising from the primitive mesenchymal tissues. The satellite cells that play a role in skeletal muscle embryogenesis have been hypothesized as the origin of the lesion (Lund et al. 2013). The malignant tumour accounts for 8–19% of all soft tissue sarcomas and approximately 40% of the head and neck region sarcomas (Grieman et al. 1988). The tumour is more common in children. The majority of the tumours are in the paranasal sinus; however, the maxillary sinus is the least common sinus (Grieman et al. 1988). The three major subtypes of rhabdomyosarcoma are embryonal, alveolar, and pleomorphic (Lund et al. 2013). Due to the rapid growth and aggressive characteristics, the tumour presents with a wide range of presentations, such as pain, facial swelling, nasal obstruction, proptosis, headache, and paresthesia, among others. Invasion into adjacent structures such as the pterygomaxillary region, orbit, and skull base is common with rhabdomyosarcoma. Although histological examination does help with the diagnosis, it is not always sufficient and can be misleading (Grieman et al. 1988). Therefore, immunohistochemical stains such as desmin, muscle-specific actin, and skeletal muscle-specific myo-regulatory protein can provide valuable insight (Lund et al. 2013). Treatment with surgery alone is only sufficient if negative margins can be obtained without resulting in significant morbidity. However, tumours presenting late with extensions attaining negative margins with surgery alone becomes more challenging. A case of sinonasal rhabdomyosarcoma with maxillary sinus extension can be seen in Fig. 8.7. Therefore, a combination of surgery, chemotherapy, and radiotherapy is generally preferred for rhabdomyosarcomas (Thompson et al. 2013).

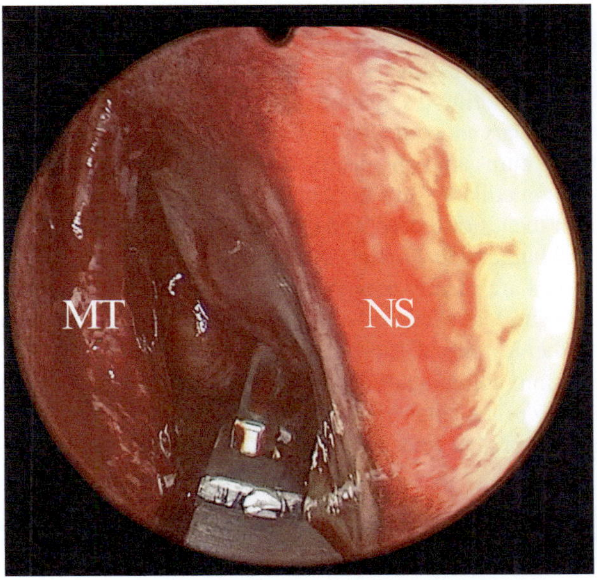

Fig. 8.7 This is an intraoperative video of a patient undergoing Endoscopic Sinus Surgery for rhabdomyosarcoma extending to the maxillary sinus. As can be seen in the thumbnail (left side nasal cavity), maxillary sinusotomy is done to remove the tumour. (*NS* nasal septum, *MT* middle turbinate) (Audio 8.3 and Video 8.2)

Spindle Cell Carcinoma

This tumour is a mixture of squamous cell carcinoma combined with larger malignant spindle cells. Although the spindle cells have a mesenchymal appearance, they have an epithelial origin, making them more prone to misdiagnosis (Lund et al. 2013). It is highly aggressive and occurs mostly in the glottic region of the larynx, rarely occurring in the sinonasal complex, especially within the maxillary sinus (AlNoury 2014; Lund et al. 2013). There is a male predominance with a mean age of 54.3 years. Unilateral nasal obstruction is the most common presentation. The mass has a polypoid shape on examination. Histologically, the lesion is commonly referred to as sarcomatoid. The main component dominating is the spindle cell pattern, whereas the squamous portion can be either intrusive or in situ. Regarding treatment, due to the limited number of cases reported, no standardized treatment has been established. The majority of the tumours are surgically excised, with some cases requiring further treatment with radiotherapy and chemotherapy. Regardless of the therapeutic approach of choice, the prognosis of the lesion is not favourable (Lund et al. 2013).

Mucoepidermoid Carcinoma

Mucoepidermoid carcinoma is a tumour of the minor salivary gland. The lesion very rarely occurs in the maxillary sinus, and it is characterized by epidermoid, mucus-secreting intermediate cells (Lund et al. 2013; Simpson et al. 1988). Extension to adjacent structures is common, and no definite aetiology has been established. Mucoepidermoid carcinoma accounts for 13% of all maxillary sinus malignant lesions (Daryani et al. 2012).

Although the features are non-specific on histology, it is possible to see complete obliteration of the maxillary sinus in radiology due to the growth of the tumour. The aggressiveness of the lesion varies, and the tumour is histologically divided into low, intermediate, and high grade. Goblet cells predominate low-grade tumours, whereas high-grade tumours are mainly composed of squamous cells. The main therapeutic approach is wide surgical excision. Although the tumour is not very radiosensitive, additional radiotherapy has still been attempted (Lund et al. 2013). The overall prognosis of the carcinoma is not desirable. Many attribute this to the location and the close proximity of the sinus to vital adjacent structures, such as the orbit and the skull base, making surgical resection more challenging (Daryani et al. 2012).

Fibrosarcoma

Any malignant mesenchymal tumour where the proliferating cells resemble that of normal fibroblasts is referred to as fibrosarcoma. The term mostly holds a historical value as the majority of the tumours that were considered fibrosarcoma are now reclassified to other lesions such as leiomyosarcoma, rhabdomyosarcoma, and peripheral nerve sheath tumours, among others (Lund et al. 2013). Fibrosarcomas of the nasal cavity and the paranasal sinuses are very rare. The lesion mostly occurs in males and presents within the third to fourth decade of life (Ekinci et al. 2018). Due to its rarity, very limited information is available on the lesion. Although its aetiology is yet to be established, irradiation has been suggested to play a role. Most of the patients with this tumour complain of nasal obstruction that may or may not be associated with epistaxis. Furthermore, for lesions within the sinus, signs and symptoms such as facial mass and swelling, tooth loosening, facial numbness, and proptosis can also be present (Lund et al. 2013). Similarly to the other malignant paranasal sinuses, there is no characteristic specific to fibrosarcoma on imaging. Regarding its histological appearance, the tumours appear as a well-circumscribed mass with no capsule. Based on the grade of the tumour, varying degrees of infiltration is observed. Different amounts of collagen are visualized, separating compact fascicles of spindle cells. Surgery remains the primary mode of treatment. With recent advancements, endoscopic surgeries have taken over for more conventional techniques. Resection by pieces is advised over en bloc resection (Ekinci et al. 2018). Assuming the lesion is low-grade and has remained localized, the prognosis is relatively better, with the overall long-term survival being 75% (Lund et al. 2013).

Leiomyosarcoma

Leiomyosarcoma is a rare malignant tumour that mostly presents within the uterine myometrium, followed by the gastrointestinal tract. The tumour is a mesenchymal tumour of smooth muscle cells that rarely presents within the head and neck region (Lund et al. 2013). Not only do they make up 6.5% of all sarcomas, but only 3.5% of them are of the head and neck region (Sah et al. 2018). Like other sarcomas, leiomyosarcoma has been linked to prior irradiation exposure, along with cyclophosphamide. Although the mean age is 52 years, the age of patients ranges from 18 to 75 years. On examination, the tumour can be described as either bulky, polypoidal or nodular. Similar to other paranasal malignancies, the tumour presents with obstruction and epistaxis. Although there are no specific characteristics on imaging, the lesion can show significant bony destruction on imaging (Lund et al. 2013). Varying degrees of infiltration can be histologically observed based on the grade of the tumour. Another valuable tool used for the diagnosis is immunohistochemistry. Among the commonly positive stains are vimentin, actin, desmin and calponin. Complete resection of the tumour with a clean margin of at least 1 cm is advisable. Although radical resection is preferred, this is not always possible due to the vital adjacent structures (Sah et al. 2018).

Extramedullary Plasmacytoma of the Maxillary Sinus

Plasmacytoma is a malignant tumour of monoclonal plasma cell accumulation. If localized to the bone marrow, the tumour is referred to as solitary bone plasmacytoma

(Jeyaraj et al. 2015). Localized aggregation of monoclonal plasma cells in an extraskeletal site is called extramedullary plasmacytoma (Megat Shiraz et al. 2008). It is very rare for the tumour to occur in the head and neck region and more specifically, in the maxillary sinus. Either via a bone marrow examination, bone scan, serum, and urine electrophoresis, it is crucial to rule out multiple myeloma before making the diagnosis of extramedullary plasmacytoma (Chandrasekharan et al. 2015). The average age of diagnosis is 55 years, and the tumour has a 3:1 male to female gender predominance. For tumours of the sinonasal region, the presenting signs and symptoms will mostly include nasal obstruction and a nasal mass. To confirm the diagnosis of extramedullary plasmacytoma, magnetic resonance imaging, flow cytometry, and polymerase chain reaction is required. Histological analysis should demonstrate monoclonal plasma cells while the bone marrow plasma cell infiltration must exceed 5% of all nucleated cells. Since the majority of plasma cell neoplasms are highly radiosensitive, the treatment of choice is radiation therapy while the role of surgery is limited to biopsy and resection of any remaining tumour following other therapeutic approaches (Jeyaraj et al. 2015).

References

Abdelmeguid AS (2018) Olfactory neuroblastoma. Curr Oncol Rep 20. https://doi.org/10.1007/s11912-018-0661-6

Adouly T, Adnane C, Oubahmane T et al (2015) Uncommon presentation of non-Hodgkin's lymphoma of maxillary sinus: a case report. Am J Med Case Rep 3:410–412. https://doi.org/10.12691/ajmcr-3-12-7

AlNoury MK (2014) Management of spindle cell carcinoma of the maxillary sinus: a case report and literature review. Am J Case Rep 15:454–458. https://doi.org/10.12659/ajcr.891007

Al-Osaimi SM, Hameed AA, Alsufyani AA et al (2021) Olfactory neuroblastoma managed with endoscopic sinus surgery. J Pharm Bioallied Sci 13:1728. https://doi.org/10.4103/jpbs.jpbs_62_21

Andrade MF, De Faria PR, Cardoso SV et al (2014) Adenoid cystic carcinoma of the maxillary sinus: a clinical–pathological report of 10 years of experience from a single institution. Int J Oral Maxillofac Surg 43:1313–1318. https://doi.org/10.1016/j.ijom.2014.06.016

Arnold PM, Habib A, Newell K, Anderson KK (2009) Esthesioneuroblastoma metastatic to the thoracic intradural and extradural space. Spine J 9:e1–e5. https://doi.org/10.1016/j.spinee.2008.08.010

Ascierto PA, Accorona R, Botti G et al (2017) Mucosal melanoma of the head and neck. Crit Rev Oncol Hematol 112:136–152. https://doi.org/10.1016/j.critrevonc.2017.01.019

Bachar G, Loh KS, O'Sullivan B et al (2008) Mucosal melanomas of the head and neck: the Princess Margaret Hospital experience. Head Neck 30:1325–1331. https://doi.org/10.1002/hed.20878

Bashir A, Khan ZA, Maqsood A et al (2023) The evaluation of clinical signs and symptoms of malignant tumours involving the maxillary sinus: recommendation of an examination sieve and risk alarm score. Healthcare 11:194. https://doi.org/10.3390/healthcare11020194

Bhattacharya A, Adwani D, Arora R, Bhagat B (2013) Non-Hodgkin's lymphoma of maxillary sinus: an unusual presentation. Ann Maxillofac Surg 3:95. https://doi.org/10.4103/2231-0746.110079

Sah BP, Chettri ST, Karki S, Shah SP, Manandhar S, Jaiswal RK (2018) Leiomyosarcoma of maxillary sinus – a rare clinical entity. Heighpubs Otolaryngol Rhinol 2:001–005

Bracigliano A, Tatangelo F, Perri F et al (2021) Malignant sinonasal tumours: update on histological and clinical management. Curr Oncol 28:2420–2438. https://doi.org/10.3390/curroncol28040222

Bradley PJ, Jones NS, Robertson I (2003) Diagnosis and management of esthesioneuroblastoma. Curr Opin Otolaryngol Head Neck Surg 11:112–118. https://doi.org/10.1097/00020840-200304000-00009

Cancer Council (2024) Lymphoma | causes, symptoms & treatments. https://www.cancer.org.au/cancer-information/types-of-cancer/lymphoma. Accessed 31 Jul 2024

Chandrasekharan R, Ashish G, Parmar H (2015) A rare case of sinonasal extramedullary plasmacytoma with orbital involvement. Int J Head Neck Surg 6:121–124. https://doi.org/10.5005/jp-journals-10001-1239

Choi KY (2024) Malignant tumours of the sinuses: practice essentials, epidemiology, etiology. https://emedicine.medscape.com/article/847189-overview?form=fpf#a1

Chundru NSV, Amudala R, Thankappan P, Nagaraju CD (2013) Adenoid cystic carcinoma of palate: a case report and review of literature. Dent Res J 10:274. https://doi.org/10.4103/1735-3327.113372

Cleveland Clinic (2024) Mucosal melanoma: a rare cancer that affects your mucous membrane. https://my.clevelandclinic.org/health/diseases/24643-mucosal-melanoma. Accessed 31 Jul 2024

Daryani D, Gopakumar R, Nagaraja A (2012) High-grade mucoepidermoid carcinoma of maxillary sinus. J Oral Maxillofac Pathol 16:137. https://doi.org/10.4103/0973-029x.92993

De Fátima Bernardes V, Cardoso SV, Mesquita RA et al (2006) Carcinoma adenóide cístico sólido em palato e seio maxilar. Rev Bras Otorrinolaringol 72:573. https://doi.org/10.1590/s0034-72992006000400023

DePeña CA, Van Tassel P, Lee Y-Y (1990) Lymphoma of the head and neck. https://www.semanticscholar.org/paper/Lymphoma-of-the-head-and-neck.-DePe%C3%B1a-Tassel/580ef0aea4250cbf4c36050af1ce9c9ffe327351

Devaiah AK, Andreoli MT (2009) Treatment of esthesioneuroblastoma: a 16-year meta-analysis of 361 patients. Laryngoscope 119:1412–1416. https://doi.org/10.1002/lary.20280

Dierks EJ (1999) Treatment of malignant tumours of the maxillary sinus. Oral Maxillofac Surg Clin North Am 11:125–136. https://doi.org/10.1016/s1042-3699(20)30289-2

Du Cancer CCS/SC (2020) Cancerous tumours of the nasal cavity and paranasal sinuses. Canadian Cancer Society. https://cancer.ca/en/cancer-information/cancer-types/nasal-and-paranasal-sinus/what-is-nasal-cavity-and-paranasal-sinus-cancer/cancerous-tumours#:~:text=the%20salivary%20gland.-

Dubal PM, Bhojwani A, Patel TD et al (2015) Squamous cell carcinoma of the maxillary sinus: a population-based analysis. Laryngoscope 126:399–404. https://doi.org/10.1002/lary.25601

Dulguerov P, Allal AS, Calcaterra TC (2001) Esthesioneuroblastoma: a meta-analysis and review. Lancet Oncol 2:683–690. https://doi.org/10.1016/s1470-2045(01)00558-7

Ekinci A, Karataş D, Yetiş A et al (2018) Destructive fibrosarcoma of the maxillary sinus. J Craniofac Surg 29:e226–e228. https://doi.org/10.1097/scs.0000000000004173

Faragalla H, Weinreb I (2009) Olfactory neuroblastoma. Adv Anat Pathol 16:322–331. https://doi.org/10.1097/pap.0b013e3181b544cf

Fiani B, Quadri SA, Cathel A et al (2019) Esthesioneuroblastoma: a comprehensive review of diagnosis, management, and current treatment options. World Neurosurg 126:194–211. https://doi.org/10.1016/j.wneu.2019.03.014

Fliss DM (2012) Open surgical approaches to the anterior skull base and paranasal sinuses. Tel Aviv Sourasky Medical Center, Tel Aviv

Fukuda K, Kojiro M, Hirano M et al (1989) Predominance of squamous cell carcinoma and rarity of adenocarcinoma of maxillary sinus among Japanese. Kurume Med J 36:1–6. https://doi.org/10.2739/kurumemedj.36.1

Gautam K, Tiwari SB, Shrestha S et al (2022) Sinonasal mucosal melanoma presenting as a maxillary sinus mass: a case report. Clin Case Reports 10:e05374. https://doi.org/10.1002/ccr3.5374

Gill KS, Frattali MA (2015) An unusual presentation of adenoid cystic carcinoma. Case Rep Otolaryngol 2015:1–4. https://doi.org/10.1155/2015/826436

Goel S, Sachdev R, Mohapatra I et al (2016) Unusually aggressive primary testicular diffuse large B cell lymphoma with post therapy extensive metastasis. J Clin Diagn Res. https://doi.org/10.7860/jcdr/2016/17441.8074

Grieman RB, Katsikeris NF, Symington JM (1988) Rhabdomyosarcoma of the maxillary sinus: review of the literature and report of a case. J Oral Maxillofac Surg 46:1090–1096. https://doi.org/10.1016/0278-2391(88)90456-9

Gurung S, Pathak BD, Karki S et al (2022) Adenoid cystic carcinoma of maxillary antrum: a case report. Int J Surg Case Rep 94:107055. https://doi.org/10.1016/j.ijscr.2022.107055

Higgins TS, Thorp B, Rawlings BA, Han JK (2011) Outcome results of endoscopic vs craniofacial resection of sinonasal malignancies: a systematic review and pooled-data analysis. Int Forum Allergy Rhinol 1:255–261. https://doi.org/10.1002/alr.20051

Holmes M, Su SY, Bell D (2016) Ectopic primary olfactory neuroblastoma of the maxillary sinus. Ann Diagn Pathol 22:45–48. https://doi.org/10.1016/j.anndiagpath.2016.04.001

Yoon JH, Chun YC, Park SY, Yang WI, Lee SJ, Kim J (2001) Malignant lymphoma of the maxillary sinus manifesting as a persistent toothache. J Endod 27(12):800–802

Howell JY, Hadian Y, Ramsey ML (2024) Squamous cell skin cancer. In: StatPearls—NCBI Bookshelf. https://www.ncbi.nlm.nih.gov/books/NBK441939/

Jeyaraj P, Venkatesan M, Nijhawan VS (2015) Solitary extramedullary plasmacytoma of the maxillary sinus, progressing to smoldering multiple myeloma with multifocal skeletal involvement, which resolved completely following chemotherapy alone. J Maxillofac Oral Surg 15:229–239. https://doi.org/10.1007/s12663-015-0742-0

Kato H, Kanematsu M, Sakurai K et al (2013) Adenoid cystic carcinoma of the maxillary sinus: CT and MR imaging findings. Jpn J Radiol 31:744–749. https://doi.org/10.1007/s11604-013-0247-z

Kim GE, Park HC, Keum KC et al (1999) Adenoid cystic carcinoma of the maxillary antrum. Am J Otolaryngol 20:77–84. https://doi.org/10.1016/s0196-0709(99)90015-7

Kondo M, Ando Y, Inuyama Y et al (1986) Maxillary squamous cell carcinomas staged by computed tomography. Int J Radiat Oncol Biol Phys 12:111–116. https://doi.org/10.1016/0360-3016(86)90424-4

Lahjaouj M, Berrada O, Rayhane A et al (2021) Advanced adenoid cystic carcinoma of maxillary sinus: rare case report and review of literature. Int J Surg Case Rep 80:105622. https://doi.org/10.1016/j.ijscr.2021.02.008

Li Y, Hao D, Song X, Zhang C (2021) Computed tomography and magnetic resonance imaging of adenoid cystic carcinoma in the maxillary sinus: a retrospective study with radiologic-histopathologic correlations. Oral Surg Oral Med Oral Pathol Oral Radiol 131:111–121. https://doi.org/10.1016/j.oooo.2020.06.019

Lund VJ, Howard DJ, Wei WI (2013) Tumours of the nose, sinuses and nasopharynx. Thieme Medical Publishers, Stuttgart

Mayo Clinic (2023) Melanoma—symptoms and causes—Mayo Clinic. https://www.mayoclinic.org/diseases-conditions/melanoma/symptoms-causes/syc-20374884#:~:text=Melanoma%20is%20a%20kind%20of

Megat Shiraz M, Jong Y, Primuharsa Putra S (2008) Extramedullary plasmacytoma in themaxillary sinus. Singapore Med J 49:e310–e311

Meyer C, Hamersley ERS, Manosalva RE et al (2017) Olfactory neuroblastoma with divergent differentiation: an unusual histologic finding in a rare tumour. Head Neck Pathol 11:531–536. https://doi.org/10.1007/s12105-017-0781-6

Michel G, Joubert M, Delemazure AS et al (2013) Adenoid cystic carcinoma of the paranasal sinuses: retrospective series and review of the literature. Eur Ann Otorhinolaryngol Head Neck Dis 130:257–262. https://doi.org/10.1016/j.anorl.2012.09.010

National Cancer Institute (2024) Olfactory neuroblastoma—NCI. https://www.cancer.gov/pediatric-adult-rare-tumour/rare-tumours/other-rare-tumours/olfactory-neuroblastoma. Accessed 31 Jul 2024

Peng KA, Kita AE, Suh JD et al (2014) Sinonasal lymphoma: case series and review of the literature. Int Forum Allergy Rhinol 4:670–674. https://doi.org/10.1002/alr.21337

Rahmani K, Zahir ST, Yazdi MB, Navabazam A (2017) Aggressive adenoid cystic carcinoma of maxillary sinus in a 43-year-old male: rare case report and review of literature. Case Rep Med 2017:1–5. https://doi.org/10.1155/2017/2324717

Rhee C, Won T, Lee CH et al (2006) Adenoid cystic carcinoma of the sinonasal tract: treatment results. Laryngoscope 116:982–986. https://doi.org/10.1097/01.mlg.0000216900.03188.48

Santos MRM, Servato JPS, Cardoso SV et al (2014) Squamous cell carcinoma at maxillary sinus: clinicopathologic data in a single Brazilian institution with review of literature. PubMed Central (PMC). https://www.ncbi.nlm.nih.gov/pmc/articles/PMC4313952/

Sapkota S, Shaikh H (2023) Non-Hodgkin lymphoma. In: StatPearls—NCBI Bookshelf. https://www.ncbi.nlm.nih.gov/books/NBK559328/

Sharma RK, Irace AL, Overdevest JB et al (2022) Association of race, ethnicity, and socioeconomic status with esthesioneuroblastoma presentation, treatment, and survival. OTO Open 6. https://doi.org/10.1177/2473974x221075210

Sheikh Y, Bickle I (2017) Squamous cell carcinoma of the maxilla. Radiopaedia.org. https://doi.org/10.53347/rid-52181

Sigal R, Monnet O, De Baere T et al (1992) Adenoid cystic carcinoma of the head and neck: evaluation with MR imaging and clinical-pathologic correlation in 27 patients. Radiology 184:95–101. https://doi.org/10.1148/radiology.184.1.1319079

Simpson RJ, Hoang K, Hyams VJ, Jarchow RC (1988) Mucoepidermoid carcinoma of the maxillary sinus. Otolaryngol Head Neck Surg 99:419–423. https://doi.org/10.1177/019459988809900412

Song J-Y (2016) Non Hodgkin lymphoma in the maxillary sinus mimicking dental abscess: a case report. J Dent Rehabil Appl Sci 32:130–134. https://doi.org/10.14368/jdras.2016.32.2.130

Stern SJ, Goepfert H, Clayman G et al (1993) Squamous cell carcinoma of the maxillary sinus. Arch Otolaryngol Head Neck Surg 119:964–969. https://doi.org/10.1001/archotol.1993.01880210052008

Thompson CF, Kim BJ, Lai C et al (2013) Sinonasal rhabdomyosarcoma: prognostic factors and treatment outcomes. Int Forum Allergy Rhinol 3:678–683. https://doi.org/10.1002/alr.21157

Tosoni A, Di Nunno V, Gatto L et al (2023) Olfactory neuroblastoma: diagnosis, management, and current treatment options. Front Oncol 13. https://doi.org/10.3389/fonc.2023.1242453

Usuda D, Izumida T, Terada N et al (2021) Diffuse large B cell lymphoma originating from the maxillary sinus with skin metastases: a case report and review of literature. World J Clin Cases 9:6886–6899. https://doi.org/10.12998/wjcc.v9.i23.6886

Vasudevan V, Kailasam S, Venkatappa M et al (2012) Well-differentiated squamous cell carcinoma of maxillary sinus. https://www.semanticscholar.org/paper/Well-differentiated-squamous-cell-carcinoma-of-Vasudevan-Kailasam/87162ab9e7b4e612a882b3b62dd26ba98d3ec8a3

Yasumoto M, Taura S, Shibuya H, Honda M (2000) Primary malignant lymphoma of the maxillary sinus: CT and MRI. Neuroradiology 42:285–289. https://doi.org/10.1007/s002340050887

Other Pathologies of Maxillary Sinus

9

Goran Latif Omer, Vivek Sasindran, Mithra Sara, Pier Giorgio Giacomini, Sahand Soran Ali, Aland Salih Abdullah, Gianluca Velletrani, Beatrice Francavilla, and Riccardo Maurizi

Silent Sinus Syndrome

Introduction

The silent sinus syndrome was first described by Montgomery in 1964. Thirty years later, Soparkar proposed the term "Silent Sinus Syndrome" (SSS) and systematised the diagnosis as spontaneous enophthalmos and hypoglobus on the ipsilateral hypoplastic maxilla, secondarily causing orbital floor resorption (Stryjewska-Makuch et al. 2022). SSS, also known as imploding antrum syndrome, is a very rare condition, usually represented by asymptomatic spontaneous collapse of the sinus walls and floor of the orbit. There is great confusion around its definition, diagnosis, and proper management as a result of the rare mention of the condition in the literature.

The terms SSS and Chronic Maxillary Sinus Atelectasis (CMA) have been used interchangeably in the past; the latter can be defined as a persistent and progressive decrease in maxillary sinus volume because of inward curving of the antral walls (Rosso et al. 2022). The fundamental difference between CMA and SSS is the absence of sinusitis symptoms and facial pain. According to literature analysis,

Supplementary Information The online version contains supplementary material available at https://doi.org/10.1007/978-3-031-83468-4_9.

G. L. Omer (✉) · S. S. Ali · A. S. Abdullah
Department of Clinical Sciences, College of Medicine, University of Sulaimani, Sulaymaniyah, KRI, Iraq

V. Sasindran · M. Sara
KM Cherian Institute of Medical Sciences, Chengannur, Kerala, India

P. G. Giacomini · G. Velletrani · B. Francavilla · R. Maurizi
Department of Otorhinolaryngology, University of Rome Tor Vergata, Rome, Italy

© The Author(s), under exclusive license to Springer Nature Switzerland AG 2025

G. L. Omer, S. Di Girolamo (eds.), *Maxillary Sinus: A Comprehensive Guide*,
https://doi.org/10.1007/978-3-031-83468-4_9

Brandt claims that stage III of CMA and SSS are two different manifestations of the same illness (Stryjewska-Makuch et al. 2022). Silent sinus syndrome can make a challenge in the diagnosis of the condition. The patient may present with unilateral ptosis or retraction, a deep superior sulcus or even orbital asymmetry (Health Jade 2020).

Aetiology

The aetiology of SSS remains debatable. Patients usually deny pre-existing underlying sinus disease or trauma to the orbitofacial structures. Most researchers agree that the collapse of the inferior orbital wall is induced by the negative pressure generated by the resorption of gas after a natural ostium occlusion, which may occur during the first or second decade of life (Rosso et al. 2022).

Epidemiology

Silent sinus syndrome typically presents in the third to fifth decade of life with no gender predilection. Overall, the condition is idiopathic; however, trauma to the lateral nasal wall and ostiomeatal complex may be the cause in a small proportion of patients, e.g., endonasal intubation (Cleveland Clinic 2023).

Pathophysiology

Understanding the underlying pathophysiology is quite important for the ideal management of silent sinus syndrome. It was first suggested to be an idiopathic disorder. Nowadays, it is thought that an inciting event causes occlusion of the ostiomeatal complex through which the maxillary sinus drains into the middle meatus of the nasal antrum. As a result of the occlusion, there will be an accumulation of secretions that are eventually resorbed, resulting in a vacuum-like effect. Hypoventilation of the sinus and sub-atmospheric pressure for a long period of time results in negative pressure, which leads to the inward migration of the sinus walls. Along with the orbital floor being pulled downward, there may also be thinning and remodelling of the bony structures because of increased osteoclast activity. Usually, the periosteum is not affected (Health Jade 2020).

Clinical Feature

Typically, the patients present with painless asymmetry of the face relatively for a long period of time (months to years), enophthalmos of 2–5 mm, and hypoglobus. It is not always necessarily associated with sinusitis-related symptoms. Patients could develop diplopia if the disease progresses and it is severe enough to cause significant deformity of the orbital floor. However, extraocular movements usually remain normal (Cleveland Clinic 2023) (Fig. 9.2).

Silent sinus syndrome diagnostic criteria include (Illner et al. 2002):

- Spontaneous enophthalmos and/or hypoglobus.
- Absence of symptoms of sinonasal inflammatory disease.
- CT imaging showed a contraction of the maxillary sinus.
- Absence of history of orbital trauma and absence of enophthalmos due to another aetiology.
- Absence of documented congenital deformity.

Radiographic Features

Despite the fact that otolaryngologists and ophthalmologists typically make the diagnosis clinically, imaging of the sinuses can help to confirm it. Sometimes, the condition is diagnosed incidentally by imaging the region for other pathology.

Plain Radiograph

Plain radiographs are no longer considered sufficiently sensitive or specific for the assessment of paranasal sinus disease. However, they are still not infrequently performed. The findings are the same as those seen on computerised tomography (CT).

Computerised Tomography

Computerised tomography is preferably performed as a volumetric acquisition with three-plane orthogonal reformats and is able to elegantly demonstrate changes in the sinus and the adjacent structures.

The sinus is fully developed; however, it is completely opaque, smaller in size, and has inward bowing on all four of its walls. This manifests as:

- Inferior bowing of the roof (orbital floor): Increased orbital volume and enophthalmos.
- Lateral bowing of the medial wall: lateral displacement of the middle and inferior turbinate.
- Posterior bowing of the anterior wall: flattening of the malar eminence.
- Anteromedial bowing of the posterolateral wall.

The uncinate process is typically shifted laterally and superiorly, in direct contact with the inferomedial wall of the orbit and the ostiomeatal complexes occluded. These are seen in Fig. 9.1.

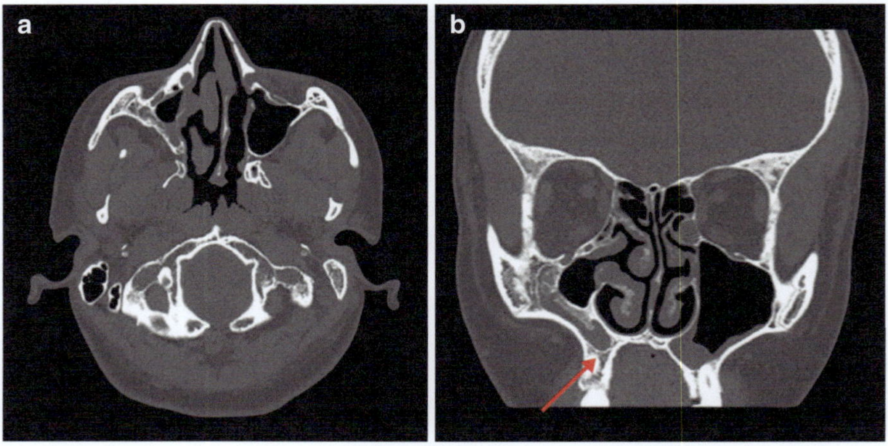

Fig. 9.1 Small size right maxillary with compensatory increased alveolar height (arrow, **a**: Axial, **b**: Coronal)

Magnetic Resonance Imaging

Magnetic resonance imaging (MRI) is not necessary for the diagnosis; however, if it is performed, it will demonstrate a fully opacified sinus with an increase in the thickness and enhancement of the mucosa in addition to the aforementioned structural changes. The secretions are of variable intensity (Cleveland Clinic 2023).

Treatment

The treatment of silent sinus syndrome can be definitively achieved by creating an outlet for mucus drainage from the obstructed sinus. The treatment is performed endoscopically by creating a nasal antral window or a maxillary antrostomy. After surgery, the sinus arrangement may remain unchanged, improve slightly, or gradually return to a close to normal form. Regardless of how the sinus ultimately looks after endoscopic sinus surgery, disease progression is stopped without the emergence of new deformities. It is possible to restore the orbital floor in addition to or after functional endoscopic sinus surgery, but this repair is usually reserved for patients suffering from diplopia or severe cosmetic deformity as well as for those patients with little improvement after functional endoscopic sinus surgery (Sharma and Gaillard 2010).

Prognosis

Whenever surgery is performed to provide ideal drainage, further volume loss will be arrested. However, any deformity at the time of surgery will be permanent and may require surgical correction, especially if diplopia is present (Cleveland Clinic 2023).

Agenesis of the Maxillary Sinus

Introduction

The maxillary sinus is one of the paranasal sinuses, and it lies within the maxillary bone (Ilie et al. 2022). The paranasal sinuses are spaces filled with air and lined by mucosa in the maxillofacial region, and they consist of four pairs: Frontal, Ethmoid, Sphenoid, and Maxillary sinus (Whyte and Boeddinghaus 2019). The maxillary sinus and the ethmoid sinus are the only two paranasal sinuses that are present at birth, even though the development of all paranasal sinuses begins in utero (Duncavage and Becker 2011). Embryologically, the development of the maxillary sinus begins in the 10th week (Nuñez-Castruita et al. 2012). At about the 16th week, the primordial structure of the maxillary sinus arises from the inferior aspect of the ethmoidal infundibulum (Duncavage and Becker 2011). The sinus continues to enlarge from the maxillary infundibulum throughout the second and third trimester, reaching a size of 7.0 mm in anteroposterior depth, 4.0 mm in height, and a width of 2.7 mm (Duncavage and Becker 2011). The size of the sinus increases with the growth of the nasal cavity. There is a 2 mm increase in the maxillary antrum laterally and vertically each year, with a 3 mm anteroposterior annual growth as well. After the eruption of the maxillary teeth, the final pneumatisation of the maxillary sinus happens in the inferior direction, and it reaches adult size by the age of 15–18 (Dedeoglu and Duman 2020). Cessation of this process at any of the stages can result in agenesis, Aplasia or hypoplasia.

Agenesis refers to the lack of the organ primordium; Aplasia indicates the presence of the primordium but the failure of its development; and lastly, hypoplasia describes a case where the primordium has started its growth but has failed to complete it (Maggs et al. 2008).

In terms of the development of the paranasal sinuses, hypoplasia is characterised as a delay in sinus pneumatisation after the age of 8, whilst Aplasia is defined as a complete absence of pneumatisation in persons aged 10 years and older (Hasan 2022).

Maxillary sinus hypoplasia (as seen in Fig. 9.2) has been divided into three different types, including mild, significant, and profound maxillary sinus hypoplasia. Significant and profound maxillary sinus hypoplasias are the types that are associated with abnormalities of the uncinate process (Duncavage and Becker 2011).

Aetiology

Infection, trauma, surgical procedure, irradiation, and congenital anomalies are all among the causes of maxillary sinus hypoplasia. Treacher-Collins syndrome is among the congenital anomalies that are seen to be associated with unilateral maxillary sinus hypoplasia (Khanduri et al. 2014). Even though severe Aplasia and hypoplasia of the maxillary sinus are not common, it has been seen with increased frequency in patients with cystic fibrosis since they usually suffer from recurrent and chronic infections with poor aeration and ultimately limited sinus expansion (Duncavage and Becker 2011).

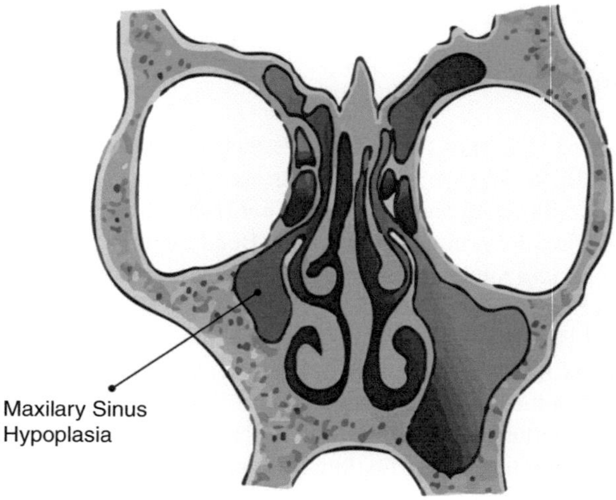

Fig. 9.2 Hypoplasia of the left maxillary sinus

Epidemiology

With reports of only eight cases in the world medical literature, agenesis or Aplasia of the maxillary sinus is considered an extremely rare condition (De Alencar Pierre and Santana 2000). Maxillary sinus hypoplasia is another rare abnormality with an incidence of 0.73% to 10.4% among patients with symptoms of the sinus, and it is usually associated with other anomalies such as that of the infundibular passage and the uncinate process (Yousif Ali Hasan et al. 2017). In a retrospective study on cone beam computed tomography (CT) images of dental patients with maxillary sinus hypoplasia, the average age was found to be 37.1 ± 14.1 (Alsufyani et al. 2021). Most studies show unilateral hypoplasia of the maxillary sinus than the bilateral form (Wake et al. 1993).

Pathophysiology

By the fourth month of pregnancy, a mucosal evagination within the middle meatus begins to form the maxillary sinus. Any disruption or cessation of this process could result in Aplasia (Yousif Ali Hasan et al. 2017).

Clinical Feature

Even though some patients with Aplasia and hypoplasia of the maxillary sinus may suffer from voice problems, facial pain, and chronic headaches, the majority are asymptomatic and are unaware of the condition until it is found incidentally on routine radiographs (Jafari-Pozve et al. 2014). If there is obstruction of the osteomeatal complex, maxillary sinus hypoplasia could be seen to result in sinusitis (Weed and Cole 1994).

Diagnosis

Either a CT scan (as seen in Fig. 9.3) or a cone beam CT (CBCT) scan using thin cuts is required for a proper diagnosis of maxillary sinus aplasia. A bone scan could also confirm the complete absence of the maxillary sinus (Carrasco Rueda et al. 2019). Most hypoplasias of the maxillary sinus are incidentally detected on

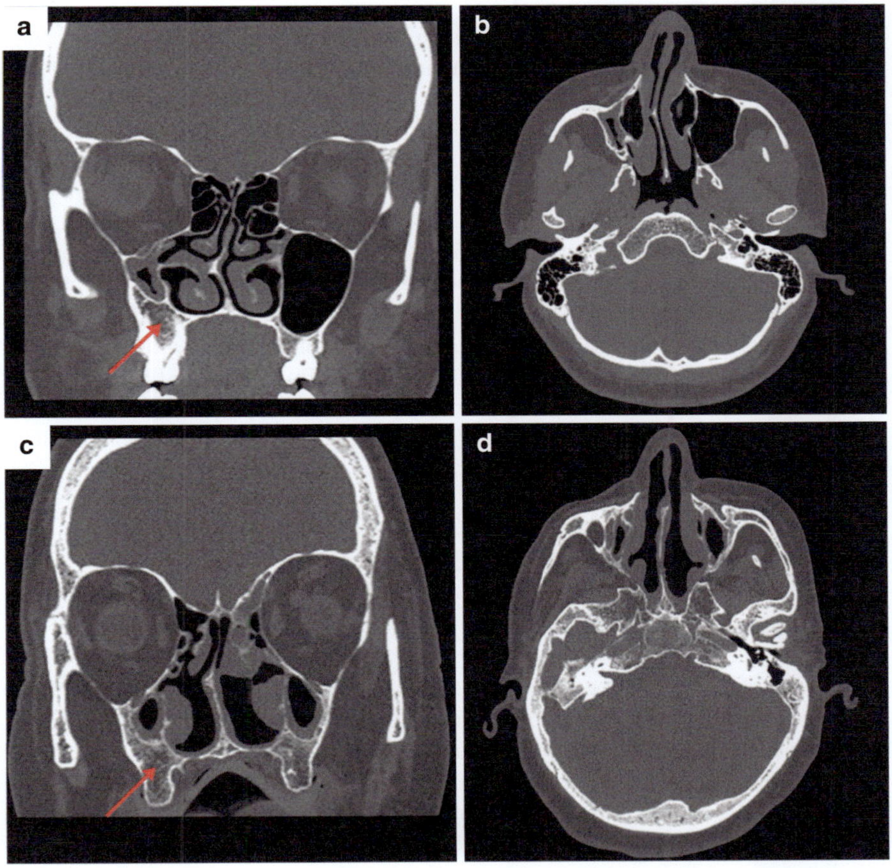

Fig. 9.3 Right maxillary sinus atelectasis with partial opacifications and peripheral thick rim of calcification associated with inferior bowing of the orbital floor with mild enophthalmos, posterior bowing of the anterior wall with flattening of the malar eminence and lateral bowing of the medial wall (**a** and **c**: Coronal, **b** and **d**: Axial view)

conventional X-ray since patients are usually asymptomatic (Jafari-Pozve et al. 2014). Apart from aiding in differentiating maxillary sinus hypoplasia from other diseases, such as infections and neoplasms, a CT scan can also serve as a guide for the surgeon to figure out the surgical plan and avoid unfortunate surgical complications (De Alencar Pierre and Santana 2000).

Differential Diagnosis

CT scan can help differentiate maxillary sinus hypoplasia from the following (De Alencar Pierre and Santana 2000):

- Infections
- Neoplasms
- Any opacified maxillary antrum on plain films could also be a differential diagnosis for maxillary sinus aplasia (Alnafisah and Hameed 2020).

Management

Since maxillary sinus hypoplasia is liable to mucus retention, this makes them more prone to persistent maxillary sinusitis, for which endoscopic surgery has been recommended as an effective treatment modality. It is worth pointing out that usually, maxillary sinus hypoplasia is associated with other abnormalities, such as those of the lateral nasal wall, and in those cases, the surgical approach of choice is a posteriorly placed middle meatal antrostomy (Salib et al. 2001). For most patients, apart from being informed about the condition in case of future symptoms, no additional therapeutic approach is taken since most are asymptomatic and have no complications (Jafari-Pozve et al. 2014).

Missed Maxillary Sinus Ostium Syndrome

Introduction

Despite an increase in the number of functional endoscopic sinus surgery (FESS) operations done for patients with medically refractory chronic rhinosinusitis (CRS), a considerable proportion of surgical failures remain with persistent disease. Even though success rates ranging from 76% to 98% are claimed, a significant proportion of patients continue to present with symptoms (Meechor and Javer 2008). In the maxillary sinus, secretion transmission originates in the floor of the sinus in a stellate like pattern. The mucus is transmitted through the anterior, medial, posterior, and lateral walls of the sinuses as well as along the roof. All of these secretory pathways come together at the natural ostium of the maxillary sinus. After passing through the maxillary sinus ostium, secretions are delivered into the narrow ethmoid infundibulum. The secretions from the maxillary sinus unite with those from the frontal and anterior ethmoid sinuses to approach the nasopharynx. Whenever the natural maxillary sinus ostium is missed, what is known as the maxillary sinus recirculation phenomena results (Christmas et al. 2003).

Pathophysiology

The missed ostium sequence, as informed by Parons et al., happens when the most anterior part of the uncinate process is not completely removed, which consequently obscures the site of the natural maxillary sinus ostium. This obstruction inhibits the middle meatal antrostomy from interacting with the natural ostium, leading to recirculation. In the present scenario, mucociliary flow causes mucus to re-enter the sinus, resulting in a functional blockage of the maxillary sinus and continued sinus disease (Fig.) (Duncavage and Becker 2011). This drainage pathway may be sufficient during periods of well-being and not pose complications; however, it is when nasal oedema occurs that the ostium/infundibulum interface becomes insufficient which inhibits appropriate ventilation and drainage (Parsons et al. 1996).

Some authors, on the other hand, contend that mucus recirculation in the postoperative period may be caused by excessive trauma and scarring of the natural ostium and natural mucus pathways, which likely leads to mucus stagnation. As the final common pathway is damaged, this mucus is directed towards the accessory ostium (Kaluskar and Sachdeva 2006).

Clinical Feature

The recirculation phenomenon in the maxillary sinus may be the cause of recurrent sinusitis in people who have had endoscopic sinus surgery.

Examination with a 0° or 30° telescope will reveal mucus originating from the region of the natural ostium of the maxillary sinus and flowing back into the maxillary sinus through a surgically made middle meatal window. (As seen in the figure below).

This may leave the patient vulnerable to:

- post-nasal discharge
- nasal obstruction
- and persistent or recurrent sinus complaints (Christmas et al. 2003).

Prevention

Failure to identify and incorporate the natural maxillary sinus ostium is a common error during a maxillary antrostomy.

Proper identification and incorporation of the natural ostium in the surgically constructed antrostomy is crucial.

The creation of a posterior antrostomy is going to result in mucus recirculation and put the patient at risk for recurrent sinusitis.

By identifying the infundibulum that leads to the natural maxillary ostium, the surgeon is able to incorporate the natural ostium into the surgical antrostomy, preventing recirculation (Batra and Han 2015).

Treatment

The intervention performed during surgery is to resect the intervening tissue, which removes the bridge that causes the recirculation. A 70° scope can be utilised to inspect these areas and ensure that there is no residual uncinate or scarring present (Christmas et al. 2003).

Maxillary Sinus Fracture

Introduction

Paranasal sinuses are air-filled cavities that surround the nose, usually lined with paper-thin bone with a high tendency to sustain a fracture during trauma. Although not functionally as debilitating as other fractures of the facial bones, sinus fractures can lead to a lifetime of sinus disease. Furthermore, forces greater than paranasal sinus resistance may result in traumatic brain injury.

Maxillary sinus fractures are a common and serious type of facial fracture. They can cause a variety of symptoms, including pain, swelling, and breathing difficulty. In some cases, they can also lead to complications, such as infection or vision problems.

The diagnosis of maxillary sinus fractures is based on a physical examination, imaging studies, and medical history. Treatment depends on the location and severity of the fracture. In most cases, maxillary sinus fractures can be treated successfully with conservative or surgery treatment.

Epidemiology and Aetiology

Among paranasal sinus fractures, the maxillary sinus fracture is the most frequent, accounting for approximately 10% of all facial fractures. Males in their 20–30s are the most common group to sustain facial trauma. The most common mechanism of injury is a high-energy trauma to the eyeball; other causative factors include blunt trauma, penetrating trauma, and surgical procedures (Bell and Ye 2017; Brasileiro et al. 2005; Zhang et al. 2012).

Maxillary sinus injury can be a consequence of either facial trauma or iatrogenic damage (e.g., displaced dental implant).

The aetiology for facial trauma causing paranasal and maxillary fractures varies geographically: in urban regions, assaults and motor vehicle accidents are the main reasons for facial trauma; by contrast, in rural regions, animal-related accidents are the main cause of facial trauma (Batista et al. 2012; Bell and Ye 2017; Zhang et al. 2012).

Clinical Presentation

Signs and symptoms of maxillary sinus fractures vary according to the location and severity of the fracture; the most common injuries and fracture sites are the floor of orbit/roof of the sinus (blow-out fracture) and the inferior sinus wall (iatrogenic injury) (Bell and Ye 2017; Ramstead et al. 2008).

The chief complaint is usually facial pain and, in some instances, deformity, although facial swelling can make the assessment of sinus wall depression difficult.

Symptoms can include:

- Facial Pain
- Numbness or tingling in the face, especially hypoesthesia of the upper lip and upper dental arch.
- The difficulty of breathing through the nose.
- Double vision and/ or loss of vision.

Signs can include:

- Facial deformities
- Swelling of the face
- Nose and/ or mouth bleeding
- Subcutaneous Emphysema

Anatomy and Pathology

Traumatic forces directed towards the facial skeleton are transmitted and absorbed by a bony framework that surrounds paranasal sinuses. Disruption of the bony framework results in paranasal sinus fractures.

Although possible, isolated fractures of the sinus walls are a rare entity: most commonly, maxillary sinus wall fracture is a sign of a more complex and extensive facial trauma.

The Le Fort classification system, which can be seen in Fig. 9.4, categorises common types of bony framework disruption along "lines of weakness" and can be associated with certain types of paranasal sinus fractures (Ibrahim and Gaillard 2008).

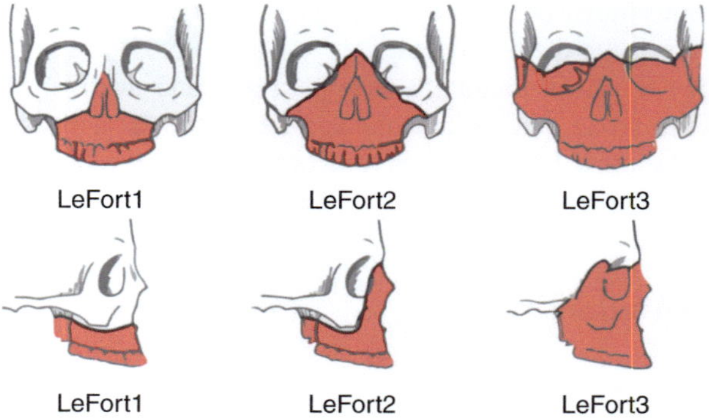

Fig. 9.4 Le Fort's classification for fractures

Le Fort 1, also known as a Guerin fracture, is a horizontal maxillary fracture separating the teeth from the upper face; the fracture line passes through the alveolar ridge, lateral nose and inferior wall of the maxillary sinus.

Le Fort 2 is like a pyramidal fracture with the teeth at the base and the nasofrontal suture as its apex; the fracture arch passes through the posterior alveolar ridge, lateral walls of maxillary sinuses, inferior orbital rim and nasal bones.

Le Fort 3, also known as craniofacial disjunction, is a transverse fracture in which the fracture arch passes through the nasofrontal suture, maxillo-frontal suture, orbital walls and zygomatic arch/zygomatic frontal suture.

In addition to the Le Fort classification system, other classifications have been devised for facial fractures that are too complex for the Le Fort fracture lines, which focus on anatomical subunits of the mid-face, including zygomaticomaxillary complex (ZMC), the naso-orbitoethmoidal complex (NOE), and the dentoalveolar complex (DAC).

- Le Fort I and II fractures, ZMC fractures: associated with maxillary sinus fracture.
- Le Fort II and III fractures: associated with ethmoid sinus fracture.
- NOE fractures: associated with frontal/ethmoid sinus fractures (Bell and Ye 2017).

Physical Examination

The signs and symptoms of maxillary sinus fractures may vary according to the location and severity of the fracture (Flint et al. 2014).

First and foremost, the initial assessment must address the so-called ABCs of trauma management and any other potentially life-threatening injuries.

While assessing the extent of the patient's disabilities, a detailed neurologic exam should be performed to calculate a Glasgow Coma Scale Score and, in a cooperative patient, cranial nerves assessments should be performed.

Firstly, the general facial appearance should be examined.

When lacerations are present, a sterile examination of the wound may yield information about the status of the underlying bone and the presence of foreign bodies.

If any fluid discharge is evident, the possibility of epistaxis, purulent drainage, cerebrospinal fluid leakage, otorrhoea, and/or rhinorrhoea should be considered.

Often, the most severe bleeding is from the nose and sinuses, and this can be managed by tamponade with packing. However, laceration of the internal carotid artery in the skull base may require immediate angiography and balloon occlusion above and below the arterial laceration, although such injuries are rarely compatible with survival.

Furthermore, visual status should be evaluated as soon as possible; a progressive loss of vision usually indicates increasing intraorbital pressure or optic nerve injury. In this case, an early intervention is required to prevent permanent vision loss.

The main factors that may affect the result of a physical evaluation are the amount of time that has passed since the trauma occurred, the severity of oedema and/or hematoma of the cervical-facial region, and the presence of treatment-related devices (e.g., packing, tubes, and cervical collars).

Radiographic Features

Though physical examination may be enough to diagnose Maxillary sinus fractures, at other times, imaging will be required to exclude other injuries and assist with presurgical planning. The numerous overlapping shadows of the plain film X-ray make it easier to miss fractures that would be found on a CT scan; for this reason, most ENT and maxillofacial trauma surgeons have abandoned the plain radiographic imaging even as a screening tool (Flint et al. 2014; Lenkeit et al. 2023).

Nowadays, computed tomography of the maxillofacial bones without contrast is the gold standard imaging study needed in facial trauma injuries (Roselló et al. 2020). Modern high-speed, high-resolution CT scanners allow to assess of the presence of fractures and dislocated bone fragments, hemosinus, pneumocephalus, soft tissue damage and foreign bodies, thus creating a more efficient and faster diagnosis and treatment of the maxillary sinus fracture (Lambert et al. 1997).

A less commonly used imaging modality is magnetic resonance imaging, which tends to be indicated as a complement to initial CT scans, specifically with suspected CSF leaks and orbital soft tissue injuries such as herniation of orbital fat versus entrapment of orbital muscle (Roselló et al. 2020).

Treatment and Prognosis

In most cases, maxillofacial fractures are non-emergent and can be treated up to 2 weeks following the initial trauma (Lenkeit et al. 2023).

The treatment of maxillary sinus fractures depends on the location and severity of the fracture.

- Simple fractures may be treated with conservative measures, such as pain medication, ice, and elevation.
- Displaced fractures may require surgery to reposition the bone fragments. Surgical indications for maxillary sinus fractures are similar to the indications for LeFort fractures, which include poor facial aesthetics, restoration of midfacial height, correction of malocclusion, and repair of mid-face projection.
  If surgical indications are met, basic treatment of the anterior sinus wall should be based on repositioning the fracture segments with fixation using plates, screws, mesh grafts, or resorbable foils. Most surgeons will plan for open reduction and internal fixation (ORIF) via a Caldwell-Luc (gingival buccal) incision or an endoscopic nasal approach, depending on the provider's preference.

There is a lack of evidence for antibiotic prophylaxis in patients with basal skull fractures involving the paranasal sinuses (Bell and Ye 2017; Ratilal et al. 2015).

Complications

Noted complications in the literature include different districts (Da Silva De Menezes et al. 2016; Lenkeit et al. 2023):

- Ocular manifestations of maxillary sinus fractures may include extraocular eye muscle entrapment (inferior rectus and inferior oblique muscles), orbital cellulitis, orbital abscess, orbital emphysema, enophthalmos, and hypophthalmos.
- Nasal cavity and maxillary sinus manifestations of fractures may include impairments in sinus drainage, maxillary sinusitis and sinus mucocele, epistaxis and CSF rhinorrhea.
- Oral cavity and dental problems: oromaxillary fistula, dental malocclusion, tooth loss or root damage.
- General concerns: infection, facial asymmetry, pressure sensitivity, chronic facial pain, infraorbital nerve paraesthesia.

Foreign Body in the Maxillary Sinus

Cases of foreign bodies entering the sinuses are rare. Maybe that's why, when unusual symptoms appear, the thought that a foreign object may be in the maxillary sinus does not always come to mind. However, if sinusitis does not go away for a long time, it is worth taking an X-ray to look and see if it is caused by a foreign body (Shenoy and Maller 2013).

The anatomic conditions of the maxillary sinus carry the risk of complications when medical procedures are performed in this region. Iatrogenic displacement of the foreign body into the maxillary sinus shows an increasing tendency, especially in regard to the raising amount of dental implant installation procedures and their further accidental migration. Foreign bodies may penetrate the maxillary sinus by different mechanisms, such as apical migration of filling fragments, accidental rough handling, or an oroantral fistula (Wojtera et al. 2020).

Other types of objects dislocated into the sinus during medical procedures include fractured teeth roots, whole teeth, endodontic materials and tools, dental filling materials, dental burs, or dental impression materials. Apart from dental procedures that might induce a foreign body into the sinus, the complication can be caused by otorhinolaryngologists by accidental leaving of gauzes used for nasal or sinus packing or other materials (Hallak et al. 2021). Foreign bodies are frequently encountered in ENT practice and are commonly found in the nasal cavities, ears, and pharynx. However, a foreign body in the paranasal sinuses is rare, about 80% of which occurs in the maxillary sinus.

There are two main causes of paranasal sinus foreign bodies. The most common is iatrogenic, which is a consequence of dental, ophthalmic, and otorhinolaryngological procedures and makes up 60% of cases. The causes of this complication include incorrect extraction technique, poor anatomical information, reduced visualisation of the surgical field, and complications experienced during sinus lifting operations (Alrasheed et al. 2021). The other cause is traumatic incidents, which account for 25% of cases. The maxillary sinus is the most commonly affected site (75%), followed by the frontal sinus (18%) (Wojtera et al. 2020).

However, case reports about migrated implants into ethmoid and sphenoid sinuses are also available in the literature (Alrasheed et al. 2021). Traumatic foreign bodies can be a result of direct external trauma to the sinus or indirectly through orbital or palate injuries (Şahin 2019). These foreign bodies may consist of various substances such as wooden sticks, plastic, glass, metal, and bullets. These are usually detected when a patient has unexplained rhinosinusitis or as an accidental finding during a radiological examination. If the foreign body is not removed from the sinus, it can lead to serious complications such as sinusitis, inflammatory reactions, and fungal infections (Şahin 2019). Foreign bodies' impaction in paranasal sinuses is an unusual clinical condition. The majority of impacted foreign bodies are found in the maxillary sinus and come from an odontogenic source. Of these, only approximately 10% will cause maxillary sinusitis. Oroantral fistulas, secondary to dental manipulations, are the most common entry point for foreign bodies into the maxillary sinus. Unilateral maxillary sinusitis is usually related to specific underlying causes, such as facial trauma with maxillary injury, tumours, fungal infections, dental affections, or foreign bodies (Wojtera et al. 2020).

The anatomical proximity between the maxillary sinus and teeth makes the odontogenic origin the most common source of maxillary sinusitis (Wojtera et al. 2020). Maxillary molar or premolar tooth extractions are considered the most common causes of oroantral communications. This is the reason why a careful inspection for an eventual oroantral communication, using the Valsalva manoeuvre, especially after maxillary molar and premolar tooth extractions or endodontic surgery performed on maxillary teeth, is recommended (Wojtera et al. 2020).

It is known that the presence of foreign bodies in a sinus induces chronic physical and chemical irritation of the mucosa, promotes some degree of ciliary insufficiency and leads to secondary infections; this is the reason why the removal of all foreign bodies in the paranasal sinus is widely recommended (Wojtera et al. 2020).

The largest of paranasal sinuses, maxillary sinuses, are the pyramidal-shaped cavities localised within the maxillary bone bilaterally. This pyramidal base, an apex of which points towards the zygomatic process, forms by the lateral wall of the nasal cavity. The upper wall is bounded by the base of the orbit, and the lower wall is bounded by the maxillas processus alveolaris. The lowest part of the lower wall is 3–5 mm below the nasal cavity and close to the first molar and the second premolar. Maxillary sinus volume has a natural tendency to increase among life, and especially when premolars and molar teeth are extracted, the maxillary sinus may expand downward (Alrasheed et al. 2021). Factors that play a role in the process of pneumatisation of the maxillary sinus are the absence of tooth roots after tooth extraction and atrophic resorption of the maxillary alveolar crest. Resorption of the bones can occur in the toothless alveolar crest with wide maxillary sinuses. In such cases, dental implant application is needed together with the sinus lift procedure (Alrasheed et al. 2021).

Because of the anatomical proximity of the upper teeth and dental implant placement in this area, maxillary sinuses are the most important among the paranasal sinuses for clinicians and surgeons in dentistry. Because of this close anatomic relationship, a careful clinical and radiological examination is needed before surgeries are made in this area. Maxillary sinus-related complications in dentistry are maxillary sinusitis, oroantral fistula formation and migration of foreign bodies into the maxillary sinus (Alrasheed et al. 2021). Dental implant foreign bodies can be displaced and migrate into the maxillary sinus due to poor bone density and/or poor initial stability in the posterior maxilla. Other foreign bodies, such as tooth roots or metallic objects, can migrate into the sinus due to the doctor's inexperience (Sohn et al. 2011). Sinonasal ectopic teeth are uncommon. The aetiology of teeth in the maxillary sinus is most commonly secondary to trauma, including iatrogenic/dental procedures. Supernumerary teeth can also erupt idiopathically into the nasal cavity (Levin and Sommer 2019). A literature search revealed only two British' and two Japanese-published reports of dental burs displaced into the maxillary antrum; all four of these cases are published in the dental literature (Smith and Emko 2007). Patients with this complication would likely be referred to an otolaryngologist for treatment. Therefore, it is important to be familiar with this complication and its management. The natural history of foreign bodies in the paranasal sinuses is only anecdotal and is not truly known. "Reported sequelae include chronic sinusitis, cutaneous fistula, rhinolith formation (an approach to maxillary sinus rhinolith can be seen in Fig. 9.5), and chronic pain". Likewise, metallic foreign bodies have been associated with malignancy, and when the metal is lead, there is concern for an increased risk of lead poisoning, particularly in children. For these reasons, the removal of metallic foreign bodies is indicated (Smith and Emko 2007).

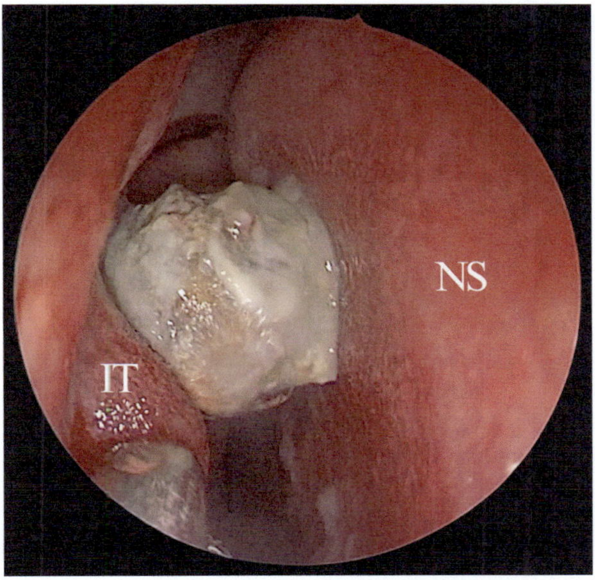

Fig. 9.5 This is an intraoperative video of a patient undergoing Endoscopic Sinus Surgery for rhinolith inside the maxillary sinus ostium. As can be seen in the thumbnail (right side nasal cavity), the stone was taken out of the ostium. (*NS* nasal septum, *IT* inferior turbinate) (Audio 9.1 and Video 9.1)

Penetration Routes

For a foreign body to make its way into the maxillary sinus is quite rare and not so easy. These sinuses are hollow formations over the upper jaw and are lined with mucous membranes. They perform several important functions, including warming up the air entering the nasal passage, resonating sound, creating an individual timbre and also helping to recognise smells (Shenoy and Maller 2013). A foreign body entering the sinus could be due to the result of unprofessional dental procedures, trauma, or a gunshot wound, all usually leading to an inflammatory process. This is not always the case since sometimes a foreign body in the maxillary sinus may not manifest itself for a long time (if it is small enough and not infected). Most often, dental materials can get into the maxillary sinuses. This can happen during root canal filling when the material is inserted too deeply. In this case, it is extremely rare for the inflammatory process to occur. Often, the presence of a foreign body can only be noticed incidentally on an X-ray (Shenoy and Maller 2013). Foreign bodies (FBs) can be presented in the maxillary sinus by traumatic or non-traumatic causes. Gurkan et al. found ectopic third molar teeth in the right maxillary sinus as a non-traumatic cause. The traumatic causes can be classified as accidental or iatrogenic. The presence of pieces of glass, a ballpoint pen, and multiple wood and plastic pieces are considered accidental causes (Şahin 2019).

Clinical Presentation

The extent of the inflammation within the maxillary sinus will be deepened on features of the foreign object, such as its size, sterility, and the individual characteristics of the organism. Sometimes, all that occurs is simply a mucous membrane forming around it without the object bothering anyone, but more often, the rejection response is activated, triggering an inflammatory process (Shenoy and Maller 2013).

- A feeling of heaviness in the sinuses.
- Pain felt during chewing which radiates to the upper jaw.
- The pain was sensed with sharp tilts of the head.
- Elevated body temperature (Up to 38 °C).
- Purulent nasal discharge, often odourless.
- Signs of general intoxication: nausea, weakness and dizziness.

Due to the similarity of the symptoms to sinusitis, it's usually the first suspicion. In principle, this is not wrong since the only difference between them is that the usual sinusitis most often has an infectious nature. In this case, eradicating all symptoms is not possible unless the foreign object is removed from the sinus (Shenoy and Maller 2013).

Patients with FB in the sinuses can present with mild fever, facial pain, headache, nasal obstruction, and chronic nasal discharge. Some patients have been found to have an FB in the sinuses without any symptoms. However, the FB should be removed to avoid tissue reactions and prevent sinusitis. The mechanism of sinusitis caused by FBs is unknown. It has been suggested that FBs can lead to ciliary insufficiency by causing tissue reaction and producing chronic irritation of the mucosa (Şahin 2019).

Diagnostics

If you find yourself having the symptoms listed above or if you have chronic sinusitis, which you cannot get rid of in any way, it is worth undergoing a diagnostic examination.

It consists of several stages:

- Initial consultation with a therapist to provide a complete history of the disease.
- Visual inspection of the nasal passages followed by palpation of the sinuses.
- Laboratory tests: blood (general and biochemistry) and nasal sputum (for microflora).
- Rhinoscopy or internal examination of the nasal passages with an endoscope.
- If teeth were previously treated, consult with a dentist.
- X-ray of the upper jaw and sinuses.
- If necessary, computed tomography could also be used (Shenoy and Maller 2013).

Only after analysing all the results obtained during the examination a final decision can be made regarding whether or not it is necessary to remove the foreign bodies from the maxillary sinus or to have a more conservative approach to treatment (Shenoy and Maller 2013).

Management

Conservative Treatment

Conservative treatment is used in the preoperative period to reduce inflammation and remove pus from the maxillary sinus. These treatments are also used in the postoperative to avoid the activation of the inflammatory process. It is also necessary to heal the sinuses when, for some reason, surgical removal of a foreign body is currently impossible (Shenoy and Maller 2013).

The standard course of treatment consists of the following drugs:

- antibacterial—help fight pathogenic microflora;
- anti-inflammatory—stop active inflammatory processes, lower body temperature;
- Antihistamines—relieve puffiness, reduce the amount of mucous secretions, and prevent allergies to antibiotics; antiseptics—used to flush the sinuses to remove excess mucus from them (Shenoy and Maller 2013).

A good effect is given by nasal drops with antibiotics or essential oils, for example, the natural drug "Pinosol". But all these measures help for a while; sooner or later it will be necessary to remove a foreign body (Shenoy and Maller 2013).

Surgical Treatment

Removal of the displaced foreign body might cause major difficulties regarding a method of management and the ability to perform certain procedures. There is a deficiency of reliable guidelines on how to treat the displaced object (Hallak et al. 2021). There are different methods used to extract foreign bodies from the sinus. The type of management is determined by the size, shape, and location of the foreign body. The Caldwell-Luc procedure, the lateral window approach, and endoscopic sinus surgery are common procedures used for the removal of foreign bodies (Şahin 2019). If a foreign body in the maxillary sinus provokes inflammation and becomes the cause of chronic sinusitis, it must be removed. Otherwise, it can cause serious complications: prolonged intoxication of the body, inflammation of the facial bones (with their subsequent destruction), periodontal disease and loss of healthy teeth (Shenoy and Maller 2013). Regarding the maxillary sinus, small foreign bodies can be expelled spontaneously. Several surgical techniques have been reported for the removal of foreign bodies in the maxillary sinus, such as transnasal endoscopic approach oral antrostomy via the anterior maxillary wall, mainly by means of the Caldwell-Luc procedure or a combined approach in some cases. The choice of the appropriate approach depends on multiple factors, such as the size and location of the foreign bodies in the sinus.

A transoral approach to the maxillary sinus may be indicated in cases of small foreign bodies without sinusitis because of the limited field of vision and accessibility. The transnasal endoscopic approach (FESS) is minimally invasive and carries more advantages, such as allowing for simultaneous treatment of sinusitis involving the maxillary, ethmoidal, or frontal sinuses (Wojtera et al. 2020).

Accurate management of odontogenic foreign body-induced maxillary sinusitis requires not only total removal of the foreign body but also the closure of any oroantral communications by establishing a physical barrier between the oral cavity and the maxillary sinus. Small defects less than 5 mm usually heal spontaneously, defects larger than 5 mm need to be closed, and several surgical techniques have been described (Wojtera et al. 2020).

Simuntis et al. report an incidence of oroantral communications as a complication of dental extractions in the posterior maxillary area of up to 80% of cases. In a study of 121 cases of odontogenic maxillary sinusitis reported by Mattias et al., 12 bone substitutes and root canal filling were the most frequently detected foreign bodies in the maxillary sinus (Wojtera et al. 2020). Surgeries using the standard Caldwell-Luc approach are under local anaesthesia. With this method, the sinusoid approach is essential by opening a window on the lateral wall of the maxillary sinus. The approach is direct from the opened window, and this method is advantageous for the experienced clinician (Alrasheed et al. 2021; Şahin 2019).

Comparing Caldwell-Luc surgery with endoscopic sinus surgery, the main disadvantage of endoscopic sinus surgery is the need for general anaesthesia. If the foreign bodies are close to the anterior or inferior wall of the maxillary sinus, it is almost impossible to obtain these objects with a transnasal approach (Alrasheed et al. 2021). Conservative Caldwell-Luc operation should be performed for foreign body removal only if other techniques are not available; it brings a 15–18% risk of postoperative sinusitis. Frequent symptoms appear, such as facial numbness, cheek pain, cheek swelling, teeth numbness, and gingival problems associated with damage to the bone and infraorbital nerve (Hallak et al. 2021). However, when the Caldwell-Luc or lateral window approach is performed without a sinus graft, the access window may not be replaced by a new bony wall in the lateral wall of the sinus. To remove foreign bodies, the use of endoscopy is definitely effective; but this procedure, which requires specific training and equipment, has some disadvantages (Sohn et al. 2011). The Caldwell-Luc approach has some disadvantages, such as postoperative numbness, paraesthesia, facial asymmetry, and dental problems (Sohn et al. 2011). The lateral window approach provides better direct vision to verify the foreign body in the sinus than an approach through the alveolar socket, and sinus bone grafting could be followed after the removal of the foreign body from the sinus (Sohn et al. 2011). However, the lateral window or Caldwell-Luc approach for the retrieval of a foreign body violates the integrity of the lateral wall of the sinus and the access window may not be replaced by a bony wall if the sinus bone graft is not performed at the same time (as shown after the classic Caldwell-Luc operation). In addition, a sinus graft is not indicated in all patients after the removal of a foreign body from the sinus. Sinus grafting is contraindicated when the patients have a history of sinus-related pathology or severely perforated sinus membranes. In addition, except for displaced dental implants into the sinus, a bone graft is not required in most patients after the removal of a foreign body from the sinus. The replaceable bony window maintains the integrity of the lateral wall of the sinus after the removal of the foreign body (Sohn et al. 2011). A piezoelectric saw insert-assisted osteotomy has some advantages, such as speed, precision, and minimal bone loss. The lateral bony window made by the piezoelectric saw inserted with a thin blade is precisely repositioned, whether bone grafting in the sinus was performed because of the tilted osteotomy into the sinus and the minimal bone loss during osteotomy. The replaceable bony window acts as a homologous barrier over the bone graft in the sinus. Replaceable bony windows not only prevent soft tissue invasion into the grafted site as a barrier but also act as osteoinductive/osteoconductive substrates for new bone formation in the sinus and new bony wall in the lateral wall of the sinus (Sohn et al. 2011).

Previous studies reported the potency for new bone formation with replaceable bony windows in the maxillary sinus without bone grafts in humans (Sohn et al. 2011). Histological evidence to confirm new bone formation in human sinuses, with replaceable windows and no bone grafts for sinus augmentation, has been previously reported. As an alternative to bone grafting for sinus augmentation, the patient's blood, gelatin sponges, platelet-rich plasma, and platelet-rich fibrin blocks with concentrated growth factors grafted in the new compartment under the elevated sinus membrane have shown successful new bone formation in the sinus (Sohn et al. 2011). Endoscopic surgery is less invasive than the Caldwell-Luc approach and effectively verifies the presence of a foreign body in the sinus. However, endoscopic surgery is limited to a specialist with special training, and requires special equipment. Saline irrigation through a small incision site of sinus mucosa into the sinus cavity mobilises displaced foreign bodies in the sinus, and a surgical suction apparatus aspirates the saline and foreign body at the same time. This technique is a simple and quick method to retrieve a foreign body out of the sinus and does not require special instruments, as endoscopy does (Sohn et al. 2011). In the past, Caldwell-Luc (trans-antral) type approaches were most commonly performed to remove foreign bodies from the maxillary sinus.

In recent years, endoscopic removal of maxillary sinus foreign bodies has become an often preferred technique. Compared to the Caldwell-Luc procedure, the endoscopic removal of maxillary sinus foreign bodies can reduce perioperative morbidity and complications and shorter operating times. Despite the widespread applicability of endoscopic techniques, surgeons are still reporting using the trans-antral approach for maxillary sinus ectopic tooth removal. This can be combined with endoscopic techniques both as a second portal and to achieve more lateral/anterior access, although this may also be achieved by endoscopic access anterior to the lacrimal duct (Levin and Sommer 2019). Chronic maxillary rhinosinusitis caused by various foreign bodies such as dental implants, dental impressions and even toothpicks, among others, have been described. Despite the benefits of the endoscopic approach, very few case reports describe the endoscopic removal of ectopic maxillary sinus or nasal cavity teeth causing chronic rhinosinusitis or nasal obstruction. While there have previously been reviews regarding literature on ectopic maxillary sinus teeth, none of these have specifically focused on endoscopic removal of paranasal sinus and nasal cavity teeth. It is thus beneficial to highlight the role of the endoscopic approach for the removal of ectopic paranasal sinus teeth through this systematic review. Hence, this review aims to summarise the literature on the endoscopic removal of sinonasal ectopic teeth. By systematically reviewing the literature and understanding these technical and clinical details, otolaryngologists and oral maxillofacial surgeons may be able to better diagnose and stratify patients and select their management method from an evidence-based perspective (Levin and Sommer 2019). Despite these advantages of endoscopic sinus surgery, open approaches are better suited for the removal of larger objects or those located anteriorly in the sinus (Smith and Emko 2007). If the foreign body is large, has sharp edges, is traumatised, etc., it is often necessary to perform a full-fledged surgical intervention. Contraindications to its implementation are pregnancy, acute inflammatory processes, weakened immunity, blood clotting disorders, and tolerance to anaesthesia. In this case, chronic inflammation is relieved with drug therapy. But this course will have to be repeated several times a year until the problem is solved radically (Shenoy and Maller 2013).

Preventive Measures

No one is immune from accidental injury, as a result of which a foreign body appears in the maxillary sinus. But you are quite capable of preventing other reasons for hitting it. Preventive measures, as always, are simple (Shenoy and Maller 2013):

- regularly and properly taking care of one's teeth, visiting the dentist at least twice a year,
- it is obligatory to treat a runny nose to the end to prevent the development of chronic sinusitis;
- closely monitoring compliance with sterility during dental procedures;
- do not ignore preventive examinations at the dentist and otolaryngologist;
- avoiding drafts, hypothermia, and not staying near operating air conditioners for a long time;
- taking measures to strengthen immunity.

Even if you do not have sinusitis yet but only have chronic rhinitis, the nature of which is not clear, especially if it appears sometimes after visiting the dentist, consult a doctor. The sooner a foreign body trapped in the maxillary sinus is detected, the lower the risk of various complications (Shenoy and Maller 2013).

Oroantral Fistula

Introduction

An abnormal communication between the maxillary antrum and the oral cavity is referred to as an Oro-Antral fistula. This communication or fistula is epithelialised

(Verma and Verma 2021). The fistula occurs when appropriate management is not provided, such as following a surgical operation of the maxillary posterior region (Khandelwal and Hajira 2017). It could also occur following the extraction of antral or sinus teeth. Whistling sounds while speaking, unilateral nasal discharge, bad taste in the mouth, and difficulty sucking through a straw are among the complaints patients can present with (Konate et al. 2021). Small lesions, especially those less than 2 mm, could potentially self-resolve; however, the abnormality still requires immediate attention to prevent complications. Other etiologies include different infections of the maxillary sinus (Khandelwal and Hajira 2017). If not appropriately managed, it can impact the patient's quality of life and result in maxillary sinusitis (Konate et al. 2021). The sinusitis itself could make it harder to close the fistula and make management more challenging. To manage the abnormality, the maxillary sinus is first cleared of the disease, and then a graft is used to cover the defect (Verma and Verma 2021). Compilations generally arise if the fistula persists for more than 3 weeks and doesn't heal. The type of flap used and the treatment approach taken are mostly dependent on the size.

Epidemiology

The population impacted the most by Oroantral fistula are those aged between 30 and 60 years old (Salari et al. 2023). Although not a very significant difference, there seems to be a slight male gender predominance (Borgonovo et al. 2012).

Aetiology

Molar and premolar tooth extraction are the most common causes of oroantral fistula. This is because the bone partition between the maxillary sinus and the posterior tooth is thin. This permits the apex of the posterior teeth to reach the maxillary sinus and makes it more prone to the development of the fistula (Verma and Verma 2021). Premolar and molar tooth extraction account for 48% of the cases (Khandelwal and Hajira 2017). Moreover, other etiological factors are infections, both bacterial and fungal, osteomyelitis, malignancy, Paget's disease, granulomatous disease, and maxillofacial trauma (Verma and Verma 2021). Trauma accounts for 7.5% of the cases, whereas maxillary cysts and tumours were responsible for 18.5% of the cases (Khandelwal and Hajira 2017).

Clinical Presentation

Lesions smaller than 2 mm with no infection heal spontaneously by secondary healing following the clot formation. Complications and complaints occur in patients who suffer from a persistent fistula. Although some patients do remain asymptomatic, the majority complain of unilateral nasal discharge, whistling while talking, issues with sucking through a straw, nasal regurgitation of liquid, and an unpleasant taste (Khandelwal and Hajira 2017). Furthermore, other symptoms include alterations in voice and free drainage of fluid through the oral fistula. As the disease reaches a more advanced stage, the antral polyps can be seen through the defect (Azzouzi et al. 2022). In certain cases, patients with large defects can remain asymptomatic because of a concurrent antral polyp closing the gap (Parvini et al. 2019). Regarding pain, if present, it will be from the malar region (Khandelwal and Hajira 2017).

Diagnosis and Imaging

As previously touched, more advanced large defects can be directly visualised on inspection; however, smaller defects require the nose-blowing test, also known as a Valsalva test. In this test, the patient is asked to keep his mouth open and the nostril closed while concurrently blowing gently down the nose. In patients with oroantral fistula, a whistling sound will be heard with this test due to air going down and through the fistula into the oral cavity. Other ways to confirm the escape of air through the nostril is via using a mouth mirror at the oroantral fistula that becomes foggy or by using a cotton wisp placed at the fistula (Khandelwal and Hajira 2017). A negative result is not enough to exclude or rule out the fistula, especially since smaller defects are harder to detect (Parvini et al. 2019). To further strengthen the diagnosis, radiographic means such as CT scans can be used. Blond CT scans and panoramic radiographs can be used to figure out the characteristics of the defect such as its size, location and extent of sinus involvement (Parvini et al. 2019). Radiographic means can demonstrate the discontinuity in the floor of the maxillary sinus. Apart from the defect, CT scans can also show the fluid in the ipsilateral sinus or the soft tissue opacification. Furthermore, due to their susceptibility to sinus infections, CT and Cone Beam Computed Tomography (CBCT) are considered the gold standard for excluding maxillary sinusitis (Parvini et al. 2019).

Histopathology

The abnormal communication between the oral cavity and the maxillary antrum is lined by epithelial cells.

Treatment and Prognosis

Both surgical and non-surgical approaches can be taken to manage oroantral fistula. Non-surgical means include placing certain materials into the fistula to act as a mechanical barrier (Verma and Verma 2021). Surgical methods generally indicate using different types of flaps, possibly in combination, to close the defect (Verma and

Verma 2021). Local flaps, distant flaps, and grafting can all be utilised to cover the defect. The flaps used are rotating or advancing soft tissues such as the palatal flap, buccal flap, submucosal flap and buccal fat pad, among others (Khandelwal and Hajira 2017). In most of the cases, a resultant flap is advanced into the fistula to correct the defect. For cases where a buccal mucoperiosteal flap is chosen, straight-advancement flap, transverse flap, rotation-advancement flap and sliding flap techniques can be used. This is in contrast to those using a palatal mucoperiosteum flap, where a straight-advancement flap, rotational advancement flap, island flap, and hinged flap procedures are used (Waldrop and Semba 1993). Recently, innovative approaches with bone grafts have shown to be successful in moderate to large fistulas. It does provide better predictable results than xenograft (Konate et al. 2021). Other materials, such as platelet-rich fibrin, gel foam, fat, bone, and cartilage, can be added as a means of providing further support (Verma and Verma 2021). If the fistula is complicated by bacterial and fungal sinusitis, it is essential to manage the sinusitis with the fistula to ensure complete resolution and prevent recurrences and complications (Kodur et al. 2017). Postoperative management is very crucial for patients with oroantral fistula. Patients are advised to eat soft food, drink from the opposite side and avoid hard food items. Furthermore, until further healing occurs, excessive strenuous exercises should be avoided to not increase intra-sinusoidal pressure. Moreover, patients are instructed to open their mouths when they cough or sneeze and to avoid blowing their noses with their mouths closed (Khandelwal and Hajira 2017).

References

Alnafisah AM, Hameed S (2020) Aplasia of the maxillary sinus, a large periapical cyst in the maxillary arch, and a swimming and kissing molar: a rare case report. Curēus. https://doi.org/10.7759/cureus.6859

Alrasheed MA, Alhaddad MS, Almuhainy NA, Almohammedali AA (2021) An unusual maxillary sinus foreign body: a case report. Am J Case Rep 22. https://doi.org/10.12659/ajcr.928534

Alsufyani N, El-Hakim H, Major P (2021) Prevalence of maxillary sinus hypoplasia and association with variations in the sinonasal complex: a cone beam CT study. Clin Oral Investig 25:5463–5471. https://doi.org/10.1007/s00784-021-03854-3

Azzouzi A, Hallab L, Chbicheb S (2022) Diagnosis and management of oro-antral fistula: case series and review. Int J Surg Case Rep 97:107436. https://doi.org/10.1016/j.ijscr.2022.107436

Batista AM, Marques LS, Batista AE et al (2012) Urban-rural differences in oral and maxillofacial trauma. Braz Oral Res 26:132–138. https://doi.org/10.1590/s1806-83242012000200008

Batra PS, Han JK (2015) Practical medical and surgical management of chronic rhinosinusitis. Springer, Cham

Bell D, Ye L (2017) Paranasal sinus fractures. Radiopaedia.org. https://doi.org/10.53347/rid-56923

Borgonovo AE, Berardinelli FV, Favale M, Maiorana C (2012) Surgical options in oroantral fistula treatment. Open Dent J 6:94–98. https://doi.org/10.2174/1874210601206010094

Brasileiro BF, Cortez ALV, Asprino L et al (2005) Traumatic subcutaneous emphysema of the face associated with paranasal sinus fractures: a prospective study. J Oral Maxillofac Surg 63:1080–1087. https://doi.org/10.1016/j.joms.2005.04.007

Christmas DA, Mirante JP, Yanagisawa E (2003) The missed maxillary sinus ostium syndrome. Ear Nose Throat J 82:546–548. https://doi.org/10.1177/014556130308200803

Cleveland Clinic (2023) Silent sinus syndrome: symptoms, causes & treatment. Cleveland Clinic. https://my.clevelandclinic.org/health/diseases/25192-silent-sinus-syndrome. Accessed 1 January 2024

Da Silva De Menezes JD, Moura L, Pereira-Filho V, Hochuli-Vieira E (2016) Maxillary sinus mucocele as a late complication in zygomatic-orbital complex fracture. Craniomaxillofac Trauma Reconstr 9:342–344. https://doi.org/10.1055/s-0036-1582453

De Alencar Pierre JHA, Santana EA (2000) Maxillary sinus agenesis—report of two cases. https://inis.iaea.org/search/search.aspx?orig_q=RN:31028033

Dedeoglu N, Duman S (2020) Clinical significance of maxillary sinus hypoplasia in dentistry: a CBCT study. Dent Med Probl 57:149–156. https://doi.org/10.17219/dmp/114982

Duncavage JA, Becker SS (2011) The maxillary sinus. Thieme, Stuttgart

Flint PW, Haughey BH, Lund VJ et al (2014) Cummings otolaryngology—head and neck surgery E-Book. Elsevier Health Sciences, Amsterdam

Hallak B, Teiga P, Bühler J, Bouayed S (2021) Unexpected foreign body induced refractory maxillary sinusitis. Clin Case Rep 9:2185–2188. https://doi.org/10.1002/ccr3.3976

Hasan TS (2022) Total aplasia of the paranasal sinuses and nasal cavity: the first case report. Egypt J Otolaryngol 38. https://doi.org/10.1186/s43163-022-00224-y

Health Jade (2020) Silent sinus syndrome. https://healthjade.net/silent-sinus-syndrome/#footnote_5_43065

Ibrahim D, Gaillard F (2008) Le Fort fracture classification. Radiopaedia.org. https://doi.org/10.53347/rid-1317

Ilie AC, Jianu AM, Rusu MC, Mureşan AN (2022) Anatomical changes in a case with asymmetrical bilateral maxillary sinus hypoplasia. Medicina 58:564. https://doi.org/10.3390/medicina58050564

Illner A, Davidson HC, Harnsberger HR, Hoffman J (2002) The silent sinus syndrome. Am J Roentgenol 178:503–506. https://doi.org/10.2214/ajr.178.2.1780503

Jafari-Pozve N, Sheikhi M, Ataie-Khorasgani M, Jafari-Pozve S (2014) Aplasia and hypoplasia of the maxillary sinus: a case series. PubMed Central (PMC). https://www.ncbi.nlm.nih.gov/pmc/articles/PMC4241618/

Kaluskar S, Sachdeva S (2006) Complications in endoscopic sinus surgery diagnosis, prevention and management. Jaypee Brothers, Medical Publishers Pvt. Limited, Chennai

Khandelwal P, Hajira N (2017) Management of oro-antral communication and fistula: various surgical options. PubMed Central (PMC). https://www.ncbi.nlm.nih.gov/pmc/articles/PMC5339603/

Khanduri S, Agrawal S, Chhabra S, Goyal S (2014) Bilateral maxillary sinus hypoplasia. Case Rep Radiol 2014:1–3. https://doi.org/10.1155/2014/148940

Kodur S, Kiran HY, Shivakumar AM (2017) Odontogenic fungal maxillary sinusitis: a case report of a displaced dental foreign body. Indian J Otolaryngol Head Neck Surg 71:1805–1809. https://doi.org/10.1007/s12070-017-1167-5

Konate M, Sarfi D, Bouhairi ME, Benyahya I (2021) Management of oroantral fistulae and communications: our recommendations for routine practice. Case Rep Dent 2021:1–6. https://doi.org/10.1155/2021/7592253

Lambert DM, Mirvis SE, Shanmuganathan K, Tilghman DL (1997) Computed tomography exclusion of osseous paranasal sinus injury in blunt trauma patients: the “clear sinus” sign. J Oral Maxillofac Surg 55:1207–1210. https://doi.org/10.1016/s0278-2391(97)90167-1

Lenkeit CP, Lofgren DH, Shermetaro C (2023) Maxillary sinus fracture. In: StatPearls—NCBI Bookshelf. https://www.ncbi.nlm.nih.gov/books/NBK557455/

Levin M, Sommer DD (2019) Endoscopic removal of ectopic sinonasal teeth: a systematic review. J Otolaryngol Head Neck Surg 48. https://doi.org/10.1186/s40463-019-0353-8

Maggs DJ, Miller PE, Ofri R, Slatter DH (2008) Slatter’s fundamentals of veterinary ophthalmology. Elsevier, Amsterdam

Meechor B, Javer AR (2008) Revision endoscopie sinus surgery: the St. Paul's Sinus Centre experience. Can Soc Otolaryngol Head Neck Surg. 37:676–680

Nuñez-Castruita A, López-Serna N, Guzmán-López S (2012) Prenatal development of the maxillary sinus. Otolaryngol Head Neck Surg 146:997–1003. https://doi.org/10.1177/0194599811435883

Parsons DS, Stivers F, Talbot A (1996) The missed ostium sequence and the surgical approach to revision functional endoscopic sinus surgery. https://www.semanticscholar.org/paper/The-missed-ostium-sequence-and-the-surgical-to-Parsons-Stivers/9cf91450da59c04688416ecd9a7a6dfeb4c4dc36

Parvini P, Obreja K, Begic A et al (2019) Decision-making in closure of oroantral communication and fistula. Int J Implant Dent 5. https://doi.org/10.1186/s40729-019-0165-7

Ramstead C, McCabe J, Alkahtani M et al (2008) Traumatic dislocation of the globe into the maxillary sinus. Can J Ophthalmol 43:364–366. https://doi.org/10.3129/i08-045

Ratilal BO, Costa J, Pappamikail L, Sampaio C (2015) Antibiotic prophylaxis for preventing meningitis in patients with basilar skull fractures. Cochrane Database Syst Rev 2015. https://doi.org/10.1002/14651858.cd004884.pub4

Roselló EG, Granado AMQ, Garcia MA et al (2020) Facial fractures: classification and highlights for a useful report. Insights Imaging 11. https://doi.org/10.1186/s13244-020-00847-w

Rosso C, Saibene AM, Felisati G, Pipolo C (2022) Silent sinus syndrome: systematic review and proposal of definition, diagnosis and management. Acta Otorhinolaryngol Ital 42:305–316. https://doi.org/10.14639/0392-100x-n1598

Carrasco Rueda CA, Vinitzky Brener I, Rodríguez Colín E, Ornelas Zárate A (2019) Aplasia of the maxillary sinus: a case report. Rev Mex Ortodon 7(3):159–162

Şahin O (2019) Removal of foreign bodies from maxillary sinus: a report of three cases. Ann Clin Anal Med 10. https://doi.org/10.4328/jcam.5992

Salari A, Rasoul TK, Norouzi V (2023) Review paper: the prevalence, etiology & management of oroantral fistula. https://3dj.gums.ac.ir/article-1-586-en.html

Salib RJ, Chaudri SA, Rockley TJ (2001) Sinusitis in the hypoplastic maxillary antrum: the crucial role of radiology in diagnosis and management. J Laryngol Otol 115. https://doi.org/10.1258/0022215011908612

Sharma R, Gaillard F (2010) Silent sinus syndrome. Radiopaedia.org. https://doi.org/10.53347/rid-9443

Shenoy V, Maller V (2013) Maxillary antrolith: a rare cause of the recurrent sinusitis. Case Re Otolaryngol 2013:1–4. https://doi.org/10.1155/2013/527152

Smith JL, Emko P (2007) Management of a maxillary sinus foreign body (Dental Bur). Ear Nose Throat J 86:677–678. https://doi.org/10.1177/014556130708601120

Sohn D-S, Jung H-S, Kim K-H et al (2011) Removal of displaced foreign body from the maxillary sinus using replaceable bony windows and saline irrigation, followed by suctioning of the foreign body. Implant Dent 20:112–117. https://doi.org/10.1097/id.0b013e31820faf53

Stryjewska-Makuch G, Goroszkiewicz K, Szymocha J et al (2022) Etiology, early diagnosis and proper treatment of silent sinus syndrome based on review of the literature and own experience. J Oral Maxillofac Surg 80:113.e1–113.e8. https://doi.org/10.1016/j.joms.2021.08.166

Verma RR, Verma R (2021) Oro-antral fistulas and their management: our experience. Indian J Otolaryngol Head Neck Surg 74:1576–1583. https://doi.org/10.1007/s12070-021-02739-x

Wake M, Shankar L, Hawke M, Takeno S (1993) Maxillary sinus hypoplasia, embryology, and radiology. Arch Otolaryngol Head Neck Surg. 119:1353–1357. https://doi.org/10.1001/archotol.1993.01880240091011

Waldrop TC, Semba SE (1993) Closure of oroantral communication using guided tissue regeneration and an absorbable gelatin membrane. J Periodontol 64:1061–1066. https://doi.org/10.1902/jop.1993.64.11.1061

Weed DT, Cole RR (1994) Maxillary sinus hypoplasia and vertical dystopia of the orbit. Laryngoscope 104:758–762. https://doi.org/10.1288/00005537-199406000-00019

Whyte A, Boeddinghaus R (2019) The maxillary sinus: physiology, development and imaging anatomy. Dentomaxillofac Radiol 48:20190205. https://doi.org/10.1259/dmfr.20190205

Wojtera B, Woźna A, Komisarek O (2020) The management of foreign body displacement into the maxillary sinus as a complication of maxillofacial interventions: systematic review. Indian J Otolaryngol Head Neck Surg 74:1088–1093. https://doi.org/10.1007/s12070-020-02153-9

Yousif Ali Hasan H, Prabhu S, Mohammed A (2017) Hypoplastic maxillary antra. Bahrain Med Bull 39:150–153

Zhang Q-B, Zhang B, Zhang Z-Q, Chen Q (2012) The epidemiology of cranio-facial injuries caused by animals in southern-central China. J Craniomaxillofac Surg 40:506–509. https://doi.org/10.1016/j.jcms.2011.08.012

Anaesthesia in Maxillary Sinus Surgery 10

Goran Latif Omer, Amir Murad Khudadad,
Ahmed Qadir Ahmed, Attar Abdul Kareem Nadir,
Stefano Di Girolamo, and Beatrice Francavilla

Introduction

Maxillary sinus surgery, often performed as part of functional endoscopic sinus surgery (FESS), requires careful consideration of anaesthetic techniques to ensure patient safety and optimal surgical outcomes. The choice between local and general anaesthesia depends on the complexity of the procedure and the patient's medical status. This chapter provides a detailed examination of anaesthetic considerations specific to maxillary sinus surgeries, emphasizing the importance of patient preparation, intraoperative management, and postoperative care.

Initially, topical anaesthesia combined with sedation was employed for sinus surgery, particularly in minor procedures. However, more extensive resections necessitate general anaesthesia. This approach not only provides adequate airway protection and cardiovascular control but also ensures a stable, immobile patient, facilitating a superior view of the surgical field. The benefits of general anaesthesia in FESS include enhanced analgesia, reduced patient movement, and better overall surgical conditions.

FESS is generally considered a low-risk procedure, with an overall complication rate of approximately 0.5%. Specific complications include cerebrospinal fluid leaks (0.09%), meningitis, haemorrhage (0.1%), and orbital injuries (0.09%) (Suzuki et al. 2015). The anaesthetic management should be tailored to the needs of head and neck surgery, with particular attention to the specific challenges of endoscopic sinus surgery.

G. L. Omer (✉) · A. M. Khudadad
Department of Clinical Sciences, College of Medicine, University of Sulaimani, Sulaymaniyah, KRI, Iraq

A. Q. Ahmed · A. A. K. Nadir
Royal Hospital, Sulaymaniyah, KRI, Iraq

S. Di Girolamo · B. Francavilla
Department of Otorhinolaryngology, University of Rome Tor Vergata, Rome, Italy

© The Author(s), under exclusive license to Springer Nature Switzerland AG 2025
G. L. Omer, S. Di Girolamo (eds.), *Maxillary Sinus: A Comprehensive Guide*, https://doi.org/10.1007/978-3-031-83468-4_10

Preoperative Evaluation and Patient Preparation

A comprehensive preoperative assessment is essential for optimizing patient outcomes in maxillary sinus surgery. This assessment includes a detailed medical history, physical examination, and review of relevant investigations. Key components of the history include present and past medical conditions, regular medications, previous surgical experiences, allergies, ASA classification, lifestyle factors (smoking, alcohol use), and exercise tolerance. The patient should be thoroughly informed about the planned surgical procedure, the anaesthetic plan, and postoperative care arrangements. Informed consent must be obtained after addressing all patient queries.

Hypertension Management

Uncontrolled hypertension significantly increases the risk of cerebrovascular events, myocardial infarction, and end-organ damage, particularly to the kidneys. It also heightens the risk of intraoperative bleeding and postoperative hematoma formation (Aronow 2017). According to the AoA/BHS guidelines, patients with blood pressure readings below 160/100 mmHg can proceed to surgery without further delay. If preoperative clinic measurements exceed 180/110 mmHg, surgery should be postponed to allow for better blood pressure control (Hartle et al. 2016). Special consideration is needed for patients on ACE inhibitors and ARBs, as these medications should be discontinued 24 h prior to surgery and resumed 48 h postoperatively to avoid intraoperative hypotension (Duceppe et al. 2017). Diuretics should also be withheld on the day of surgery unless contraindicated by conditions such as congestive heart failure or liver disease (Miller et al. 2015; Tagawa et al. 2015). The continuation of beta-blockers is generally recommended, but high doses should be avoided due to the risk of severe bradycardia and other complications (Devereaux 2008; Fleisher et al. 2014).

Cardiac Assessment

Following the 2022 ESC guidelines, a thorough cardiovascular assessment is necessary for patients with known cardiac conditions to optimize their status before surgery. This includes a multidisciplinary discussion involving the patient's cardiologist and the surgical team to evaluate the need for additional tests and to plan perioperative management. Recognizing patients with fixed cardiac output who cannot tolerate hypotension is crucial for developing an appropriate anaesthetic strategy, including the potential need for invasive monitoring.

Diabetes Management

Diabetes mellitus poses significant perioperative risks, including metabolic derangements, delayed wound healing, and infections. Stress responses from anaesthesia and surgery, combined with steroid use, can exacerbate hyperglycaemia. Diabetic patients should have their surgeries scheduled early in the day to facilitate blood glucose management. Preoperative blood glucose and HbA1c levels should guide the timing of surgery, with postponement recommended if severe hyperglycaemia or diabetic ketoacidosis is present (Dhatariya et al. 2012). The target blood glucose range is 108–189 mg/dl, with a broader acceptable range of 72–198 mg/dl.

Asthma and Respiratory Considerations

The relationship between chronic sinusitis and asthma is well-documented, with FESS often resulting in symptomatic improvement for asthmatic patients (Nair et al. 2010). Asthma is prevalent among patients undergoing sinus surgery, and perioperative respiratory events such as bronchospasm and laryngospasm are potential risks (Woods and Sladen 2009). A history of uncontrolled asthma increases the risk of postoperative complications, including pneumonia and mortality (Lin et al. 2016). Preoperative optimization includes a detailed history, pulmonary function testing, and medication adjustments to reduce perioperative respiratory risks (Tirumalasetty and Grammer 2006).

Management of Regular Medications and Anticoagulation

Effective perioperative management of regular medications is crucial, especially concerning anticoagulants and drugs that influence haemostasis. Table 10.1 outlines the recommended discontinuation times for various anticoagulants before surgery, which is critical to minimizing intraoperative bleeding risks.

Preoperative Airway Assessment

An essential component of the preoperative evaluation is assessing the airway to identify potential difficulties in intubation or oxygenation. A history of previous anaesthesia or airway-related issues, combined with physical assessments (e.g., Mallampati classification, thyromental distance), helps predict airway challenges. A comprehensive airway assessment allows the anaesthesiologist to prepare appropriate equipment and strategies, ensuring patient safety.

Laboratory and Other Investigations

Routine preoperative laboratory tests, including a complete blood count, coagulation profile, and renal function tests, are standard. Additional investigations such as EKGs, chest X-rays, and CT scans of the sinuses may be indicated based on the patient's medical history and planned surgical procedure. Special attention is

Table 10.1 Discontinuation guidelines for anticoagulants before surgery (Horlocker et al. 2018; Yeung et al. 2016)

Anticoagulant	Discontinuation time before surgery	Notes
Unfractionated heparin	6 h	
Low molecular weight heparin (LMWH)	• Prophylactic dose: 12 h • Treatment dose: 24 h	
Xa inhibitors such (e.g., Rivoxanaban, Apixaban, edoxaban)	24–48 h	Cr Cl > 30: 48 h Cr Cl 30–50: 72 h Cr Cl 30–50: 48 h
IIa inhibitor (dabigatran)	48 h	Cr Cl 50–80 72 h
Warfarin	Five days	
Aspirin and Clopidogrel	Seven days	
Stents: Bare metal stents Drug-eluting stents	Bare metal: Delay surgery for 6 weeks Drug-eluting: Delay for 6–12 months	

required for patients with cardiovascular or pulmonary conditions to tailor anaesthesia management to their specific needs.

Causes for Postponement and Cancellation of Surgery

Advancements in anaesthetic agents and monitoring technologies have reduced the need for postponing surgeries. However, common reasons for cancellation include upper respiratory infections, uncontrolled systemic diseases, and failure to adhere to preoperative fasting guidelines. A detailed evaluation and discussion with the patient and surgical team are necessary to determine the best course of action.

Local Anaesthesia Versus General Anaesthesia in Maxillary Sinus Surgery

In major maxillary sinus surgeries, general anaesthesia is often preferred due to its comprehensive advantages, which include ensuring patient relaxation and minimizing anxiety, which are crucial for procedural cooperation. Additionally, general anaesthesia allows surgeons to operate without distraction, particularly in delicate procedures requiring microscopy, as it provides complete immobility at the surgical site. This approach also offers better control over haemodynamics, especially important in procedures necessitating controlled hypotension, and it secures the airway, thereby minimizing the risk of pulmonary aspiration.

In contrast, local anaesthesia is an alternative primarily considered when patients refuse general anaesthesia or have contraindications to it due to severe systemic diseases such as advanced cardiac or pulmonary conditions. Local anaesthesia avoids the need for airway instrumentation and the use of inhalational agents, thereby reducing the risks associated with positive pressure ventilation. Additionally, it is generally less expensive than general anaesthesia and reduces postoperative complications like coughing or straining, which are beneficial in certain patient populations.

Nowadays, the approach often combines local and general anaesthesia to optimize patient outcomes. After the induction of general anaesthesia and securing the airway, local anaesthetics with vasoconstrictors (e.g., lidocaine with epinephrine at a 1/80,000 concentration) are used to achieve complete analgesia and reduce intraoperative bleeding.

Local anaesthesia with sedation, or monitored anaesthesia care (MAC), is suitable for various nasal sinus procedures. The choice of local anaesthetic and its administration depends on the specific anatomy to be numbed. Common side effects, such as itching, numbness, and a burning sensation, are typically mild and short-lived. Patients are advised to avoid alcohol before the procedure to prevent postoperative nausea and vomiting, which can delay discharge. Additionally, patients should refrain from driving or operating heavy machinery postoperatively due to potential dizziness.

The maxillary division of the trigeminal nerve provides sensory innervation to the mid-face, including the lower eyelid, upper lip, maxillary sinus, nasal cavity, and palate. For maxillary sinus surgery, the infraorbital nerve and the sphenopalatine ganglion can be targeted for anaesthesia (Sim et al. 2013). Topical decongestants, such as cocaine with phenylephrine, and local anaesthetic injections, like lidocaine with epinephrine, are used to reduce mucosal swelling and bleeding.

Induction and Maintenance of Anaesthesia

The choice of anaesthetic technique depends on the type of surgery, the patient's age, and overall health. Preoperative preparation includes patient positioning and monitoring, such as the insertion of an arterial line for continuous blood pressure monitoring (Fig. 10.1), which is crucial for procedures involving controlled hypotension. Anaesthesia induction typically involves preoxygenation, followed by administration of opioids like fentanyl and sedatives like propofol or thiopentone. Muscle relaxants such as rocuronium or cisatracurium are used to facilitate intubation and ensure immobility.

During surgery, maintenance of anaesthesia is typically achieved using TIVA, combining propofol and remifentanil for optimal hemodynamic control and minimal postoperative nausea. The use of NSAIDs is generally avoided due to the increased risk of postoperative bleeding.

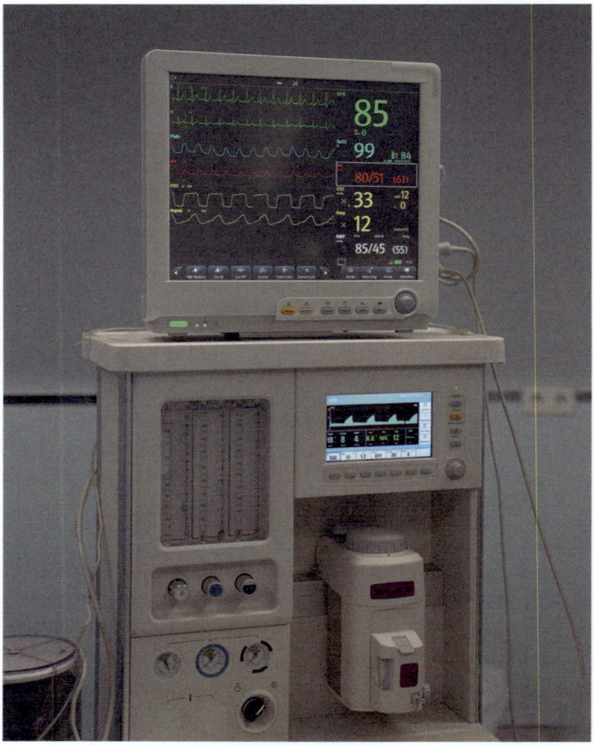

Fig. 10.1 Controlled hypotension technique mandates using invasive blood pressure monitoring, which facilitates beat to beat blood pressure monitoring and arterial blood sampling for arterial blood gas analysis

For maxillary sinus surgery, the choice of airway management—whether using an endotracheal tube (ETT) or a laryngeal mask airway (LMA)—is critical to both surgical and anaesthetic outcomes. The airway device is typically positioned in the midline, with the tube directed downward, minimizing interference with the surgical team. This positioning is essential for providing a clear surgical field and maintaining effective ventilation.

In terms of setup, the anaesthesia machine is usually placed on the left side of the patient, near the patient's feet, to keep it out of the surgeon's way and reduce the risk of contamination in the sterile field. When an endotracheal tube is used, a tap water-soaked pack may be placed in the patient's throat. This practice helps absorb any blood that might drain into the throat during surgery, thereby reducing the risk of blood entering the stomach, which can cause postoperative nausea and vomiting. This precaution is particularly important in reducing the incidence of emetogenic complications, contributing to a smoother recovery phase for the patient.

Measures to Decrease Blood Loss During Maxillary Sinus Surgery

Excessive bleeding, common due to the rich vascular supply of sinonasal mucosa, can obscure the surgical field and increase complications. Several strategies are employed to minimize blood loss:

(a) **Preoperative Preparation:** Optimizing systemic illnesses and discontinuing medications that increase bleeding risk.
(b) **Patient Positioning:** A 20° reverse Trendelenburg position (Fig. 10.2) helps reduce venous pressure in the surgical area (Gan et al. 2013).
(c) **Pharmacologic Interventions:** The prophylactic administration of tranexamic acid, an antifibrinolytic agent, may reduce blood loss without increasing thrombotic risks (Kim et al. 2018).
(d) **Body temperature:** Maintaining normothermia is critical to prevent coagulopathy and hypothermia-related complications (Díaz and Becker 2010).
(e) **Premedication:** Medications such as beta-blockers (e.g., metoprolol), calcium channel blockers (e.g., nifedipine), and alpha-2 agonists (e.g., clonidine) can help manage blood pressure and reduce intraoperative bleeding (Hassanein and Talaat 2015; Sadek et al. 2019; Tugrul et al. 2016).

Controlled Hypotension in Anaesthesia

Controlled hypotension is a deliberate reduction of blood pressure during surgery to minimize blood loss and improve the surgical field's visibility. This technique is particularly valuable in maxillary sinus surgeries, where a clear surgical field is crucial for precision and reducing operative time. The target is usually to lower the systolic blood pressure to 80–90 mmHg, maintain a mean arterial pressure (MAP)

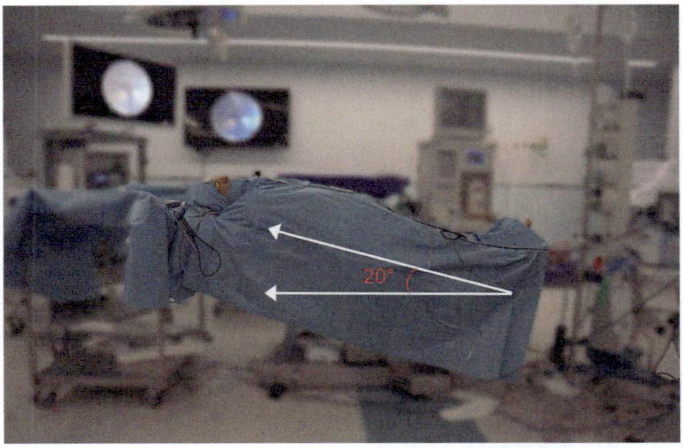

Fig. 10.2 20° reverse Trendelenberg position helps by pooling blood to the lower body and reducing upper body blood congestion, hence more clearer surgical field

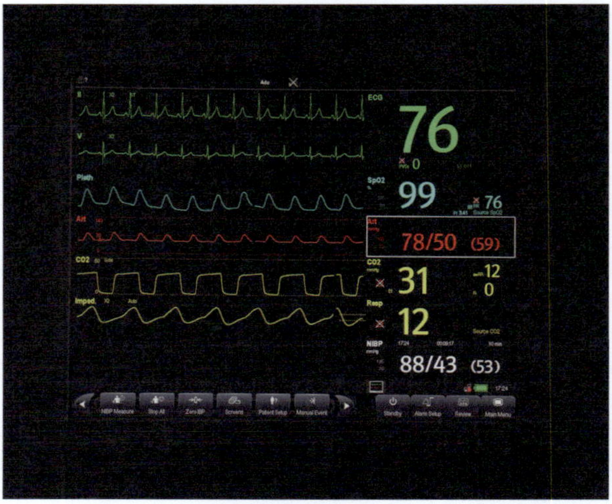

Fig. 10.3 Controlled hypotension to decrease blood loss in maxillary sinus surgery, by keeping MAP between 50 and 60 mmHg. Keep in mind that $EtCO_2$ and $PaCO_2$ change with hypotension, so arterial blood gas determination should be carried out intermittently to make sure that the $PaCO_2$ is within the desired range

between 50 and 60 mmHg, or achieve a 30% reduction from the patient's baseline MAP (Fig. 10.3).

Commonly used agents include inhalational anaesthetics, beta-adrenergic antagonists, vasodilators, and alpha-2 agonists like dexmedetomidine (Naaz and Ozair 2014). Continuous monitoring of oxygen saturation, end-tidal CO_2, and blood pressure is essential to avoid hypoperfusion and hypoxia. Invasive blood pressure monitoring is recommended for accuracy. Hypothermia management includes pre-warming the patient and maintaining room temperature.

Pharmacologic Agents Used in Controlled Hypotension

Inhalational Anaesthetics

Agents such as isoflurane, sevoflurane, and desflurane are commonly used due to their potent vasodilatory effects, which help reduce systemic vascular resistance and induce controlled hypotension. These agents also provide muscle relaxation, enhancing surgical conditions. However, their use must be balanced with the potential for increased bleeding, as their vasodilatory effects can increase tissue perfusion in the surgical area, potentially leading to higher blood loss. Additionally, high concentrations of inhalational anaesthetics may pose risks of nephrotoxicity, hepatotoxicity, and postoperative nausea and vomiting.

Beta-Adrenergic Antagonists

Drugs like esmolol and metoprolol are used to reduce heart rate and myocardial contractility, contributing to lower cardiac output and thus lowering blood pressure.

These agents are particularly useful in patients with cardiovascular risks, as they provide hemodynamic stability with minimal side effects.

Vasodilators

Sodium nitroprusside, nitroglycerin, and hydralazine are effective in reducing blood pressure by causing direct vasodilation. These drugs are potent and allow for rapid titration, making them suitable for achieving precise blood pressure control. However, their use requires careful monitoring due to potential side effects such as excessive hypotension and reflex tachycardia.

Alpha-2 Adrenergic Agonists

Agents like clonidine and dexmedetomidine are increasingly used due to their ability to provide sedation, anxiolysis, and analgesia without respiratory depression. These drugs also contribute to controlled hypotension by reducing sympathetic outflow, which decreases heart rate and vascular resistance. Dexmedetomidine, in particular, is valued for its ability to reduce anaesthetic and analgesic requirements during surgery, helping to maintain a stable hemodynamic state (Naaz and Ozair 2014).

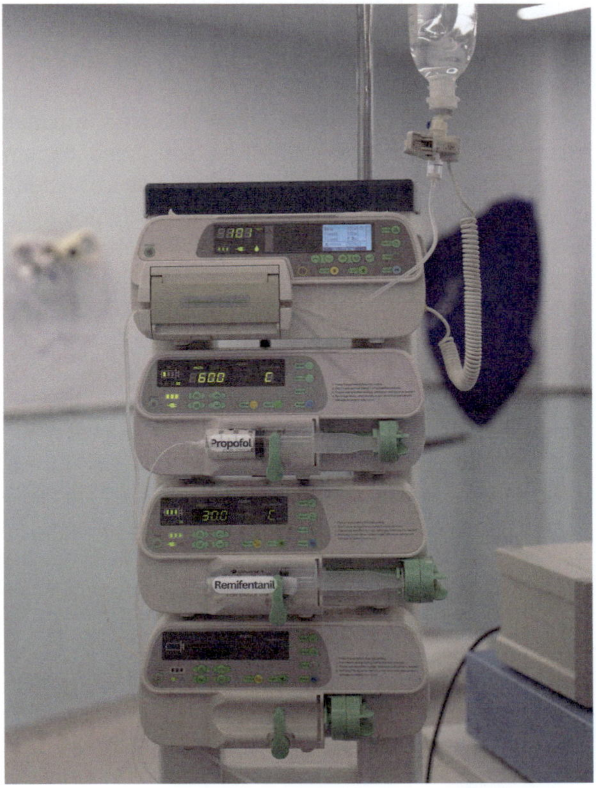

Fig. 10.4 Two main agents (propofol and remifentanil) were used during the TIVA (Total Intravenous Anaesthesia) technique for FESS

Total Intravenous Anaesthesia (TIVA)

TIVA, often using propofol and remifentanil (Fig. 10.4), offers several advantages for controlled hypotension. Propofol reduces cerebral metabolism and blood flow, aiding in minimizing blood loss in sinus surgeries by reducing blood flow via the ethmoidal and supraorbital arteries. Remifentanil, a potent and ultra-short-acting opioid, is effective in managing the hemodynamic response to surgical stimuli, offering rapid titration and minimizing postoperative pain. This combination provides precise control over anaesthesia depth and cardiovascular parameters, which is essential for achieving and maintaining controlled hypotension (Mertens et al. 2003; Eleveld et al. 2020).

Monitoring, Contraindications, and Risks of Controlled Hypotension

The use of controlled hypotension necessitates stringent monitoring to avoid complications such as hypoperfusion and hypoxia. Continuous monitoring of oxygen saturation, end-tidal CO_2, and electroencephalogram (EEG) is crucial to ensure adequate tissue perfusion and detect any signs of ischemia or other complications. Blood pressure should be closely monitored, preferably with invasive arterial monitoring, to provide real-time data and enable prompt adjustments.

Hypothermia is another concern during controlled hypotension, as it can exacerbate coagulopathy and increase the risk of surgical bleeding. Measures to maintain normothermia include pre-warming the patient, maintaining an appropriate ambient temperature in the operating room, and warming intravenous fluids and irrigation solutions.

Controlled hypotension is contraindicated in patients with significant ischemic heart disease, cerebrovascular accidents, and certain haematological conditions such as severe anaemia or sickle cell disease. Additionally, patients with poorly controlled hypertension may not tolerate hypotension well due to compromised autoregulation of vital organs, making them susceptible to complications such as renal or cerebral ischemia. In such cases, the benefits of controlled hypotension must be carefully weighed against the risks, and the technique should only be employed if the anaesthesiologist is experienced and the necessary monitoring is available (Sharrock et al. 1991; Upadhyay et al. 2015).

The primary risks associated with controlled hypotension include inadequate tissue perfusion leading to organ dysfunction, prolonged recovery from anaesthesia, and increased postoperative cognitive dysfunction. There is also a risk of surgical field bleeding and insufficient haemostasis, which can complicate the procedure and prolong operative time (Perez-Chrzanowska et al. 2022). Therefore, controlled hypotension should be employed with caution, ensuring that the patient's medical status and the surgical team's experience support its use.

Emergence from Anaesthesia

The goal during emergence from anaesthesia is a smooth recovery without respiratory complications such as coughing or straining, which could lead to increased intranasal bleeding. Awake extubation for functional endoscopic sinus surgery (FESS) allows the return of laryngeal reflexes, protecting the airway from blood and secretions. However, it carries risks such as laryngospasm, coughing, bucking, oxygen desaturation, and increased bleeding. Conversely, deep extubation facilitates a smoother emergence from anaesthesia, with reduced coughing and movement. Still, it poses higher risks of laryngospasm and airway obstruction, especially in patients at risk of aspiration from blood in the airway. Nasal packing further complicates maintaining airway patency, so preoperative counselling should include instructions for patients to breathe through their mouth upon awakening.

Postoperative Care

Postoperative nausea and vomiting (PONV) and post-discharge nausea and vomiting (PDNV) are common and can delay recovery and discharge, increasing healthcare costs. Patients undergoing endoscopic sinus surgery are at high risk for PONV due to blood ingestion, uvula inflammation, and opioid use. Prevention strategies include a multimodal approach with antiemetics like dexamethasone and 5HT3 antagonists (ondansetron). TIVA also reduces PONV incidence. If vomiting occurs, positioning the patient laterally can prevent aspiration pneumonia, and hydration and antiemetics are necessary. Rarely, readmission may be required.

Postoperative pain following maxillary sinus surgery is generally mild to moderate, primarily due to surgical trauma and nasal packing. Local anaesthesia used preoperatively may not suffice for pain control. Acetaminophen is typically effective, supplemented by non-opioid analgesics if necessary. NSAIDs are usually avoided in the immediate postoperative period to reduce the risk of bleeding.

References

Aronow WS (2017) Management of hypertension in patients undergoing surgery. Ann Transl Med 5:227. https://doi.org/10.21037/atm.2017.03.54

Devereaux P (2008) Effects of extended-release metoprolol succinate in patients undergoing noncardiac surgery (POISE trial): a randomised controlled trial. Lancet 371:1839–1847. https://doi.org/10.1016/s0140-6736(08)60601-7

Dhatariya K, Levy N, Kilvert A et al (2012) NHS diabetes guideline for the perioperative management of the adult patient with diabetes*. Diabet Med 29:420–433. https://doi.org/10.1111/j.1464-5491.2012.03582.x

Díaz M, Becker DE (2010) Thermoregulation: physiological and clinical considerations during sedation and general anesthesia. Anesth Prog 57:25–33. https://doi.org/10.2344/0003-3006-57.1.25

Duceppe E, Parlow J, MacDonald P et al (2017) Canadian Cardiovascular Society guidelines on perioperative cardiac risk assessment and management for patients who undergo noncardiac surgery. Can J Cardiol 33:17–32. https://doi.org/10.1016/j.cjca.2016.09.008

Eleveld DJ, Colin P, Absalom AR, Struys MMRF (2020) Target-controlled-infusion models for remifentanil dosing consistent with approved recommendations. Br J Anaesth 125:483–491. https://doi.org/10.1016/j.bja.2020.05.051

Fleisher LA, Fleischmann KE, Auerbach AD et al (2014) 2014 ACC/AHA guideline on perioperative cardiovascular evaluation and management of patients undergoing noncardiac surgery. J Am Coll Cardiol 64:e77–e137. https://doi.org/10.1016/j.jacc.2014.07.944

Gan EC, Habib AR, Rajwani A, Javer AR (2013) Five-degree, 10-degree, and 20-degree reverse Trendelenburg position during functional endoscopic sinus surgery: a double-blind randomized controlled trial. Int Forum Allergy Rhinol 4:61–68. https://doi.org/10.1002/alr.21249

Hartle A, McCormack T, Carlisle J et al (2016) The measurement of adult blood pressure and management of hypertension before elective surgery. Anaesthesia 71:326–337. https://doi.org/10.1111/anae.13348

Hassanein A, Talaat M (2015) Oral nifedipine as a premedication for induced hypotension in functional endoscopic sinus surgery (FESS). Egypt J Anaesth 31:291–295. https://doi.org/10.1016/j.egja.2015.06.005

Horlocker TT, Vandermeuelen E, Kopp SL et al (2018) Regional anesthesia in the patient receiving antithrombotic or thrombolytic therapy. Reg Anesth Pain Med 43:263–309. https://doi.org/10.1097/aap.0000000000000763

Kim DH, Kim S, Kang H et al (2018) Efficacy of tranexamic acid on operative bleeding in endoscopic sinus surgery: a meta-analysis and systematic review. Laryngoscope 129:800–807. https://doi.org/10.1002/lary.27766

Lin C-S, Chang C-C, Yeh C-C et al (2016) Postoperative adverse outcomes in patients with asthma. Medicine 95:e2548. https://doi.org/10.1097/md.0000000000002548

Mertens MJ, Olofsen E, Engbers FHM et al (2003) Propofol reduces perioperative remifentanil requirements in a synergistic manner. Anesthesiology 99:347–359. https://doi.org/10.1097/00000542-200308000-00016

Miller RD, Eriksson LI, Fleisher LA, Wiener-Kronish JP, Cohen NH, Young WL (2015) Miller's Anesthesia. 8th ed. Philadelphia: Elsevier Saunders. ISBN: 978-0-7020-5283-5.

Naaz SA, Ozair E (2014) Dexmedetomidine in current anaesthesia practice—a review. J Clin Diagn Res. https://doi.org/10.7860/jcdr/2014/9624.4946

Nair S, Bhadauria RS, Sharma S (2010) Effect of endoscopic sinus surgery on asthmatic patients with chronic rhinosinusitis. Indian J Otolaryngol Head Neck Surg 62:285–288. https://doi.org/10.1007/s12070-010-0086-5

Perez-Chrzanowska H, Mendez PS, Otero RP (2022) Intraoperative controlled hypotension—a review of the literature and 60 years of personal experience from the point of view of anesthesiologists. www.alliedacademies.org. https://doi.org/10.35841/aajptr-6.3.111

Sadek AA, Mostafa M, Abdel-Monem T (2019) Metoprolol significantly improves visual clarity and hemodynamic parameters during functional endoscopic sinus surgery. Biomed Hub 4:1–8. https://doi.org/10.1159/000497045

Sharrock NE, Mineo R, Urquhart B (1991) Haemodynamic effects and outcome analysis of hypotensive anaesthesia in controlled hypertensive patients undergoing total hip arthroplasty. Br J Anaesth 67:17–25

Sim AJ, Levine AI, Govindaraj S (2013) Functional nasal and sinus surgery. In: Anesthesiology and Otolaryngology. Vol. 9781461441847. Springer New York. p. 197–216. https://doi.org/10.1007/978-1-4614-4184-7_13

Suzuki S, Yasunaga H, Matsui H et al (2015) Complication rates after functional endoscopic sinus surgery: analysis of 50,734 Japanese patients. Laryngoscope 125:1785–1791. https://doi.org/10.1002/lary.25334

Tagawa M, Ogata A, Hamano T (2015) Pre- and/or intra-operative prescription of diuretics, but not renin-angiotensin-system inhibitors, is significantly associated with acute kidney injury after non-cardiac surgery: a retrospective cohort study. PLoS One 10:e0132507. https://doi.org/10.1371/journal.pone.0132507

Tirumalasetty J, Grammer LC (2006) Asthma, surgery, and general anesthesia: a review. J Asthma 43:251–254. https://doi.org/10.1080/02770900600643162

Tugrul S, Dogan R, Senturk E et al (2016) Effect of the premedication with oral clonidine on surgical comfort in patients undergoing fess due to advanced nasal polyposis: a randomized double blind clinical trial. Am J Otolaryngol 37:538–543. https://doi.org/10.1016/j.amjoto.2016.08.008

Upadhyay SP, Samant U, Tellicherry SS, Mallik S, Saikia PP, Mallick PN (2015) Controlled hypotension in modern anaesthesia: a review and update. Int J Biol Pharm Res 6(7):532–542
Woods BD, Sladen RN (2009) Perioperative considerations for the patient with asthma and bronchospasm. Br J Anaesth 103:i57–i65. https://doi.org/10.1093/bja/aep271
Yeung LYY, Sarani B, Weinberg JA et al (2016) Surgeon's guide to anticoagulant and antiplatelet medications part two: antiplatelet agents and perioperative management of long-term anticoagulation. Trauma Surg Acute Care Open 1:e000022. https://doi.org/10.1136/tsaco-2016-000022

11 Approaches to Maxillary Sinus

Goran Latif Omer, Stefano Di Girolamo, Kosar Hama Noori, Karwan Shahin, Saman W. Boskani, Avar Fuad Ahmed, Sahand Soran Ali, Aland Salih Abdullah, and Riccardo Maurizi

Endoscopic Approaches

Introduction

Ancient Egyptians were the first to identify the maxillary sinus (MS), and it has been extensively researched with regard to its anatomy, vascular system and connection to the dentition. During the 10th week of embryonic development, the maxillary sinus begins to form as a result of invagination of ethmoid infundibulum mucosa. Up to the 37th week of gestation, the sinus continues to grow and ossify.

The maxillary sinus grows throughout infancy until it reaches adult size between the ages of 18 and 21. Anatomically, the floor of the maxillary sinus is formed by the alveolar and palatine processes of the maxilla, and the roots of the posterior maxillary dentition lie in close relation to the floor of the sinus, with the molars having closer contact than the premolars. As a result, a variety of diseases involving the maxillary sinus are of dentoalveolar origin. Surgery is usually necessary when medical treatment fails to manage maxillary sinusitis or inflammation or in situations of malignancy (McCormick et al. 2020). In the past three decades, endoscopic sinus surgery has replaced open sinus surgery as the standard of treatment. Caldwell-Luc

Supplementary Information The online version contains supplementary material available at https://doi.org/10.1007/978-3-031-83468-4_11.

G. L. Omer (✉) · S. S. Ali · A. S. Abdullah
Department of Clinical Sciences, College of Medicine, University of Sulaimani, Sulaymaniyah, KRI, Iraq

S. Di Girolamo · R. Maurizi
Department of Otorhinolaryngology, University of Rome Tor Vergata, Rome, Italy

K. H. Noori · K. Shahin · S. W. Boskani · A. F. Ahmed
Royal Hospital, Sulaymaniyah, KRI, Iraq

© The Author(s), under exclusive license to Springer Nature Switzerland AG 2025
G. L. Omer, S. Di Girolamo (eds.), *Maxillary Sinus: A Comprehensive Guide*, https://doi.org/10.1007/978-3-031-83468-4_11

and lateral rhinotomy are examples of procedures that are relatively invasive, have a considerable risk of morbidity and disregard the sinuses' normal physiology. Even when considering surgery for sinonasal tumours, where maintaining sinus functioning is not the main goal, there are several endoscopic techniques that can substitute for conventional open procedures.

Functional endoscopic sinus surgery (FESS) was first introduced by Professor Heinz Stammberger, who popularised the Messerklinger technique, and it is the maxillary sinus that is most frequently undergone operation when there is an inflammatory sinus illness, such as chronic rhinosinusitis (CRS) (Sama and Philpott 2018).

Techniques and Classifications

Middle Meatal Antrostomy and Maxillary Sinusotomy

Middle meatal antrostomy is the standard approach to the maxillary sinus. It is the first step in endoscopic sinus surgery and is often regarded as the *relatively* simplest part of the procedure. However, technical failure and the requirement for revision surgery might result from a failure to comprehend the anatomy and natural drainage pathway of the maxillary sinus. It may not be necessary to enlarge the maxillary sinus ostium in CRS patients, particularly in those without nasal polyps. It may only be essential to expose the natural ostium if the aim of the operation is to provide drainage, irrigation of the maxillary contents or better therapeutic drug delivery to the sinuses, such as intranasal corticosteroids (Sama and Philpott 2018). The natural ostium of the maxillary sinus must be found and incorporated into the surgical antrostomy because it is the key point in endoscopic maxillary antrostomy surgery. The initial step in locating the natural ostium is to detect and completely remove the uncinate process. Because of the anterolateral position of the natural sinus maxillary ostium in relation to the uncinate process, it will not be possible to see the ostium without its removal in most cases. In addition, when both the mucosa and bone of the uncinate are diseased, the remnant tissue may result in persistent symptoms and prevent adequate medication delivery to the ostiomeatal complex. Prior to excision, radiographic evaluation should be used to assess the variations in the uncinate anatomy, paying special attention to its superior attachment and its connections to the orbit. The three common sites of attachment of the uncinate process are:

- Lamina papyracea leads to the formation of a recessus terminalis
- Skull base/ethmoid "roof"
- Middle turbinate

There are a variety of techniques for the removal of uncinate processes that largely fall into anterograde and retrograde dissection. Those advocates for anterior to posterior fashion start incising the uncinate process with a sickle knife just posterior to the maxillary line, a curvilinear mucosal eminence that corresponds to the junction of the uncinate process and the maxilla. Alternatively, those advocating for posterior to anterior fashion start dividing the uncinate at the junction of the inferior third and superior two-thirds by using backbiter (paediatric if required). The superior component can be dissected and removed, for example, with a paediatric 90° forceps or through cutting forceps. The inferior component can then be individually excised at its junction with the inferior turbinate using a down-biting antral punch or filleted out in its submucosal plane. This will avoid a blind entry through the lamina papyracea and thus the potential for consequent orbital injury. In any scenario, the uncinate should be removed completely to proceed to the next step. However, if the main aim is to expose the maxillary sinus ostium in a particular case, merely removing the lower third of the uncinate may be sufficient since it still produces a sufficient infundibulotomy for this purpose. When the uncinate has been adequately removed, the ideal strategy for enabling clear visualisation of the natural ostium is to use an angled endoscope; using the angled scope can also be very beneficial during the lower uncinectomy. A 30° scope can be used to remove the lower uncinate and visualise the natural ostium; however, sometimes, a 70° scope may be necessary to avoid confusing an accessory ostium for the natural one. Since the uncinate process is often considered as the entrance to the sinuses, improper completion of this step might lead to poor ESS outcomes. So that is why correctly locating the natural maxillary ostium is important in avoiding false surgical ostium formation and, therefore, goes hand in hand with the uncinectomy. Creation of a false surgical ostium is risky for mucociliary recirculation as a result of mucus flowing out of the natural ostium and in through the surgical neo-ostium.

Maxillary Sinusotomy

There is a need for extending the natural ostium of the maxillary sinus when there is an accessory ostium, the need for instrumentation within the maxillary sinus (e.g. removal of an antrochoanal polyp) and certain specific pathological causes of CRS (e.g. cystic fibrosis, Samter's triad, mycetoma, etc.). The natural ostium is expanded posteriorly and inferiorly to varying degrees in these situations (Sama and Philpott 2018). There are three types of maxillary sinusotomy (Simmen et al. 2014):

1. Type I: In this type, the sinus ostium is enlarged by up to 1 centimetre posteriorly. However, if there is an accessory ostium, it is joined to the natural ostium. This can be seen in Fig. 11.1.
2. Type II: Here, the ostium is enlarged by approximately 2 cm, both posteriorly and inferiorly. This can be seen in Fig. 11.2.
3. Type III: The ostium is enlarged even more, posteriorly extending to the level of the maxillary antrum (anterior to the lacrimal sac) and inferiorly to the base of the inferior turbinate. This can be seen in Figs. 11.3 and 11.4.

Large Antrostomy

The appropriate size for a maxillary antrostomy has long been debated. The biggest concern with large antrostomies is the drying effect on the sinus mucosa, which arises from early rabbit models that showed a cessation of maxillary mucociliary clearance in the presence of maxillary sinus airflow (Kennedy and Adappa 2011). Another major concern is the reduction of protective nitric oxide concentration

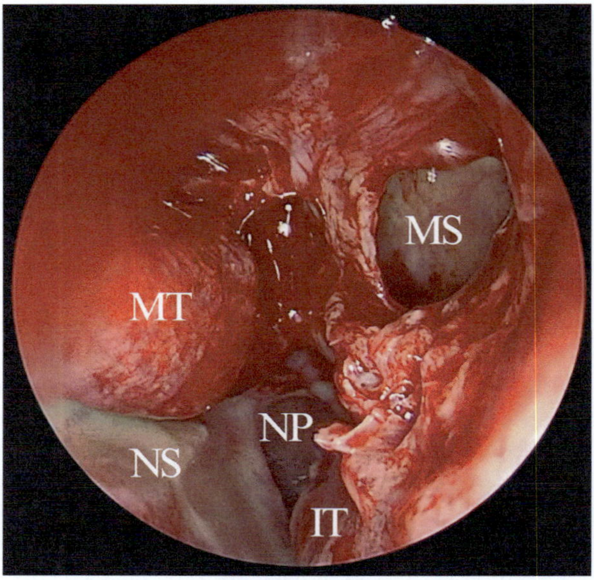

Fig. 11.1 This is an intraoperative video of a patient undergoing endoscopic maxillary sinusotomy type 1. As can be seen in the thumbnail (left side nasal cavity), the maxillary sinus ostium is opened, and the posterior wall of the maxillary sinus is visible. (*MS* maxillary sinus, *NP* nasopharynx, *MT* middle turbinate, *NS* nasal septum, *IT* inferior turbinate) (Audio 11.1 and Video 11.1)

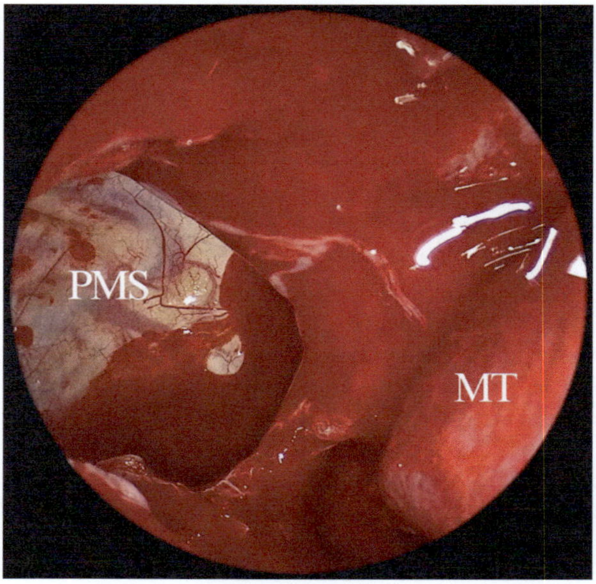

Fig. 11.2 This is an intraoperative video of a patient undergoing endoscopic maxillary sinusotomy type 2. In the thumbnail (right side nasal cavity), the posterior wall of the maxillary sinus (PMS) and middle turbinate (MT) can be seen (Audio 11.2 and Video 11.2)

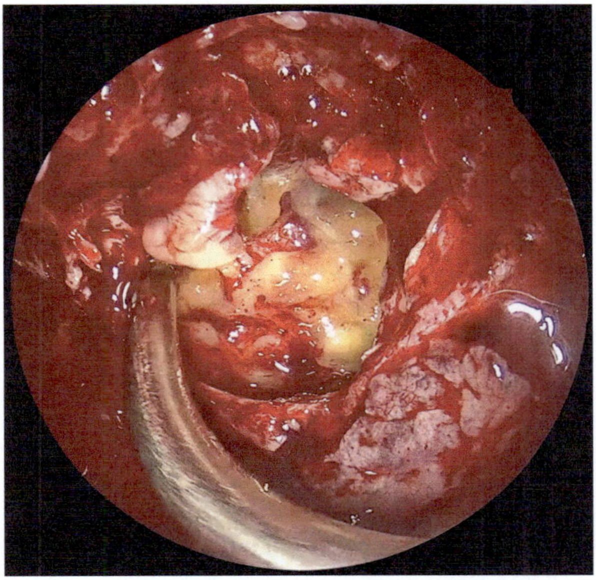

Fig. 11.3 This is an intraoperative video of a patient undergoing endoscopic maxillary sinusotomy type 3. As can be seen in the thumbnail (left side nasal cavity), the medial wall of the maxillary sinus is completely removed, up to the posterior wall of the maxillary sinus posteriorly, the nasolacrimal duct anteriorly, the superior border of the inferior turbinate inferiorly and the orbital floor superiorly (Audio 11.3 and Video 11.3)

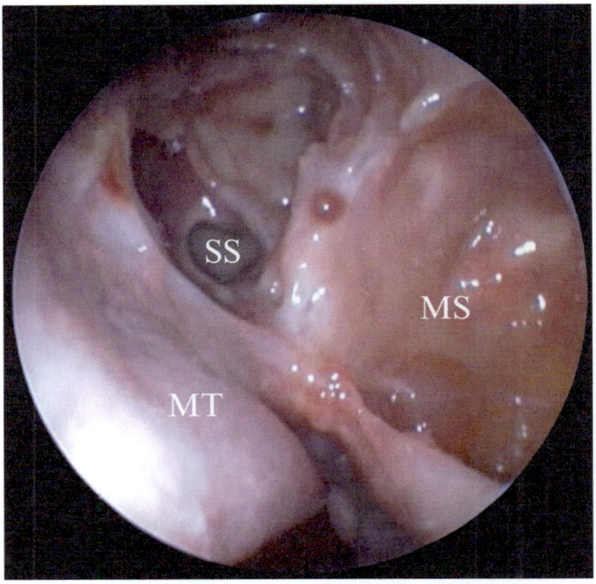

Fig. 11.4 This is a postoperative endoscopic video of a patient who underwent endoscopic maxillary sinusotomy type 3. In the thumbnail, the maxillary sinus (MS), sphenoid sinus (SS) and middle turbinate (MT) can be seen (Audio 11.4 and Video 11.4)

within the maxillary sinus. To prevent impaired mucociliary clearance, the posterior aspect of the ostium and mucosa in the ethmoid infundibulum should ideally be preserved. In some cases of CRS, particularly in those with severe nasal polyposis and allergic fungal rhinosinusitis, expanding the natural ostium at ESS will aid in the clearance of the sinus contents; however, this can be achieved by preserving the posterior aspect of the ostium and infundibulum by inferior enlargement. Other examples are antrochoanal polyps, where removal of the stalk and root is necessary to avoid recurrence, and fungal balls, where the pathology has often already damaged and distorted the normal architecture, but a larger opening will be required to discharge the bothersome contents. Mega-antrostomy is, in fact, a partial medial maxillectomy, as it involves the removal of part of the inferior turbinate so that the ostium is lowered to the nasal floor. Thus, in some cases, as dictated by underlying pathology or systemic disease, it is certainly necessary to make a larger antrostomy. Thus, in some cases, as dictated by underlying pathology or systemic disease, it is certainly necessary to make a larger antrostomy (Sama and Philpott 2018).

Endoscopic Medial Maxillectomy

Maxillectomy has not been an exception to the universalisation of endoscopy in surgeries, and many surgeons have developed new and unique ways to approach the maxilla with FESS. Endoscopic medial maxillectomy is needed in many cases where a conservative sinusotomy is not enough to control the pathology. Due to the many new techniques that are showcased in the literature, some renowned specialists have worked to provide some unity and classify endoscopic medial maxillectomy types; in this chapter, we are going to mention three of them.

Schreiber et al. Endoscopic Medial Maxillectomy (EMM) Classification

This classification is based on the volume of surgical exposure within the sinus and the percentage of posterolateral wall exposure. It is worth mentioning that within their study, Schreiber and colleagues considered many anatomic variables, including the width and height of the pyriform aperture, medial protrusion of the medial maxillary wall, sagittal position of the nasolacrimal duct, sagittal length of the maxillary sinus, height of the inferior turbinate insertion and, finally, anterior maxillary wall angulation. The classification has four types, each of which can be either through the ipsilateral nasal cavity or transseptally through the contralateral nasal cavity. The transseptal approach is through an anterior septal window and is used when adequate exposure cannot be achieved ipsilaterally (Schreiber et al. 2017). The types can be seen in Table 11.1.

Type A can be seen in Fig. 11.3 (since maxillary sinusotomy type 3 and medial wall maxillectomy type A are practically similar), Type B can be seen in Fig. 11.5, Type C in Fig. 11.6 and Type D in Figs. 7.10, 7.13 and 11.7.

Regarding the transseptal approach, first, a short 1.5–2 cm vertical incision is made on the septum just posterior to the anterior margin of the septal cartilage; however, only the mucosa and perichondrium are dissected from the nasal floor, preserving the septal cartilage posteriorly. Next, subperichondrial dissection is done 5 mm posteriorly so that a vertical incision is done on the septal cartilage, but this

Table 11.1 Schreiber's endoscopic medial maxillectomy (EMM) classification

Schreiber et al. endoscopic medial maxillectomy (EMM) classification			
Type	Volume (cm³)	Area (%)	Description
Type A	28.6	21.6	– Inferior uncinectomy – Medial maxillary wall removal to the inferior turbinate insertion, orbital floor, palatine canal and nasolacrimal duct (either ipsilaterally/transseptal)
Transseptal Type A	26.8	27.1	
Type B	30.6	50.4	Type A, in addition to: – Inferior turbinectomy – Medial maxillary wall removal posterior to the nasolacrimal duct (either ipsilaterally/transseptal) B2: Prelacrimal approach (anterior to the duct) (definition of Simmens)
Transseptal Type B	45.0	76.2	
Type C	33.7	68.0	Type B, in addition to: – Removal of the nasolacrimal duct – Removal of the residual anterior portion of the medial maxillary wall (either ipsilaterally/transseptal)
Transseptal Type C	51.8	79.4	
Type D	40.7	84.0	Type C, in addition to: – Removal of the anterior maxillary wall medial to the infraorbital foramen (either ipsilaterally/transseptal) E: Some portion of the anterior wall lateral to the infraorbital canal Some portion of the posterolateral wall in some cases of inverted papilloma of the posterolateral wall
Transseptal Type D	56.9	85.5	

This classification has four types, A–D, each of which is either ipsilateral or transseptal in approach. The area is the percentage of posterolateral wall exposure, while the volume reveals the extent of surgical exposure within the maxillary sinus (Schreiber et al. 2017)

time, the contralateral mucosa and perichondrium are preserved. Then, subperichondrial dissection is done for another 5 mm. Last, a posteriorly pedicled mucocartilagenous flap would be harvested through superior and inferior incisions from the initial "cartilage-less" incision to the bony cartilaginous junction of the nasal septum. Finally, the flap can be moved bilaterally to aid in increasing the access of FESS.

Turri–Zanoni et al. Transnasal Endoscopic Partial Maxillectomy (TEPM) Classification

To keep a balance between the scarcity of surgical exposure in maxillary sinusotomy and the complications that radical maxillectomy techniques lead to, Turri–Zanoni and colleagues worked on a 6-type classification system in a large-scale retrospective study and provided specific indications and contraindications to each type. Therefore, based on the exposure required for a specific pathology, a specific type is allocated (Turri-Zanoni et al. 2016). The types of TEPM proposed are described in Table 11.2.

With all that said, Schreiber's classification lacks a few approaches that are currently available to access the maxillary sinus and Turri–Zanoni's classification is not as straightforward. That is why the author added some of the techniques in

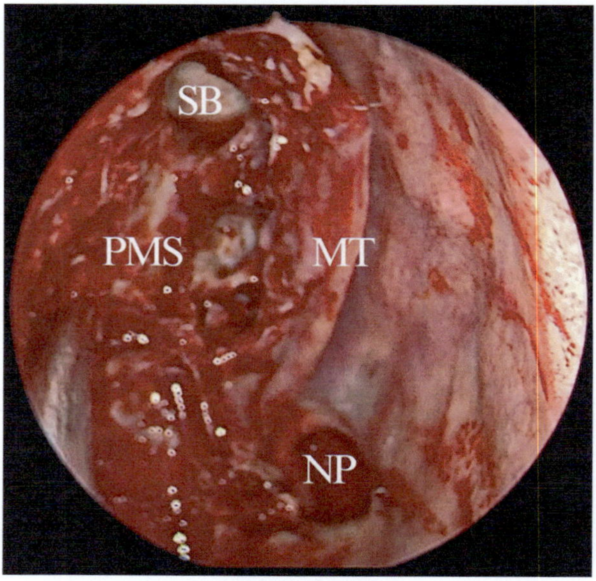

Fig. 11.5 This is an intraoperative video of a patient undergoing endoscopic medial wall maxillectomy type B (Schreiber et al.'s classification) for olfactory neuroblastoma. In the thumbnail (right side nasal cavity), the posterior wall of the maxillary sinus (PMS), middle turbinate (MT), skull base (SB) and nasopharynx (NP) can be found (Audio 11.5 and Video 11.5)

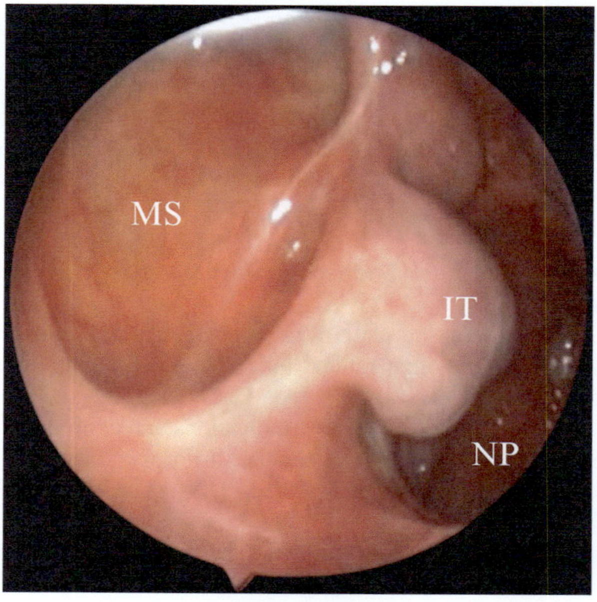

Fig. 11.6 This is a postoperative endoscopic video of a patient who underwent endoscopic medial wall maxillectomy type C (Schreiber et al.'s classification). In the thumbnail, the maxillary sinus (MS), inferior turbinate (IT) and nasopharynx (NP) can be found (Audio 11.6 and Video 11.6)

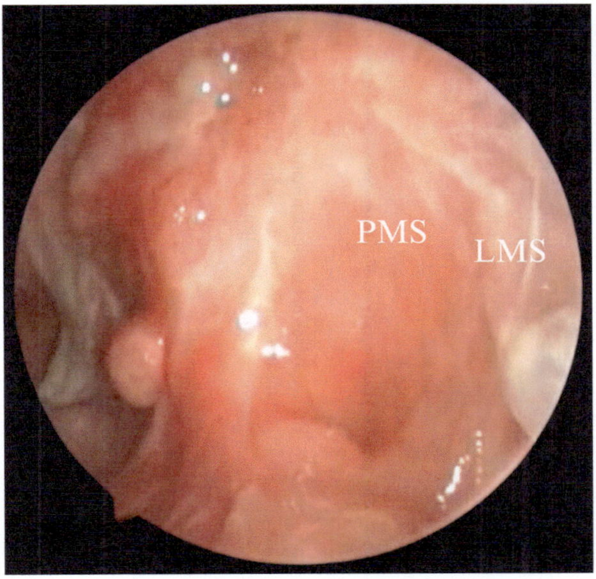

Fig. 11.7 This is a postoperative endoscopic video of a patient who underwent endoscopic medial wall maxillectomy type D (Schreiber et al.'s classification). The posterior and lateral walls of the maxillary sinus (PMS and LMS, respectively) are clearly seen in the thumbnail (Audio 11.7 and Video 11.7)

Turri–Zanoni's classification to Schreiber's, thus adding type B2 and E. Type B2 (Prelacrimal approach) was added with Simmen's medial wall maxillectomy principals in mind; this modification of the previous classification by the author can be seen in Table 11.3.

Modified Denker's Approach

The modified Denker's approach integrates the original techniques developed by Alfred Denker in 1906 with the endonasal procedure introduced by Strurmann and Canfield in 1908, which is also known as TEAMM (total endoscopic anterior medial maxillectomy) technique. This technique is frequently used for managing extensive conditions affecting the maxillary sinus and allows surgeons to get direct access to historically hard-to-reach areas of the maxillary sinus without the need for certain incisions, including a gingivobuccal or transseptal incision. It completely exposes the anterior, inferior and lateral recesses of the maxillary sinus and the entire posterior wall, making straight entry to specific areas, including to the pterygopalatine and infra-temporal fossa. It also simplifies drilling for tumours such as inverted papilloma pedicled to the lateral wall without the need for angled burrs and resection of lesions involving the anterior wall with the underlying bone without the need to get through the tumour itself. The endoscopic Denker's procedure stands out from other procedures as it does not need angled scopes or instrumentation and is not limited by the concavity of the anterior maxilla. This technique allows for improved visualisation of the anterosuperior alveolar and infraorbital nerves, aiding

Table 11.2 Turri–Zanoni et al. transnasal endoscopic partial maxillectomy (TEPM) classification

Turri–Zanoni et al. transnasal endoscopic partial maxillectomy (TEPM) classification		
Type	Description	Indication
Type 1	– Middle meatal antrostomy – The inferior portion of the uncinate process is removed – The maxillary sinus ostium is enlarged posteriorly, which is by removal of the upper portion of the medial maxillary wall until the level of the vertical process of palatine bone Type 1 leads to adequate visualisation of posterior and superior portions of the maxillary sinus	– Medically refractory inflammatory disease of the maxillary sinus (e.g. sinusitis) with a history of multiple functional endoscopic sinus surgeries – Severe and irreversible mucosal injury – Management of benign and malignant tumours with limited extension in order to preserve surgical landmarks
Type 2	Type 1, in addition to: – Partially or completely removing the medial maxillary wall with the inferior turbinate – Connecting the nasal floor to the maxillary sinus – With or without removal of the posterior wall of the maxillary sinus	
Type 3A	Type 2, in addition to: – Lacrimal bone removal – Transection of the nasolacrimal duct (a few mm distal to the lacrimal sac) Type 3A leads to better visualisation of the lateral and inferior walls of the maxillary sinus and better control of the retrolacrimal recess	– Medically refractory inflammatory disease and benign tumours on the anterolateral part of the antrum without medial wall involvement
Modified Type 3A (Prelacrimal approach)	The prelacrimal approach is different in that: – The inferior turbinate is temporarily displaced and then replaced in its position – Instead of removing/transecting the nasolacrimal duct, it is preserved but mobilised This type can NOT be used when the pathology includes the medial wall of the maxillary sinus	

(continued)

Table 11.2 (continued)

Turri–Zanoni et al. transnasal endoscopic partial maxillectomy (TEPM) classification		
Type	Description	Indication
Type 3B	Type 3A, in addition to: – Partially or completely drilling the ascending branch of the maxillary bone and thus removing the pyriform aperture Type 3B leads to complete control of all maxillary sinus walls and recesses	– Pathology in difficult areas, especially in the anterior half of the maxillary sinus, specifically the alveolar, zygomatic and retrolacrimal recesses – Endoscopic endonasal nasopharyngectomy in selected cases
Type 4	Type 3B, in addition to: – Removal of the anterior wall, which can be extended up to the zygomatic bone – The nasal vestibule is incised – The soft tissue and periosteum surrounding the anterior maxillary wall are dissected by identifying the pyriform crest and until the infraorbital foramen is reached – With or without • Drilling of the anterior maxillary wall up to the infraorbital nerve or zygomatic arch • Drilling of the lateral maxillary wall • Removal of the superior maxillary wall (orbital floor), with preserving the periorbital layer Type 4 leads to better management of pathologies of the anterior maxillary wall and is used in approaching deep lateral tumours of the infratemporal fossa, nasopharynx and upper parapharyngeal space	

This classification has six types, and with each successive type, access to the maxillary sinus is increased (Turri-Zanoni et al. 2016)

Table 11.3 This table shows how the authors have merged and modified the two classification systems mentioned above (Schreiber and Turri–Zanoni). When compared to Schreiber's, Type B2 and Type E are added

Our modification of Schreiber and Turri–Zanoni classifications	
Type	Description
Type A (Mega-antrostomy/Type 3 Maxillary Sinusotomy)	– Inferior uncinectomy – Medial maxillary wall removal to the inferior turbinate insertion, orbital floor, palatine canal and nasolacrimal duct
Type B1	Type A, in addition to: – Middle Portion Inferior turbinectomy – Medial maxillary wall removal posterior to the nasolacrimal duct, thus creating a common leveled floor for the maxillary sinus and nasal cavity
Type B2 (Pre-lacrimal Approach)	– The bone over the nasolacrimal duct is removed – The duct is retracted medially – The bone medial to the nasolacrimal duct (the bone of the posterior lacrimal fossa and part of the anterior wall of the maxilla) is removed – The inferior turbinate's superior part is dissected – Drilling of the lateral remnant of the pyriform aperture and the inferior posterior remains of the medial maxillary wall is done
Type C	Type B, in addition to: – Removal of the nasolacrimal duct – Removal of the lacrimal bone – Removal of the ascending process of the maxillary bone – Removal of the residual anterior portion of the medial maxillary wall
Type D	Type C, in addition to: – Removal of the entire medial wall of the maxillary sinus – Removal of the pyriform aperture and a portion of the anterior maxillary wall medial to the infraorbital foramen
Type E	Type D, in addition to: – Removal of the anterior wall lateral to the infraorbital canal until the zygomatic bone is reached – Drilling of the entire lateral wall of the maxillary sinus inferior to the infraorbital nerve. In cases where the infraorbital nerve must be removed, the entire lateral wall is removed. – The entire posterior wall of the maxillary sinus can be drilled out to access the pterygopalatine or infratemporal fossae or beyond them – A portion of the roof of the maxillary sinus (orbital floor) can be removed if indicated (while preserving the periorbital layer). – Limited removal of the maxillary sinus floor may be performed to excise pathology or reduce the risk of recurrence (Endoscopic Subtotal Maxillectomy).

in the preservation of these neural structures (Lee et al. 2016; Sharma et al. 2022). Initially, a mucosal incision is made at the junction of the nasal floor and lateral nasal wall, extending the incision through the periosteum. Subsequently, a second mucosal incision is performed superiorly alongside the lateral nasal wall and extended anteroinferiorly to rest just in front of the anterior head of the inferior turbinate, covering the edge of the pyriform aperture. Then, using a suction Freer elevator, a subperiosteal dissection is carried out to reveal the anterior maxilla, infraorbital foramen, its neurovascular bundle and the lateral nasal wall. A bony window is then made in the anterior maxilla using a high-speed drill or osteotome, ensuring it remains below the infraorbital nerve (Lee and Chiu 2019).

Open Approaches in ENT

Open Approaches to the Maxillary Sinus

The maxillary sinus continues to grow and ossify during embryonic development up to the 37th week of gestation. Growth continues in the maxillary sinus throughout infancy until it reaches adult size between the ages of 18 and 21 (McCormick et al. 2020).

Anatomically, the MS is located lateral to the nasal cavity, medial to the infratemporal fossa, inferior to the orbit, superior to the alveolar process of the maxilla and maxillary teeth, posterior to the anterior wall of the maxilla and anterior to the pterygopalatine fossa. The internal maxillary artery (IMAX) and branches of the trigeminal nerve provide the major blood supply and innervation to this area, respectively. Detailed knowledge of anatomy is necessary since if the anatomy of this sinus and the surrounding anatomic region is not well understood, it might be challenging for the ideal surgical intervention (Rezende et al. 2022). Surgery usually becomes necessary when medical treatment fails to manage maxillary sinusitis or inflammation, or in situations of malignancy (McCormick et al. 2020). The open approaches to the nasal cavity and paranasal sinuses are based on face, scalp and/or sublabial incisions to expose the facial bone and give appropriate space for osteotomies. Endoscopic endonasal procedures in sinus surgery have drastically decreased the need for open approaches. Nevertheless, open approaches to the facial skeleton are still used for facial trauma surgery, orthognathic surgery and external anterior ethmoidal artery ligation. In rare cases, the open approach is used in conjunction with endoscopic endonasal procedures to treat sinonasal diseases and skull base lesions. As a result, despite the advancement of endoscopic endonasal surgery, a sinonasal surgeon must be skilled with open approaches to be able to switch to an

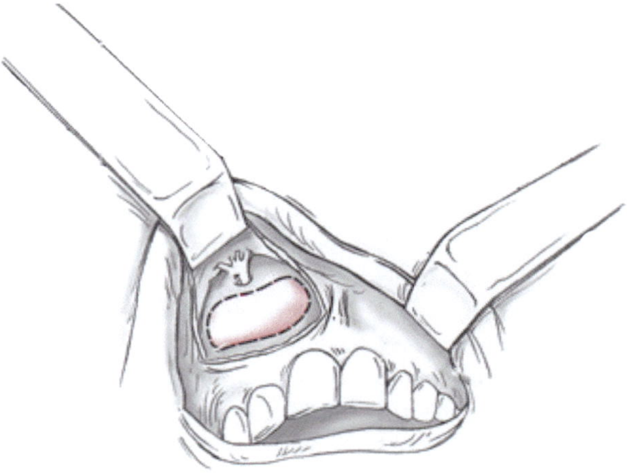

Fig. 11.8 Caldwell-Luc approach: the image demonstrates the bony opening incision

open approach whenever complications occur that cannot be controlled with endoscopic approaches (Themes 2016a).

Caldwell-Luc Approach

Prior to the discovery of endoscopic procedures, the Caldwell-Luc approach was the most commonly utilised approach to diseases in the maxillary sinus (Fig. 11.8). This approach has been used to treat chronic sinusitis, to biopsy tumours and to gain access to the pterygopalatine space for ligation of the internal maxillary artery or vidian neurectomy. The same approach can also be used to gain access to the orbital floor for fracture reduction orbital decompression and to gain access to the ethmoid and sphenoid sinuses and the pituitary fossa. When endoscopic visualisation and access are limited, such as in the inferior, lateral and anterior aspects of the maxillary sinus, it remains an effective method (Themes 2016b). It is an alternative to middle meatal antrostomy performed using endonasal endoscopic surgery (Hacking and Glick 2017). The incision is made just 3 mm above the line of reflection and extends laterally for 3.5–4 cm parallel to the teeth, beginning at the canine ridge and then raising the periosteum over the canine fossa till the infraorbital foramen is reached but while taking care not to damage the nerve.

The antrum is accessed at the canine fossa using a gouge and a hammer or a cutting burr. The bony opening should eventually be 1.5–2 cm in diameter.

Then, the surgeon will deal with the pathology and remove the nasal mucosa.

Creating a nasoantral window aids in the natural release of packing from the antrum and drainage of postoperative accumulation following pack removal and aeration.

The sinus cavity and nasal cavity are packed with a single long ribbon gauge soaked in Betadine ointment with its free end is put anteriorly in the nasal vestibule to achieve adequate hemostasis.

Lastly, the sublabial incision is sutured with chromic catgut with excellent edge approximation (Datta et al. 2015).

Lateral Rhinotomy Incision

In the case of a malignant tumour originating from the nasal cavity and maxillary sinus without palatal invasion, the lateral rhinotomy approach is performed (Fig. 11.9). Benign tumours with anterior maxillary wall involvement are treated in the same way. This approach provides a thorough exposure of the maxillary antrum, nasal cavity, ethmoidal sinuses and sphenoid sinus (Abu-Ghanem and Fliss 2013). Moure introduced a skin incision extending from the inferior portion of the frontal bone over the inner edge of the brow to the corresponding nostril. While this incision or slight variations of it may be appropriate for tumours extending up to and through the cribriform plate when performing a limited craniofacial approach, for most lesions within the nasal cavity, ethmoids, and medial maxilla, the upper limit of the incision may need to go no higher than a point just below the medial canthal

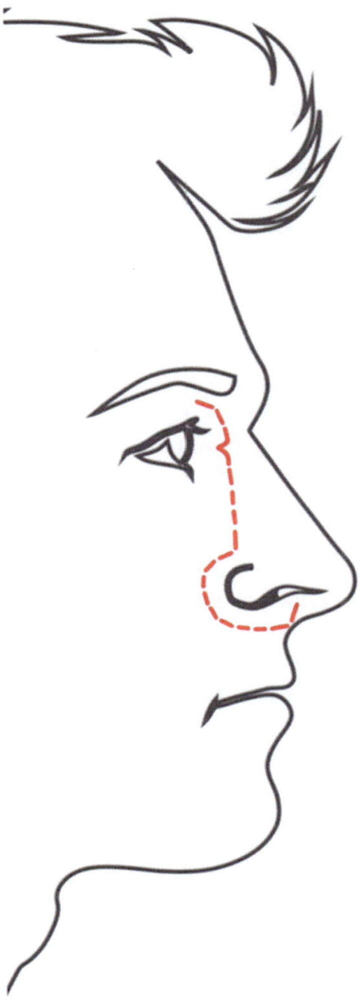

Fig. 11.9 Site of Moure's lateral rhinotomy incision along with its extension

ligament. This prevents dissociation of this critical structure and significantly enhances the aesthetic outcome. The incision may continue completely in the naso-maxillary groove, curving around the alar border to enter the nose. The nose's dorsal framework can then be separated from the pyramidal aperture and swung around medially to expose the underlying bone. The superior labial branches that flow to the vestibule in the alar section of the incision frequently require diathermy or ligation. Depending on the level of access necessary, the skin and periosteum above the nasal bone and frontonasal process are mobilised. Similarly, lateral access is achieved across the face of the maxilla and to the orbital rim. When dealing with tumours within the nasal passageways and neighbouring sinuses, it provides great access and good aesthetic effects. While midfacial degloving has frequently supplanted it in our practice, it is still a valuable and quick operation, especially in elderly patients (Lund et al. 2013).

Removal of Bone (Medial Maxillectomy)

The extent of bone removed varies depending on the underlying pathology, but it may involve both the nasal and frontonasal processes, the lacrimal fossa and lamina papyracea (while preserving the infraorbital rim). It could also include the entire lateral wall of the nose and nasal septum, and the bone of the anterior wall of the maxilla, extending as laterally as dissection of the soft tissues of the cheek allows. This is often to a site above the vertical plane from the infraorbital foramen, and in the elderly, getting to the lateral wall of the maxilla may be feasible. Of course, this approach might be coupled with endoscopic or microscopic procedures. Importantly, regardless of the degree of underlying bone removal, primary closure is always attained and typically aesthetically satisfactory in adults, but children are frequently dissatisfied in the long term. The only substantial long-term morbidity is postoperative crusting, which is considerably decreased and managed by frequent nasal douching with saline (Hacking and Glick 2017; Lund et al. 2013).

Extended Lateral Rhinotomy Approaches

The lateral rhinotomy incision can be swung laterally at the level of the medial canthal ligament, which runs across the borders of both the upper and lower parts of the palpebral fissure to the lateral canthal region. Following this dissection of both upper and lower eyelids, orbital clearing may be performed in many patients with preservation of both eyelids to seal the ensuing defect (Lund et al. 2013).

Midfacial Degloving Approach

The midface degloving approach offers broad surgical access to lesions beneath the midface while avoiding the formation of a noticeable facial scar. This approach has several key advantages: (1) Excellent accessibility to the nasal cavity, nasal septum, maxillary, ethmoid and sphenoid sinuses, nasopharynx and clivus lesions; (2) Exposure and surgical facility are equal to or even superior to the more traditional procedures requiring facial incisions; and lastly, (3) This strategy could be combined with coronal, brow, temporal and palatal incisions for extensive lesions and those involving the skull base (Price et al. 1988). To provide maximum access, a bilateral sublabial incision is made straight down to the bone, from the maxillary tuberosity to the opposite maxillary tuberosity. An incision of insufficient length makes future mobilisation of soft tissues more difficult, reducing the application and usefulness of this method. (The old surgical aphorism that wounds heal from side to side rather than end to end is especially applicable here. A little incision jeopardises the procedure and does not "improve" recovery.) The frenulum in the buccogingival sulcus is meticulously defined so that it may be precisely reconstructed after closure. The periosteum and soft tissues of the cheek are elevated as in a Caldwell-Luc approach, with care taken to expose the infraorbital nerves and clearly identify the infraorbital margin.

Intercartilaginous incisions enable access to the soft tissues on the dorsum of the nose, which are lifted with the dissection extending laterally over the anterior portion of the maxilla to meet the subperiosteal approach, as in a standard rhinoplasty. The intercartilaginous incisions are extended into a transfixion incision along the dorsal and caudal margins of the cartilaginous septum, separating it from the medial crura of the lower lateral cartilages. This incision is carried across the floor of the nose to link the intercartilaginous incision laterally. Entering the nasal cavity inferiorly from the sublabial incision allows for better positioning of the inferior incisions. At the lateral end of the intercartilaginous incision, when the intercartilaginous incision is turned downward and posteriorly to the piriform aperture, instead of continuing in a circular fashion to meet the inferior incision, this stepped incision reduces the risk of postoperative vestibular stenosis. Furthermore, careful dissection of the skin and soft tissues of the dorsum of the nose now allows for complete degloving of the middle third of the face and optimum access to both nasal cavities, maxillary sinus, ethmoids, sphenoid, pterygopalatine and infratemporal fossa, and nasopharynx. The posterior limits of the resection usually consist of the posterior wall of the sphenoid sinus, pterygoid plates and related muscles, and the posterior wall of the nasopharynx. The cribriform plate and roof of the ethmoids form the superior limitation, and laterally, exploration can proceed to the coronoid process of the mandible. The pathology will certainly dictate the degree of resection, but a bilateral radical maxillectomy can be easily performed and may be coupled with orbital clearing if necessary. When coupled with a coronal incision, this approach allows for extensive craniofacial surgery without leaving any face scars. The approach is also particularly effective for the excision of an angiofibroma, giving excellent exposure of the lesion and direct control of the internal maxillary artery and its branches before any attempted excision of the angiofibroma (Lund et al. 2013).

Weber–Fergusson Approach

This approach (Fig. 11.10) can treat a wide spectrum of benign diseases, including angiofibroma, schwannoma, odontogenic lesions and fibrous dysplasia, as well as selected malignant diseases, depending on their size and location. If the anterior soft tissues of the cheek are involved in malignant disease, then the approach is definitely contraindicated. It provides great bilateral exposure of the nasal cavities, the mid-third of the face and the central skull base, and is easily modifiable and extendable (Lund et al. 2013). The facial incision begins with a lateral rhinotomy incision, which is then prolonged towards the philtrum and down to the midline lip. The incision extends inferiorly along the gingivobuccal sulcus, laterally up to the retromolar region (Themes 2016c).

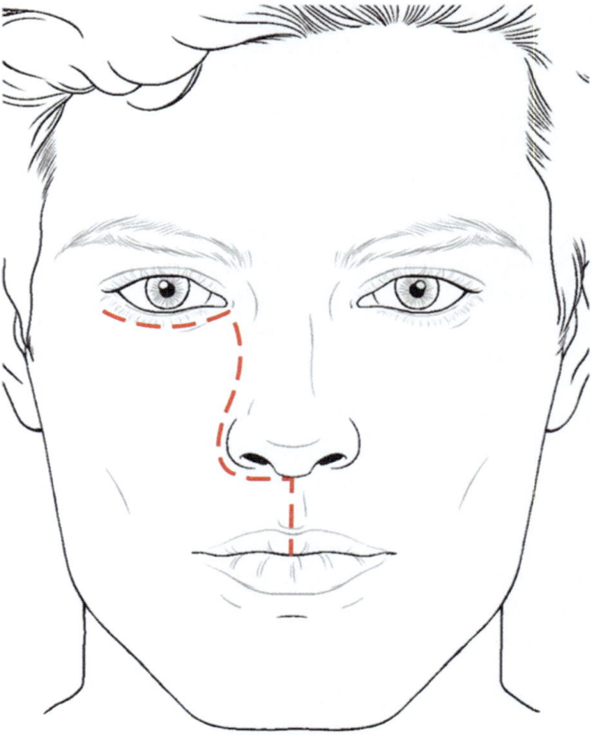

Fig. 11.10 Classic Weber–Ferguson incision

Total Maxillectomy

Total maxillectomy is a surgical resection of the whole maxilla that is typically suggested for maxillary sinus malignancies, maxillary bone (sarcomas), orbit and ethmoids that are not suitable for smaller or endoscopic resection. The term "total maxillectomy" relates to the surgical removal of the whole maxilla. The orbital floor and medial wall, as well as the ethmoid sinuses, are all resected. The procedure may be expanded to even include orbital exenteration, sphenoidectomy and pterygoid plate removal (Fagan 2017). The ordinary Weber–Fergusson incision is made 3–5 mm under the lower lash edge on the affected side, allowing the skin to be separate from the underlying orbicularis oculi. If the incision is made too low, it could lead to disfiguring oedema. Ectropion may develop if it is positioned too close to the lid edge. The incision may be prolonged below and lateral to the lateral canthus, but medially, as with a lateral rhinotomy, it continues through the nasomaxillary groove down the side of the nose, cutting straight through to the bone underneath and the nasal mucosa. The incision curves around the ala to the columella's midway before dividing the lip in the middle. Several variants of the medial and lower parts of the incision have been documented. Darts in the nasal sill and at the skin-vermilion junction, as well as extension along the philtral crest rather than through the midline, are examples. All have supporters, but none consistently produce ideal outcomes. The accuracy with which the skin vermilion line is closed is unquestionably essential. It is also essential to make the angle at the medial canthus as obtuse as feasible since the blood flow to this corner may be compromised, especially if the patient has already had radiation. Subsequent collapse can be a severe issue at this time. While the rest of the incision is being made, a retractor can be used to hold the upper part of the lip. The incision continues in the alveolar buccal sulcus, circling the maxillary tuberosity before crossing the palate at the confluence of the soft and hard palates. To reduce bleeding, a cutting diathermy could be tried. The incision is then extended from posterior to anterior through the mucous membrane of the hard palate at a place that is lateral to the midline, allowing some mucosal covering to be preserved on the medial aspect of the bone cut. However, the specific location of this component of the incision will be influenced by the degree of disease inside the maxilla, nasal cavity, neighbouring nasal cavity and nasal septum. The incision typically links to the alveolar buccal edge in the area of the first incisor, which must be removed if present. Again, which tooth is taken depends on the degree of radicality of the operation, and healthy teeth must be retained as much laterally on the disease side as feasible without jeopardising the oncological resection. This provides the finest anchoring and function for any prosthesis. The whole facial skin flap, which contains the buccinator, can now be elevated, displaying the maxillary bone, piriform aperture, zygomatic arch and malar bone laterally. The orbital rim is delineated, and the orbital periosteum is dissected meticulously to demonstrate the orbital floor. A thorough examination of this area, particularly along the infraorbital canal, is needed to determine that no tumour invasion has occurred, necessitating further orbital clearing. Similarly, the lamina papyracea and its neighbouring periosteum on the medial wall must be examined over its whole length, up to and including the orbital apex, if needed. The osteotomies can be performed using high-speed drills, but the malar bone can be separated with a Gigli saw inserted into the lateral section of the infraorbital fissure with curved forceps. The piriform aperture is joined by osteotomies through the orbital floor and the frontal process. To separate the hard palate, use a drill, a Gigli saw or a curved osteotome, beginning from the incisor socket and moving posteriorly lateral to the nasal septum attachment. Only the pterygoid plates must be separated posteriorly once the hard palate has been divided. This is most effectively done using a long, curved osteotome placed behind the tuberosity in the groove between it and the pterygoid plates. The bone may be detached with a varying amount of carefully controlled force and leverage, but the pterygoid muscle fibres must be severed with curved, powerful scissors before the specimen is free. After removing the maxilla, a heated pack (60–70 °C) should be placed in the cavity immediately to reduce bleeding from the internal maxillary artery. After a few minutes have passed, the cavity can be thoroughly examined and, if necessary, the artery ligated.

Additional removal of pterygoid muscle, arteries, nerves and pterygoid plates may be needed to completely eradicate the disease. The ethmoid labyrinth can be exenterated by opening the anterior wall of the sphenoid. It is possible that more orbital clearing or exenteration will be necessary. If this isn't the case, the maxillectomy cavity is examined for hemostasis and a 5 cm wide ribbon gauze soaked in Whitehead's varnish is inserted in, enough to line the cavity without hindering the fitting of any prosthesis.

The prosthodontist can now create a temporary obturator on the premade denture using gutta percha or other similar pliable material that connects to the existing teeth and fills the palatal defect, restoring the shape of the oral cavity roof and face. The use of Whitehead's varnish and an obturator together minimises maxillectomy cavity contracture and eliminates the necessity for cavity skin grafting. Indeed, given enough time, the cavity will mucosalise with natural mucosa, which is better than a skin graft. Therefore, normal speech and eating can be achieved in the earliest postoperative time. Some prosthodontists recommend that the skin flap be laid back and sealed with subcutaneous and skin sutures before the obturator is fashioned. This complicates the fitting but improves the accuracy of the facial shape evaluation. Skin sutures must be handled with extreme caution in the medial canthal area and at the vermilion edge.

After the tarsorrhaphy sutures have been removed, the eye is thoroughly washed of blood, chloramphenicol ointment is used, and an eye pad is put, followed by a mild pressure dressing for 24 h. Preservation of the Lockwood suspensory ligament, the medial and lateral palpebral ligaments, and frequently the posterior portion of the orbital floor gives sufficient support for the eye, leading to satisfactory function in the majority of patients (Lund et al. 2013).

Maxillectomy

Introduction

The maxilla is a bony structure that plays a significant role in craniofacial anatomy. It provides support to the orbit as well as sharing parts as oronasal and oroantral bridges. Furthermore, the main musculature framework of the face is dependent on the existence of the maxilla and the support it provides (O'Connell and Futran 2010). It laterally articulates with the zygomatic bone and centrally with the nasal and ethmoid bones.

The word maxillectomy ("ectomy" means cutting or removing) refers to the surgical cutting of the maxilla in an effort to manage certain pathologies with different degrees of severity (Bidra et al. 2012). The first surgeon who attempted maxillectomy was Lazars in 1827, but the procedure missed the mark due to excessive blood loss, which can be explained by the naturally rich blood supply of the maxilla and the associated structures (McGuirt 1995; Jategaonkar et al. 2020). These stumbling efforts continued in their gradual development with time. It reached significant advancement in 1950 when excessive blood loss was reduced with anaesthetic techniques, thus reducing morbidity, which was the main issue (McGuirt 1995). Following blood loss, non-aesthetic results from extraoral incision are also considered a main issue, which was overcome by the Weber–Ferguson approach recorded in the same year.

In the beginning, the challenge was the surgical procedure itself and its success rate. Later on, with the development of surgical techniques and equipment, the challenge shifted to what is after the surgery, which is the reconstruction part. This gave virtual surgical planning, navigation and 3D printing the important role they have in maxillectomy.

Indication and Classification of Maxillectomy

The main indication for maxillectomy is ablation of tumours (malignant and some benign) and some other specific diseases such as mucormycosis, aspergillosis (fungal infection), bisphosphonate osteonecrosis and osteoradionecrosis. All these conditions require resection of the maxillary bone, either partial or total, depending on the extent and severity of the condition. As headlines, maxillectomy is mainly done so by resection of the aimed target with a 1 cm safe margin whenever no bone perforation is detected. If detected, the complete removal with periosteum becomes a must. According to the site and the extension of defects, the Brown classification, which was introduced in 2000 (which is also called the Liverpool system), provides lucid guidelines for maxillectomy while also classifying the route of resection in the vertical and the horizontal dimensions into several classes (Bidra et al. 2012):

- Class 1: Alveolectomy or maxillectomy with no oroantral fistula: This procedure is the least invasive one with no excessive removal of bone. The resection is carried out by removing defected alveolar bone without passing the boundaries towards the palate horizontally nor creating an oronasal or an oroantral fistula vertically. According to this description, there is no need for aggressive incision to be done extraorally as the site can be reached directly.
- Class 2: Low-level maxillectomy: The vertical extension will differ from the previous type since it extends to involve the maxillary sinus without reaching or involving the orbital floor, thus resulting in an oroantral or an oronasal fistula. This still does not need an excessive amount of exposure for surgical procedures. Horizontally, it is divided into two subdivisions according to the extension:
  - Class 2A: Unilateral resection of palatal bone without involving the nasal floor.
  - Class 2B: A more extensive resection for defects that involve the nasal floor, which requires a brave decision to remove with no hesitation of being aggressive.
- Class 3: High-level maxillectomy: This is the most difficult of all types. Its vertical extension will involve the floor of the orbit as well as the medial wall (ethmoidal region) but with preservation of the orbit, which represents the pivotal challenge during surgical procedure. Here, a more invasive and extended approach should be performed to provide sufficient access that reduces any rate of complication that cannot be eliminated by any means necessary.
- Class 4: High-level maxillectomy with orbital exenteration: This procedure is much easier than the previous one because there is no need to be careful in order to protect and preserve the orbit since it will be removed completely as the defect involves it. Brown's classification system wasn't the only one produced but it is the most acceptable to be used with ease.

Techniques and Approaches

There is a gradual increase in the ferocity for choosing the surgical technique indicated in certain maxillectomy cases. It depends on the spread of the defect and the amount of tissue and structures that are involved. It is according to the Brown classification and is listed from the least aggressive to the most:

Medial Maxillectomy

Medial maxillectomy is indicated in cases of tumours or defects that involve the lateral wall of the nose, the medial wall of the maxillary sinus and the ethmoid. The word "medial" refers to the surgical site that is to be resected, which is exposing the medial part of the face by an incision that begins medially from the medial canthus extending downward along the nasomaxillary groove to the ala of the nose (Jategaonkar et al. 2020). In some cases, there may be a need to extend the incision to the upper lip for more release. In this approach, the infraorbital neurovascular bundle will remain intact (Fig. 11.11a).

Subtotal Maxillectomy

This is indicated for more extensive tumours that require more structural removal alongside the maxilla. The technique may be either infrastructure maxillectomy or suprastructure maxillectomy. The first one refers to removing the lower part of the maxilla with the teeth and the palate. This will make a hole that does not necessarily require reconstruction. The latter refers to the surgical procedure in which the parts to be removed are the superior part of the maxilla, with the possibility of including the orbital floor, orbit, tear duct and neurovascular bundle may be involved (Jategaonkar et al. 2020).

An incision of this type begins from the lateral canthus and extends to the superior or the inferior of the eye, depending on its involvement. The excision then proceeds towards the medial canthus to continue as the first approach, which requires an oral incision that extends from the labial release laterally alongside the maxillary vestibule towards the maxillary tuberosity and then from the central incisors extending palatally till the junction of hard and soft palate (Fig. 11.11b).

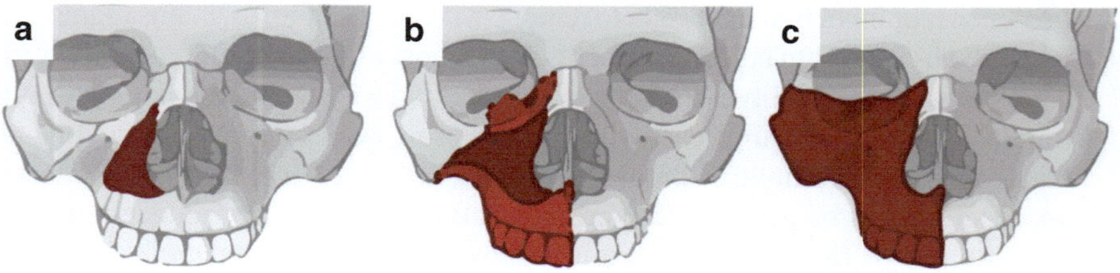

Fig. 11.11 (**a**) Medial maxillectomy: This part highlighted is removed in the medial maxillectomy approach while preserving the eye and hard palate. (**b**) Subtotal maxillectomy: A portion but not all of the maxilla is removed. (**c**) Total maxillectomy: As demonstrated by the highlight, the hard palate, orbital floor and entire maxilla are removed from one side

Total Maxillectomy

Total maxillectomy refers to the complete resection of the maxilla and the palate with the orbital floor. This is the most aggressive type which requires reconstruction of the resected parts. The incision resembles that of the subtotal type with all its extensions and releases (Fig. 11.11c) (McGuirt 1995).

Endoscopic Resection

With the gradual increase of endoscope involvement in surgical management, endoscope utilisation in maxillectomy is no exception since it is a less invasive technique with good results and prognosis.

The use of an endoscope in maxillectomy may be considered equivalent to an endonasal route which assists in the major approaches to help facilitate the procedures (Clerc et al. 2020).

For tumours that spread in a minor fashion and involve a small area, such as the lateral wall of the nose and the medial wall of the maxillary sinus, endoscopic resection may be the best conservative choice of surgical treatment.

Virtual Surgical Planning (VSP) and Navigation in Maxillectomy

The challenges in maxillectomy are the following:

- Calculate the accurate amount of structures that need to be resected in order to provide a healthy remaining tissue.
- Acknowledge the precise dimensions of the graft or alloplastic materials to be used in reconstruction.
- Predicting the rate of prognosis in each case.

The pre-surgical planning and management for any craniofacial cases gave significant improvement in obtaining the best results with fewer complications.

In VSP, the data analysis will be performed using specific computer programs applied to the CT scan of the patient. These applications are supported by the ability to define different anatomic structures, such as the normal anatomy and the important parts that need to be preserved, such as the nerves or the main blood vessels, as well as pathology.

This identification gives an obvious orientation to the surgeon and guides with the extent of the cutting. The 3D printing will produce a cutting guide in different and multiple shapes which can act as a guiding template to drive the cutting process during surgery in order to cut exactly as designed during digital planning (Clerc et al. 2020).

Another use of 3D printing is to construct the obturators and the alloplastic grafts specific to individuals. It is a remarkable challenge and also time-consuming to harvest an iliac graft and reshape it to properly fit into the surgical site, not to forget the resorption rate that cannot be calculated in autogenic and allogenic bony grafts.

Complication

Haemorrhage sores are the most frequent complication in maxillectomy, followed by infection which is a common complication in any surgical procedure. Epiphora may also occur as a late complication due to injury of the tear ducts or when it is involved in the procedure. Paraesthesia is another complication that could be temporary or permanent. Ectropion, lower lid oedema, facial contracture, notching of the lip and diplopia are among the later possible complications (Shields et al. 2001).

Reconstruction

As it is said before, the main challenge facing surgeons nowadays is the reconstruction part following the completion of surgery. This focused all the attention on answering the question, What is the patient's opinion on the result of his own surgery?" which is obviously not the surgical procedure itself but the final appearance of it. These are the main reconstruction requirements:

1. Consistently obtaining a wound that is healing.
2. Restore palatal competence and function.
3. Support the orbit or fill the orbital cavity in exenteration.
4. Obliterate the maxillectomy defect.
5. Restore facial contour and symmetry.

Depending on the surgical technique that was selected, the reconstruction technique and material will differ as well. The choices are listed below:

1. In no oral-antral communication: The small defect healing may be enough by secondary intention or a split skin graft with a plastic stent could be required. Larger defects, such as palatomaxillary extension, usually require free flap reconstruction or obturator placement (O'Connell and Futran 2010).
2. Defects with oral-antral communication reconstructed with flaps: Multiple options are available depending on the size and site of the defect, summarised as palatal transposition flap, buccal fat pad flap and facial artery myomucosal flap. The palatal transposition flap could help with small-to medium-sized defects but not with large or far-in-distance defects. This is due to its limited amount of tissue. The buccal fat pad can be considered an excellent choice for medium-sized defects due to its quick, simple and easy dissection. It can also be used under local anaesthesia, has no visible scars, a low rate of morbidity, a very low failure rate and lastly, it can be associated with other pedicled flaps. The disadvantages of the pad are that it can cover only small-to-medium defects, it is only suitable for covering because of its thinness, it provides no bulk and there is the possibility of depression occurring in the donor site (Squaquara et al. 2010). Facial

artery myomucosal flaps are mostly used to reconstruct defects from tumour ablation, but other indications such as repair of cleft palate, septal perforation and osteoradionecrosis are also included. The advantages of this flap overcome the disadvantages, making it widely used. The advantages can be summarised as no external flap, low complication rate, easy to harvest, many modifications described and primary closure of donor site if the width is under 3 cm, while the disadvantages could include limited width, bulky flap hindering the use of dental prosthesis and the requirement for a bite block to prevent biting on the flap (Ayad and Xie 2014).

3. Total maxillectomy with orbital preservation: The most important part of the reconstruction steps in this case is the orbital floor which is done by alloplastic titanium mesh, a custom implant or autogenous tissues. The alloplastic titanium mesh or the titanium implant is designed alongside the cutting guide using virtual planning to locate and calculate the exact size of the implant after accurate cutting of the defected site margin. The titanium mesh may need autogenous bone that is grafted from another site to help enhance the healing and the reconstruction journey (Clerc et al. 2020). The main disadvantage would be the cost and the high experience required to obtain maximum results.
4. Total maxillectomy with orbital exenteration: Cosmetic rehabilitation can be achieved via multiple ways of orbital cavity healing, such as healing by secondary intention, eyelid sparing technique and free skin graft, which will prepare the site for the reconstruction techniques such as paramedian forehead flap, local and regional flaps, distant pedicled flap, distant free tissue transfer with microvascular flap or non-surgical ocular and oculofacial prosthesis. Healing by secondary intention often takes several months and requires intensive postoperative care with increased morbidity and a delay in final cosmetic gratification for the patient (Shields et al. 2001). In eyelid sparing technique, the main advantage is the rapid healing, enabling the earlier fitting of a prosthesis (Shields et al. 2001), while the disadvantage may lie in the fact that a contracture would result as a final outcome, reducing the space for the prosthesis (Martel et al. 2021). Free full-thickness skin graft or split-thickness skin graft can be described as a successful choice in orbital space closure, giving a bowel shape ready for receiving the prosthesis, which is the main advantage alongside the rapid healing process. However, a second surgical site is required, which increases the perioperative morbidity (Martel et al. 2021).
5. Distraction osteogenesis plus virtual planning: This creates a dentoalveolar bone needed for a well-aligned implant placement. The importance of virtual planning lies in the construction of the cutting guide as well as the construction of obturators which fit exactly into the cavity afterwards. This will successfully allow the surgeon to close the gap of difference between what was planned preoperatively, the surgical procedure and the rehabilitation phase. The advantage of distraction osteogenesis lies in its role in minimising or eliminating the need for vascularised or non-vascularised grafts, thus eliminating donor site morbidity or graft necrosis (Fujioka et al. 2010).

References

Abu-Ghanem S, Fliss DM (2013) Surgical approaches to resection of anterior skull base and paranasal sinuses tumors. Balkan Med J 30:136–141. https://doi.org/10.5152/balkanmedj.2013.9112

Ayad T, Xie L (2014) Facial artery musculomucosal flap in head and neck reconstruction: a systematic review. Head Neck 37:1375–1386. https://doi.org/10.1002/hed.23734

Bidra AS, Jacob RF, Taylor TD (2012) Classification of maxillectomy defects: a systematic review and criteria necessary for a universal description. J Prosthet Dent 107:261–270. https://doi.org/10.1016/s0022-3913(12)60071-7

Clerc NL, Baudouin R, Carlevan M et al (2020) 3D titanium implant for orbital reconstruction after maxillectomy. J Plast Reconstr Aesthet Surg 73:732–739. https://doi.org/10.1016/j.bjps.2019.11.014

Datta RK, Viswanatha B, Harsha MS (2015) Caldwell Luc surgery: revisited. Indian J Otolaryngol Head Neck Surg 68:90–93. https://doi.org/10.1007/s12070-015-0883-y

Fagan J (2017) Open access atlas of otolaryngology, head & neck operative surgery: total maxillectomy, orbital exenteration

Fujioka M, Kanno T, Mitsugi M et al (2010) Oral rehabilitation of a maxillectomy defect using bone transport distraction and dental implants. J Oral Maxillofac Surg 68:2278–2282. https://doi.org/10.1016/j.joms.2009.12.022

Hacking C, Glick Y (2017) Caldwell-Luc operation. Radiopaedia.org. https://doi.org/10.53347/rid-51780

Jategaonkar AA, Kaul VF, Lee E, Genden EM (2020) Surgery of the palatomaxillary structure. Semin Plast Surg 34:071–076. https://doi.org/10.1055/s-0040-1709430

Kennedy DW, Adappa ND (2011) Endoscopic maxillary antrostomy: not just a simple procedure. Laryngoscope 121:2142–2145. https://doi.org/10.1002/lary.22169

Lee JT, Chiu AG (2019) Endoscopic Denker approach for anterior maxilla tumors. Elsevier, Amsterdam, pp 183–190.e1

Lee JT, Suh JD, Carrau RL et al (2016) Endoscopic Denker's approach for resection of lesions involving the anteroinferior maxillary sinus and infratemporal fossa. Laryngoscope 127:556–560. https://doi.org/10.1002/lary.26237

Lund VJ, Howard DJ, Wei WI (2013) Tumors of the nose, sinuses and nasopharynx. Thieme Medical Publishers, Stuttgart

Martel A, Baillif S, Nahon-Esteve S et al (2021) Orbital exenteration: an updated review with perspectives. Surv Ophthalmol 66:856–876. https://doi.org/10.1016/j.survophthal.2021.01.008

McCormick JP, Hicks MD, Grayson JW et al (2020) Endoscopic management of maxillary sinus diseases of dentoalveolar origin. Oral Maxillofac Surg Clin North Am 32:639–648. https://doi.org/10.1016/j.coms.2020.07.011

McGuirt WF (1995) Maxillectomy. Otolaryngol Clin N Am 28:1175–1189. https://doi.org/10.1016/s0030-6665(20)30442-4

O'Connell DA, Futran ND (2010) Reconstruction of the midface and maxilla. Curr Opin Otolaryngol Head Neck Surg 18:304–310. https://doi.org/10.1097/moo.0b013e32833b10b3

Price JC, Holliday MJ, Johns ME et al (1988) The versatile midface degloving approach. Laryngoscope 98:291–295. https://doi.org/10.1288/00005537-198803000-00010

Rezende NC, Pinheiro-Neto CD, Leonel LCPC et al (2022) Three-hundred and sixty degrees of surgical approaches to the maxillary sinus. World J Otorhinolaryngol Head Neck Surg 8:42–53. https://doi.org/10.1002/wjo2.12

Sama A, Philpott C (2018) Endonasal approaches to maxillary sinus. Int J Head Neck Surg 9:26–31. https://doi.org/10.5005/jp-journals-10001-1333

Schreiber A, Ferrari M, Rampinelli V et al (2017) Modular endoscopic medial maxillectomies: quantitative analysis of surgical exposure in a preclinical setting. World Neurosurg 100:44–55. https://doi.org/10.1016/j.wneu.2016.12.094

Sharma S, Sharma AK, Amreen N et al (2022) Sublabial approach versus modified Denker's procedure: a comparative study of pre-maxillary tissue clearance in Covid-associated mucor-

mycosis. Indian J Otolaryngol Head Neck Surg 74:3252–3258. https://doi.org/10.1007/s12070-021-03060-3
Shields JA, Shields CL, Demirci H et al (2001) Experience with eyelid-sparing orbital exenteration. Ophthalmic Plast Reconstr Surg 17:355–361. https://doi.org/10.1097/00002341-200109000-00010
Simmen D, Jones N, Balakrishnan K et al (2014) Manual of endoscopic sinus and skull base surgery. Thieme, Stuttgart
Squaquara R, Evans KK, Di Spilimbergo SS, Mardini S (2010) Intraoral reconstruction using local and regional flaps. Semin Plast Surg 24:198–211. https://doi.org/10.1055/s-0030-1255337
Themes U (2016a) The Caldwell-Luc technique. In: Ento Key. https://entokey.com/the-caldwell-luc-technique/
Themes U (2016b) External approaches in sinus surgery. In: Ento Key. https://entokey.com/external-approaches-in-sinus-surgery/
Themes U (2016c) Open surgical approaches to the paranasal sinuses. In: Plastic Surgery Key. https://plasticsurgerykey.com/open-surgical-approaches-to-the-paranasal-sinuses/
Turri-Zanoni M, Battaglia P, Karligkiotis A et al (2016) Transnasal endoscopic partial maxillectomy: operative nuances and proposal for a comprehensive classification system based on 1378 cases. Head Neck 39:754–766. https://doi.org/10.1002/hed.24676

Vascular Management of Lesions Around the Maxilla

12

Goran Latif Omer, Vivek Sasindran, Mithra Sara, Stefano Di Girolamo, Aso Khasraw Ahmed, Sahand Soran Ali, and Aland Salih Abdullah

Introduction

The posterior superior alveolar artery, infraorbital artery and posterior lateral nasal artery are three terminal branches of the maxillary artery that make up the blood supply of the maxillary sinus. Although injuries to only one of them might not be considered life-threatening, they can still limit exposure and further complicate surgeries. Among the three arteries, injuries of the posterior lateral nasal artery are the most problematic. This is due to its close relation to the sphenopalatine artery, making it more prone to anastomoses and subsequent abnormal blood flow (Flanagan 2005). Apart from direct arterial injuries, the region surrounding the maxillary sinus is vulnerable to the development of various vascular lesions that are all susceptible to bleeding. Juvenile angiofibroma, pyogenic granulomas, olfactory neuroblastoma, arteriovenous fistula and arteriovenous malformation are among the most vascular lesions of the region (Johnson 1999). Many different approaches, such as elevation of the head, electrocautery, endoscopic ligation, and arterial embolization, exist for tackling bleeding adjacent to the maxillary sinus. However, due to its less traumatic nature, endoscopic ligation is usually preferred (O'Flynn and Shadaba 2000).

G. L. Omer (✉) · S. S. Ali · A. S. Abdullah
Department of Clinical Sciences, College of Medicine, University of Sulaimani, Sulaymaniyah, KRI, Iraq

V. Sasindran · M. Sara
KM Cherian Institute of Medical Sciences, Chengannur, Kerala, India

S. Di Girolamo
Department of Otorhinolaryngology, University of Rome Tor Vergata, Rome, Italy

A. K. Ahmed
Royal Hospital, Sulaymaniyah, KRI, Iraq

© The Author(s), under exclusive license to Springer Nature Switzerland AG 2025
G. L. Omer, S. Di Girolamo (eds.), *Maxillary Sinus: A Comprehensive Guide*, https://doi.org/10.1007/978-3-031-83468-4_12

Different Techniques to Manage Vascular Lesions

Embolization

Embolization is a process whereby the blood supply to a tumour is cut off (WakeMed n.d.). It is considered the gold standard management for bleeding of paranasal lesions, and it is generally more beneficial for tumours with a single blood supply. However, due to its expensive price and financial burden, it is not always feasible (Tripuraneni et al. 2023). Another limitation of embolization is its instability in emergent cases. This is due to the 48–72 h waiting period required following embolization and prior to surgery. Embolization of tumours is usually either transarterial or percutaneous embolization. In transarterial embolization, a balloon can be used to occlude a major artery that is considered a risk for surgery. Furthermore, in preoperative transarterial embolization (PVA), particles with a size fit for occlusion of the pathological circulation can also be used. Preoperative embolization is suitable for extra-axial intracranial tumours. The procedure is not devoid of complications such as stroke, cranial nerve palsies, bleeding from perforated vessels and necrosis of tissues; however, these only occur in approximately 4% of patients. Percutaneous embolization is either performed to devascularize a tumour prior to surgery, or it is performed to relieve symptoms as a form of palliation. In this technique, the embolic agent used is either a liquid embolic or a sclerosant that is injected directly into the blood vessel of the tumour. It is highly beneficial in recurrent lesions as it can almost achieve complete tumour devascularization (Gleeson 2008). Regarding epistaxis, particles, coils and balloons can all be used.

Arterial Ligation

To cut off the blood supply in this medical procedure, the artery is tied off. This approach is generally reserved for intractable bleeding from an unknown source, unmanageable via techniques such as posterior nasal packing. Arteries that are commonly ligated are the endonasal sphenopalatine artery, the intermaxillary artery and the external carotid artery. The idea behind ligating the endonasal sphenopalatine artery is to control the bleeding as close as possible to its source. Both an operating microscope and a lens endoscope can be used for the procedure. It starts off by making an incision 8 mm anterior to and under cover of the middle turbinate's posterior end. Then, the incision is continued downward to the bone. From here, a mucosal flap is elevated posteriorly until the fibroneurovascular sleeve that arises from the sphenopalatine foramen is found. A haemostatic clip can be used to ligate the main vessel once it is identified. With regard to the internal maxillary artery ligation, either the anterior (sublabial) or combined anterior and medial (endoscopic) technique is used to transantrally reveal the artery. After exposure, an antrostomy is formed in the sublabial approach in an effort to preserve the infraorbital nerve. Then comes the elevation of the mucosa of the posterior wall of the antrum and forming a window through into the pterygopalatine fossa. Pulsation within the fat of the fossa helps identify the internal maxillary artery branches so that they can be dissected before using haemostatic clips to clip them. Lastly, despite the fact that its ligation of the external carotid artery is a step further away from the bleeding source, it is still performed in some cases, mostly due to the lack of difficulties the technique possesses. Both a skin crease incision and a longitudinal incision parallel with the anterior border of the sternocleidomastoid can be used in this technique. Firstly, the bifurcation of the carotid arteries is identified and then, after verifying the external carotid artery, it is ligated in continuity (Gleeson 2008). Based on the artery that needs to be ligated, various other external approaches can be taken.

Electrocautery

Another way to coagulate tissues is by using electrocautery. In this technique, a heated instrument is used to perform the coagulation. Cauterization with bipolar diathermy has been shown to decrease both intraoperative bleeding and the time taken to perform the operation (Gleeson 2008).

Management of Different Vascular Lesions Around the Maxilla

Juvenile Angiofibroma

The tumours are generally excised using different techniques. The technique chosen should consider the extent of the tumour, the degree of the surgeon's expertise and the tools available. Regardless of the technique used to excise the tumour, preoperative embolization is advisable due to the vascular nature of the tumour. With the advancement of endonasal endoscopic techniques, the benefits of embolization almost always outweigh its risks and are therefore advocated for. The entire vascular field is usually embolized as opposed to specific feeding arteries. This preoperative embolization helps reduce intraoperative bleeding, enhance the visual field and lower operative complications (Lund et al. 2013).

Pyogenic Granuloma

These highly vascular lesions can undergo spontaneous regression in some patients. However, in the event of recurrence, the majority of them are reduced via cautery, electrocoagulation and cryotherapy. A type of laser known to be beneficial for these vascular lesions is the neodymium-YAG laser. This is due to its high precision and its ability to haemostasis (Sharma et al. 2022). Both transarterial embolization and radiocautery have also demonstrated efficacy in pyogenic granulomas of the maxillary sinus (Abe et al. 2014; Sharma et al. 2022).

Olfactory Neuroblastoma

Although there is no standard therapeutic approach, most approaches revolve around the resection of the tumour, either endoscopically or through an open approach, followed by postoperative radiotherapy for superior results (Faragalla and Weinreb 2009). Due to the vascular nature of the tumour, both ligation and embolization of the feeding artery can be performed prior to resection of the tumour.

References

Abe M, Yamashita S, Mori Y, et al (2014) Identification of novel methylation-silenced genes in oral squamous cell carcinomas. Oral Oncology 50(7):647–653. https://doi.org/10.1016/j.oraloncology.2014.04.003

Faragalla H, Weinreb I (2009) Olfactory neuroblastoma. Adv Anat Pathol 16:322–331. https://doi.org/10.1097/pap.0b013e3181b544cf

Flanagan D (2005) Arterial supply of maxillary sinus and potential for bleeding complication during lateral approach sinus elevation. Implant Dent 14:336–339. https://doi.org/10.1097/01.id.0000188437.66363.7c

Gleeson M (2008) Scott-Brown's otorhinolaryngology, head and neck surgery. Hodder Education, London

Johnson MH (1999) Vascular lesions of the paranasal sinuses and nasal cavity. Semin Ultrasound CT MRI 20:426–444. https://doi.org/10.1016/s0887-2171(99)90025-2

Lund VJ, Howard DJ, Wei WI (2013) Tumors of the nose, sinuses and nasopharynx. Thieme Medical Publishers, Stuttgart

O'Flynn PE, Shadaba A (2000) Management of posterior epistaxis by endoscopic clipping of the sphenopalatine artery. Clin Otolaryngol Allied Sci 25:374–377. https://doi.org/10.1046/j.1365-2273.2000.00372.x

Sharma N, Rana S, Jetley S (2022) Peripheral giant cell granuloma of maxilla. J Indian Soc Periodontol 26:75. https://doi.org/10.4103/jisp.jisp_624_20

Tripuraneni SC, Gera S, Kishore GN et al (2023) Vascular control in nose and paranasal sinus tumours. Indian J Otolaryngol Head Neck Surg 75:906–914. https://doi.org/10.1007/s12070-023-03473-2

WakeMed (n.d.) Preoperative embolization. https://www.wakemed.org/care-and-services/brain-and-spine/neurosurgery/spine-tumors/preoperative-embolization#:~:text=Preoperative%20embolization%20is%20done%20to

13 Role of Chemotherapy in Management of Malignant Lesion of the Maxillary Sinus

Goran Latif Omer, Stefano Di Girolamo, Raz Haider Ahmed, Amanj Hamaamin Hamaamin, Sahand Soran Ali, Aland Salih Abdullah, and Gianluca Velletrani

Introduction

Malignant tumours of the maxillary sinus are rare, accounting for 1% of head and neck tumours. If only paranasal sinuses are considered, 80% originate from the maxillary sinus (Ashraf et al. 2010; Noronha et al. 2014). Up to 80% of these tumours are squamous cell carcinomas, with other types including adenoid cystic carcinomas, adenocarcinomas, mucoepidermoid carcinomas, sarcomas, and lymphomas. Most maxillary sinus tumours are diagnosed at later stages (Won et al. 2009).

Treatment is challenging due to the sinus's proximity to vital structures such as the eye, skull base, and nerves. Typically, treatment involves surgical resection with or without orbital exenteration, but combination therapy is often required for later-stage diagnoses. This combination usually involves surgery and postoperative radiotherapy, with chemotherapy, primarily platinum-based, added for selected patients (Watkinson and Clarke 2018).

G. L. Omer (✉) · S. S. Ali · A. S. Abdullah
Department of Clinical Sciences, College of Medicine, University of Sulaimani, Sulaymaniyah, KRI, Iraq

S. Di Girolamo · G. Velletrani
Department of Otorhinolaryngology, University of Rome Tor Vergata, Rome, Italy

R. H. Ahmed
Hiwa Hospital, Sulaymaniyah, KRI, Iraq

A. H. Hamaamin
Royal Hospital, Sulaymaniyah, KRI, Iraq

© The Author(s), under exclusive license to Springer Nature Switzerland AG 2025
G. L. Omer, S. Di Girolamo (eds.), *Maxillary Sinus: A Comprehensive Guide*, https://doi.org/10.1007/978-3-031-83468-4_13

Role of Chemotherapy in Maxillary Sinus Tumours

The literature lacks comprehensive guidelines and cited experiences regarding chemotherapy for maxillary sinus tumours. However, many authors suggest that induction chemotherapy can be effective for unresectable tumours, leading to successful surgeries in many patients (Kuo and Lin 2022). Some studies report up to 70% success rates with this neoadjuvant approach. Chemotherapy aids in organ preservation and reduces the need for radical surgery, which otherwise involves craniofacial resection, orbital exenteration and total maxillectomy, increasing morbidity and cosmetic disfigurement (Abdelmeguid et al. 2021).

Chemotherapy also works synergistically with radiotherapy, decreasing the critical tumour volume and reducing the required radiation dose post-chemotherapy (Noronha et al. 2014). Additionally, chemotherapy increases the tumour's sensitivity to radiotherapy (Niederhuber and Tepper 2019).

Chemotherapy Regimens Used in Maxillary Sinus Malignancy

The use of chemotherapy in maxillary sinus malignancies is limited. According to the National Comprehensive Cancer Network, chemotherapy is employed in the following situations (NCCN 2024):

- With radiotherapy, in T1 and T2 tumours without lymph node metastasis (N0) post-tumour resection, when there is perineural, vascular or lymphatic invasion, or when positive margins remain after re-resection, excluding adenoid cystic tumours.
- With radiotherapy, in T3 and T4, tumours without lymph node metastasis (N0) when there are positive or close margins after tumour resection.
- With radiotherapy, in T1 to T4a tumours with nodal metastasis (N+), when there are positive margins, close margins or extranodal extension post-tumour resection and neck dissection.
- In T4b tumours with or without nodal metastasis or tumours with distant metastasis (M1), chemotherapy can be used alone or with radiotherapy before tumour resection and neck dissection.

Patient characteristics such as performance status and therapy goals must be assessed before choosing the optimal regimen. Research indicates that induction chemotherapy followed by concurrent chemoradiotherapy is more successful than concurrent chemoradiotherapy alone. The recommended combinations include (NCCN 2024):

- In primary chemotherapy, high-dose cisplatin or carboplatin with 5-fluorouracil is recommended. Other agents like taxanes or hydroxyurea are used to avoid certain side effects or in advanced disease.
- In postoperative chemotherapy, only cisplatin is used.
- In induction therapy, a combination of Paclitaxel (or docetaxel), cisplatin, and 5-fluorouracil is administered.
- For recurrent or persistent disease, weekly carboplatin or cisplatin is recommended with concurrent radiotherapy (Tables 13.1 and 13.2).

Table 13.1 American Joint Committee on Cancer (AJCC) paranasal sinus cancer staging (Niederhuber and Tepper 2019)

American Joint Committee on Cancer paranasal sinus cancer staging	
Tumour	
Tx	Primary tumours cannot be assessed
T0	No evidence of a primary tumour
Tis	Carcinoma in situ
T1	Tumour limited to the maxillary sinus mucosa with no erosion or destruction of bone
T2	Tumour causing bone erosion or destruction, including extension into the hard palate and/or middle nasal meatus, except extension to the posterior wall of the maxillary sinus and pterygoid plates
T3	Tumour invades any of the following: bone of the posterior wall of the maxillary sinus, subcutaneous tissues, floor or medial wall of the orbit, pterygoid fossa or ethmoid sinuses
T4a	Tumour invades anterior orbital contents, the skin of the cheek, pterygoid plates, infratemporal fossa, cribriform plate, sphenoid sinuses or frontal sinuses
T4b	Tumour invades any of the following: orbital apex, dura, brain, middle cranial fossa, cranial nerves other than maxillary division of trigeminal nerve (V2), nasopharynx or clivus
Lymph nodes	
Nx	Regional lymph nodes cannot be assessed
N0	No regional lymph node metastasis
N1	Metastases in a single ipsilateral lymph node, ≤3 cm in greatest dimension
N2a	Metastasis in a single ipsilateral lymph node, >3 cm but ≤6 cm in greatest dimension
N2b	Metastasis in multiple ipsilateral lymph nodes ≤6 cm in the greatest dimension
N2c	Metastasis in bilateral or contralateral lymph nodes ≤6 cm in greatest dimension
N3	Metastasis in lymph node(s) >6 cm
Metastasis	
M0	No distant metastasis
M1	Distant metastasis

Table 13.2 Stage grouping of paranasal sinus tumours (Brierley et al. 2017)

Stage grouping			
Stage 0	Tis	N0	M0
Stage 1	T1	N0	M0
Stage 2	T2	N0	M0
Stage 3	T3	N0	M0
	T1, T2, T3	N1	
Stage 4A	T1, T2, T3	N2	M0
	T4a	N0, N1, N2	
Stage 4B	T4b	Any N	M0
	Any T	N3	
Stage 4C	Any T	Any N	M1

Chemotherapeutic Agents

Platinum-Based Chemotherapeutic Drugs, Particularly Cisplatin

Cisplatin is an alkylating agent within the cytotoxic medications category. It is used in solid tumours and haematological malignancies either as a single agent or in combination therapies, mostly for neoadjuvant chemotherapy. This agent is primarily used in rapidly growing tumours and works by promoting non-cell cycle cytotoxicity (Gold and Raja 2023). Cisplatin has been employed in numerous studies, especially in cases of squamous cell carcinoma of the maxillary sinus, particularly in a technique called RADPLAT, where it is administered with systemic neutralization and concomitant radiotherapy. This technique was used in a study by Homma et al. on 64 patients with T4a maxillary sinus SCC, resulting in an overall survival rate of 82.8% (Homma et al. 2024).

5-Fluorouracil

5-Fluorouracil is a chemotherapeutic drug used to treat various neoplasms. It works by impairing DNA replication and repair, leading to an imbalance in intracellular nucleotides, ultimately causing cell death (Casale and Patel 2024). In the context of maxillary sinus tumours, Nakashima and colleagues suggest FAR therapy, which includes 5-fluorouracil, vitamin A and radiotherapy. In this technique, fluorouracil and radiotherapy induce apoptosis, while vitamin A inhibits cell growth.

Taxanes, Particularly Paclitaxel

Paclitaxel is a chemotherapeutic drug primarily used for solid malignancies. Its mechanism of action is cell cycle-specific and involves the inhibition of microtubules, preventing mitosis (Ismail and Killeen 2023). In the literature, Paclitaxel has also been used in maxillary sinus tumours. For instance, in a study by Morimoto et al., the drug was used in a combination called PCE (Paclitaxel, Carboplatin, and Cetuximab), resulting in a significant decrease in tumour size. They observed a response adequate to suggest using PCE as first-line management in advanced cases of maxillary sinus carcinoma (Morimoto et al. 2024).

Immunotherapy

Recently, immunotherapy has been developed and is now used in treating non-nasopharyngeal head and neck cancers. The two immunotherapy agents approved by the FDA for use in these cancers are nivolumab and pembrolizumab, both of which are anti-PD-1 antibodies. PD-1 regulates the function of T cells and balances their cytotoxic activity; thus, blocking it enhances the immune system's response against tumour cells (Kuo and Lin 2022). Immunotherapy response is proportional to the expression of PD-L1 by the tumour, which can be identified through immunohistochemistry. It also shows great outcomes when combined with chemotherapy, especially in technically advanced cases or in patients who refuse surgery. Kuo and colleagues suggest that these agents may help in downstaging and regression of the tumour when used as the primary treatment (Kuo and Lin 2022).

References

Abdelmeguid AS, Teeramatwanich W, Roberts DB et al (2021) Neoadjuvant chemotherapy for locoregionally advanced squamous cell carcinoma of the paranasal sinuses. Cancer 127:1788–1795. https://doi.org/10.1002/cncr.33452

Ashraf M, Biswas J, Dam A, Bhowmick A, Jha A, Singh V, Nayak S (2010) Results of treatment of squamous cell carcinoma of maxillary sinus: a 26-year experience. World J Oncol 1(1):28–34. https://doi.org/10.4021/wjon2010.02.191w

Brierley JD, Gospodarowicz MK, Wittekind C (2017) TNM classification of malignant tumours. Wiley, Hoboken, NJ

Casale J, Patel P (2024) Fluorouracil. In: StatPearls—NCBI Bookshelf. https://www.ncbi.nlm.nih.gov/books/NBK549808/

Gold JM, Raja A (2023) Cisplatin. In: StatPearls—NCBI Bookshelf. https://www.ncbi.nlm.nih.gov/books/NBK547695/

Homma A, Mikami M, Matsuura K et al (2024) Dose-finding and efficacy confirmation trial of the superselective intra-arterial infusion of cisplatin and concomitant radiation therapy for locally advanced maxillary sinus cancer (JCOG1212): results of the efficacy confirmation phase in patients with T4aN0M0. Int J Radiat Oncol Biol Phys 118:1271–1281. https://doi.org/10.1016/j.ijrobp.2023.11.031

Ismail U, Killeen RB (2023) Taxane toxicity. In: StatPearls—NCBI Bookshelf. https://www.ncbi.nlm.nih.gov/books/NBK589655/

Kuo Y-H, Lin C-S (2022) Regression of advanced maxillary sinus cancer with orbital invasion by combined chemotherapy and immunotherapy: a one-year follow-up case report. Mol Clin Oncol 16:94. https://doi.org/10.3892/mco.2022.2527

Morimoto M, Takano M, Sato T, Makino S (2024) Combination treatment with paclitaxel, carboplatin and cetuximab in maxillary sinus cancer: a case report. Oncol Lett 27:93. https://doi.org/10.3892/ol.2024.14226

NCCN (2024) Head and neck cancers. https://www.nccn.org/professionals/physician_gls/pdf/head-and-neck.pdf. Accessed 31 Jul 2024

Niederhuber JE, Tepper JE (2019) Abeloff's clinical oncology. Elsevier, Amsterdam

Noronha V, Patil VM, Joshi A, Krishna MV, Dhumal S, Juvekar S, et al (2014) Induction chemotherapy in technically unresectable locally advanced carcinoma of maxillary sinus. Chemother Res Pract 2014:1–6. https://doi.org/10.1155/2014/487872

Watkinson JC, Clarke RW (2018) Scott-Brown's otorhinolaryngology and head and neck surgery. 8th ed. Boca Raton: CRC Press

Won HS, Chun SH, Kim BS, Chung SR, Yoo IeR, Jung CK, et al (2009) Treatment outcome of maxillary sinus cancer. Rare Tumors 1(2):e36. https://doi.org/10.4081/rt.2009.e36

14 Role of Radiotherapy in Maxillary Sinus Lesion

Goran Latif Omer, Stefano Di Girolamo, Sahand Soran Ali, Aland Salih Abdullah, and Beatrice Francavilla

Introduction

Radiotherapy is a mode of killing cancer cells and shrinking tumours via high-dose radiation (National Cancer Institute 2019). It aims to cure or shrink early-stage cancer, lower recurrence rate, treat symptoms caused by cancer and even treat cancer recurrences. The three main ways of administering radiotherapy are internal, external or systemic. Firstly, external radiation is when a machine directs high-energy rays from outside the body into the tumour (American Cancer Society 2024a). Internal radiation, also known as brachytherapy, is a method in which a radioactive source is inserted into the body that may or may not be removed based on the type of tumour (Patinaik et al. 2024). Lastly, systemic radiotherapy can be given either orally or intravenously (American Cancer Society).

Radiotherapy in the Maxillary Sinus

Since radiotherapy can improve both clinical and functional outcomes, it is used in the majority of head and neck cancers. It can even replace surgical resection, provided that the tumour is found in its early stages. Radiotherapy can be used in different ways. It can be used as adjuvant therapy following surgical resection, primarily to prevent recurrence (Alfouzan 2021). It can be used prior to therapy as

G. L. Omer (✉) · S. S. Ali · A. S. Abdullah
Department of Clinical Sciences, College of Medicine, University of Sulaimani, Sulaymaniyah, KRI, Iraq

S. Di Girolamo · B. Francavilla
Department of Otorhinolaryngology, University of Rome Tor Vergata, Rome, Italy

© The Author(s), under exclusive license to Springer Nature Switzerland AG 2025

G. L. Omer, S. Di Girolamo (eds.), *Maxillary Sinus: A Comprehensive Guide*,
https://doi.org/10.1007/978-3-031-83468-4_14

neoadjuvant therapy to shrink the tumour and make resection easier (American Cancer Society 2024b).

Furthermore, it can be used as a means to preserve tissues and to avoid total removal of organs, such as in cases of laryngectomy. Moreover, a combination of radiotherapy and chemotherapy can be beneficial in locally advanced diseases (Alfouzan 2021). Tumours of the paranasal sinuses generally require complete surgical resection; however, radiotherapy can still be used for tumours with positive or close surgical margins as well as locally advanced tumours (Yeh 2010). For unresectable tumours, radiotherapy can be combined with chemotherapy as a definitive treatment. In advanced tumours of the nasal cavity and paranasal sinus, radiotherapy can be used to manage symptoms, also known as palliative radiotherapy (Cancer Research UK 2024).

Radiotherapy in Benign Lesions of the Maxillary Sinus

Antrochoanal Polyp

Radiotherapy is not routinely used for antrochoanal polyps and is not part of the routine therapeutic approach. It has been tried before but its efficacy is yet to be established (Kulkarni et al. 2021).

Angiofibroma Involving the Maxillary Sinus

The mainstay therapeutic approach for juvenile nasopharyngeal angiofibroma is surgery. However, radiotherapy can still be used for tumours that recur or tumours that cannot be surgically resected. The latter could be due to the size of the tumour or its location and extension (Tork and Simpson 2023). Furthermore, radiotherapy has been shown to be beneficial as adjuvant therapy for residual tumours, especially for cases of locally advanced tumours. Local control rates as high as 90% have been reported, advocating for the success of adjuvant radiotherapy (López et al. 2017).

Regarding definitive radiotherapy for inoperable cases, long-term disease control of around 85% is achieved with shrinkage of the tumour size; however, the burden of the tumour will remain (Mallick et al. 2015). External radiotherapeutic approaches are also available, such as stereotactic radiosurgery (gamma knife surgery), intensity-modulated radiotherapy and conventional external beam radiotherapy. All radiotherapeutic approaches pose the concern of secondary neoplasm following long-term high-dose radiotherapy (Tork and Simpson 2023).

Inverted Papilloma

Although surgery is the primary treatment for inverted papilloma, it is advised to use external beam radiotherapy for inoperable cases, recurrent cases and cases associated with malignancy (Rutenberg et al. 2011). A great number of scientists advocate against this due to the risk of anaplastic transformation following radiotherapy. However, recent studies show that there is no direct relationship between radiotherapy for inverted papilloma and subsequent neoplastic formation following surgery. Among 16 cases that underwent radiotherapy for inverted papilloma, the treatment failed in only 2 of the cases. If radiotherapy is used after subtotal resection of an inverted papilloma or to prevent recurrence, then a dose of less than 60 Gy is sufficient; however, for tumours that are deemed inoperable, a dose closer to 70 Gy is preferred (Strojan et al. 2013).

Osteoblastoma

Despite surgery being the mainstay treatment, adjuvant chemotherapy and radiotherapy are still beneficial in osteoblastoma. Both radiotherapy and more aggressive resection techniques are reserved for fast-growing tumours with aggressive characteristics (Bokhari et al. 2012). The conversation about post-surgical radiotherapy holds a lot of controversy. This is partly due to the presence of facial bones around the area. Moreover, there are case reports of radiotherapy-induced osteosarcoma of the maxillary sinus, further putting its use in question (Avitia and Osborne 2007; Mouna et al. 2016).

Fibrous Dysplasia

The management of fibrous dysplasia varies widely, mainly dependent on the size of the lesion. Regarding radiotherapy, it is highly contraindicated in fibrous dysplasia and should always be avoided. This is due to the elevated risk of inducing osteosarcoma, with some reporting a 400-fold increase in the likelihood of osteosarcoma development in cases of fibrous dysplasias treated with radiotherapy (Amin and Ling 1995).

Ossifying Fibroma

Small ossifying fibromas are managed with enucleation and curettage; however, it is difficult to completely manage large ossifying fibromas with surgery alone, especially for tumours, since despite being surgically resected, negative margins will remain. Although not very common and rarely reported in the literature, there are cases of adjuvant radiotherapy following surgical resection of ossifying fibroma used for local control (Strickler et al. 2017). These are very beneficial as the tumour has a very high recurrence rate following surgical management, ranging from 30% to 56%. Other authors do consider radiotherapy a contraindication due to the high risk of malignant transformation (Tompodung and Sensusiati 2024).

Pyogenic Granuloma

There is no established standard care for pyogenic granulomas, and different treatments have different success rates (Sarwal and Lapumnuaypol 2022). Regarding radiotherapy, superficial radiotherapy (SRT-100) is among the approaches taken for pyogenic granuloma. This is primarily due to the noninvasiveness of the technique, making it suitable for inoperable cases and in patients who do not want to undergo surgery. Although in need of further research, the technique has shown desirable outcomes. Radiotherapy, in general, can be used for pyogenic granulomas as it does not result in post-surgical scarring and it has limited adverse effects; however, it might not be sufficient as a definitive curative approach and might leave signs of skin hyperpigmentation (Song et al. 2024).

Radiotherapy in Malignant Lesions of the Maxillary Sinus

Squamous Cell Carcinoma

Surgical excision is preferred since it not only removes the mass it also helps restore function. However, this is for tumours that have not metastasized. In cases of metastasis, the treatment becomes trickier as there is no optimal management (Santos et al. 2014). Many different opinions exist in the literature regarding combination therapy with radiotherapy. According to Wang et al., surgery-based comprehensive radiotherapy is preferred for maxillary sinus squamous cell carcinoma; however, Kuo et al. advocate for radiotherapy to be used as a neoadjuvant therapy (Kuo et al. 2018; Wang et al. 2020). Moreover, a combination of chemotherapy and radiotherapy as adjuvant therapy is beneficial for atypical carcinomas with positive margins (Ebara et al. 2019).

Adenocystic Carcinoma

All of surgery, chemotherapy, and radiotherapy are suitable for adenocystic carcinoma. Surgical excision is sufficient for tumours that present early with no metastasis; however, due to the subclinical expansion of the tumour necessitating wide surgical excision but the complex anatomy of surrounding structures limiting it, combination with radiotherapy is preferred. The response rate to radiation is high, sometimes reaching 96%; however, the recurrence rate following radiotherapy is also high and can reach up to around 90%. This indicates that although the tumour is radiosensitive, radiotherapy alone cannot cure it (Lahjaouj et al. 2021).

Olfactory Neuroblastoma

Although endoscopic surgical approaches are usually attempted, no established treatment approach exists for olfactory neuroblastoma of the maxillary sinus. This is primarily due to the lack of clinical trials. However, surgery combined with radiotherapy provides superior local control than surgery alone. According to Faragalla et al., the local control with surgery alone was 17%, whereas the local control achieved when surgery was combined with radiotherapy was 86% (Faragalla and Weinreb 2009). Others have also proven the efficacy of postoperative intensity-modulated radiation therapy (IMRT) following minimally invasive surgery (Cante et al. 2018). Regarding the chemo-radiation approach for locally advanced olfactory neuroblastoma, it can be effective in pre-operative settings as a means to down stage the tumour in an attempt to make the tumour more resectable. However, according to Wu et al., it can also be used as a definitive treatment.

Maxillary Sinus Lymphoma

The main approaches for non-Hodgkin's lymphoma are radiotherapy and chemotherapy. Radiotherapy is generally reserved for early stages of large tumours (Adouly et al. 2015). According to Ban et al., apart from only using radiotherapy to irradiate the mass, it can also be used to irradiate the remaining surrounding neck nodes as a prophylactic measure (Ban et al. 2012). Radiotherapy has also been proven efficacious in Hodgkin lymphomas of the maxillary sinus, especially in stages 1 and 2 (Strickler et al. 2017).

Other Rare Malignant Lesions of the Maxillary Sinus

Apart from the aforementioned malignant lesions, radiotherapy can be used, whether alone or in combination, for some other rare but malignant lesions of the maxillary sinus. Among them is adenocarcinoma of the maxillary sinus. There is very limited information available in the literature as it is an extremely rare occurrence in the maxillary sinus; however, when present, both radiotherapy and surgery can be used to tackle the tumour (Canadian Cancer Society 2020). Regarding rhabdomyosarcoma of the maxillary sinus, despite surgery being the main therapeutic approach of choice, combination with chemotherapy and radiotherapy is crucial, especially when negative margins cannot be attained with surgical excision (Thompson et al. 2013). Surgery is generally performed following initial chemotherapy followed by radiotherapy (De Melo et al. 2017).

Furthermore, another tumour where radiotherapy could be beneficial is spindle cell carcinoma of the maxillary sinus. Owing to the limited cases reported on the lesion, an established therapeutic protocol does not exist. However, surgery is usually not sufficient and postoperative chemotherapy and radiotherapy are required (Lund et al. 2014). Moreover, one malignant tumour of the maxillary sinus that is highly radiosensitive is extramedullary plasmacytoma. This is a feature that it shares with the majority of other plasma cell neoplasms (Jeyaraj et al. 2015).

References

Adouly T, Adnane C, Oubahmane T et al (2015) Uncommon presentation of non-Hodgkin's lymphoma of maxillary sinus: a case report. Am J Med Case Rep 3:410–412. https://doi.org/10.12691/ajmcr-3-12-7

Alfouzan AF (2021) Radiation therapy in head and neck cancer. Saudi Med J 42:247–254. https://doi.org/10.15537/smj.2021.42.3.20210660

American Cancer Society (2024a) How radiation therapy is used to treat cancer. https://www.cancer.org/cancer/managing-cancer/treatment-types/radiation/basics.html. Accessed 31 Jul 2024

American Cancer Society (2024b) Radiation therapy for nasal cavity and paranasal sinus cancers. https://www.cancer.org/cancer/types/nasal-cavity-and-paranasal-sinus-cancer/treating/radiation-therapy.html. Accessed 31 Jul 2024

Amin R, Ling R (1995) Malignant fibrous histiocytoma following radiation therapy of fibrous dysplasia. Br J Radiol 68:1119–1122. https://doi.org/10.1259/0007-1285-68-814-1119

Avitia S, Osborne RF (2007) Radiation-induced osteosarcoma of the maxillary sinus. Ear Nose Throat J 86:329–330. https://doi.org/10.1177/014556130708600607

Ban SB, Kim CY, Choi NS (2012) Radiation therapy of the maxillary sinus lymphoma: a case report and review of literature. Radiat Oncol J 30(4):182–185. https://doi.org/10.3857/roj.2012.30.4.182

Bokhari K, Hameed MS, Ajmal M, Togoo RA (2012) Benign osteoblastoma involving maxilla: a case report and review of the literature. Case Rep Dent 2012:1–4. https://doi.org/10.1155/2012/351241

Canadian Cancer Society (2020) Cancerous tumours of the nasal cavity and paranasal sinuses. Du Cancer CCS/SC. https://cancer.ca/en/cancer-information/cancer-types/nasal-and-paranasal-sinus/what-is-nasal-cavity-and-paranasal-sinus-cancer/cancerous-tumours#:~:text=the%20salivary%20gland.-

Cancer Research UK (2024) Having radiotherapy for nasal and paranasal sinus cancer. https://www.cancerresearchuk.org/about-cancer/nasal-sinus-cancer/treatment/radiotherapy/having. Accessed 31 Jul 2024

Cante D, Piva C, Sciacero P et al (2018) Olfactory neuroblastoma treated with minimally invasive surgery and adjuvant radiotherapy: a case report and review of the literature. BJR Case Rep 4:20170077. https://doi.org/10.1259/bjrcr.20170077

De Melo ACR, Lyra TC, Ribeiro ILA et al (2017) Embryonal rhabdomyosarcoma in the maxillary sinus with orbital involvement in a pediatric patient: case report. World J Clin Cases 5:440–445. https://doi.org/10.12998/wjcc.v5.i12.440

Ebara T, Ando K, Eishima J et al (2019) Radiation with concomitant superselective intra-arterial cisplatin infusion for maxillary sinus squamous cell carcinoma. Jpn J Radiol 37:494–499. https://doi.org/10.1007/s11604-019-00827-1

Faragalla H, Weinreb I (2009) Olfactory neuroblastoma. Adv Anat Pathol 16:322–331. https://doi.org/10.1097/pap.0b013e3181b544cf

Jeyaraj P, Venkatesan M, Nijhawan VS (2015) Solitary extramedullary plasmacytoma of the maxillary sinus, progressing to smoldering multiple myeloma with multifocal skeletal involvement, which resolved completely following chemotherapy alone. J Maxillofac Oral Surg 15:229–239. https://doi.org/10.1007/s12663-015-0742-0

Kulkarni AS, Kesari M, Patil Y (2021) Antrochoanal polyp in an unusual case of follicular ameloblastoma of maxilla: a case report. Int J Head Neck Surg 12:114–118. https://doi.org/10.5005/jp-journals-10001-1441

Kuo P, Torabi SJ, Kraus D, Judson BL (2018) Survival outcomes for induction vs adjuvant chemotherapy in squamous cell carcinoma of the maxillary sinus. Otolaryngol Head Neck Surg 160:658–663. https://doi.org/10.1177/0194599818804777

Lahjaouj M, Berrada O, Rayhane A et al (2021) Advanced adenoid cystic carcinoma of maxillary sinus: rare case report and review of literature. Int J Surg Case Rep 80:105622. https://doi.org/10.1016/j.ijscr.2021.02.008

López F, Triantafyllou A, Snyderman CH et al (2017) Nasal juvenile angiofibroma: current perspectives with emphasis on management. Head Neck 39:1033–1045. https://doi.org/10.1002/hed.24696

Lund VJ, Howard D, Wei WI (2014) Tumors of the nose, sinuses and nasopharynx. Thieme, Stuttgart

Mallick S, Benson R, Bhasker S, Mohanti BK (2015) Long-term treatment outcomes of juvenile nasopharyngeal angiofibroma treated with radiotherapy. PubMed Central (PMC). https://www.ncbi.nlm.nih.gov/pmc/articles/PMC4443565/

Mouna M, Safae K, Narimane S, Rachida D (2016) Case report: osteoblastoma of the maxillar sinus. Open J Clin Diagn 06:25–29. https://doi.org/10.4236/ojcd.2016.63005

National Cancer Institute (2019) Radiation therapy for cancer. Cancer.gov. https://www.cancer.gov/about-cancer/treatment/types/radiation-therapy

Patinaik A, Shahini R, Divya VC et al (2024) Nanomedicine in oral cancer. Int Dent J Stud Res 11:154–157. https://doi.org/10.18231/j.idjsr.2023.033

Rutenberg, Morris CG, Werning JW et al (2011) External-beam radiotherapy for inverted papillomas of the nasal cavity and paranasal sinuses: the University of Florida experience. Int J Radiat Oncol Biol Phys 81:S637. https://doi.org/10.1016/j.ijrobp.2011.06.1889

Santos MRM, Servato JPS, Cardoso SV et al (2014) Squamous cell carcinoma at maxillary sinus: clinicopathologic data in a single Brazilian institution with review of literature. PubMed Central (PMC). https://www.ncbi.nlm.nih.gov/pmc/articles/PMC4313952/

Sarwal P, Lapumnuaypol K (2022) Pyogenic granuloma. In: StatPearls—NCBI Bookshelf. https://www.ncbi.nlm.nih.gov/books/NBK556077/

Song Y-H, Chen D, Cai W-N, Zhang L (2024) Superficial radiation therapy (SRT-100) for hypertrophic neurodermatitis. Indian J Dermatol 69:107. https://doi.org/10.4103/ijd.ijd_740_23

Strickler S, Hitchcock KE, Dziegielewski PT, Mendenhall WM (2017) Radiotherapy for juvenile ossifying fibroma of the maxillary sinus: case report and literature review. Head Neck 39:E81. https://doi.org/10.1002/hed.24811

Strojan P, Jereb S, Borsos I et al (2013) Radiotherapy for inverted papilloma: a case report and review of the literature. Radiol Oncol 47:71–76. https://doi.org/10.2478/v10019-012-0045-8

Thompson CF, Kim BJ, Lai C et al (2013) Sinonasal rhabdomyosarcoma: prognostic factors and treatment outcomes. Int Forum Allergy Rhinol 3:678–683. https://doi.org/10.1002/alr.21157

Tompodung LM, Sensusiati AD (2024) Ossifying fibroma of the maxilla: a case report with literature review. Radiol Case Rep 19:915–921. https://doi.org/10.1016/j.radcr.2023.10.059

Tork CA, Simpson DL (2023) Nasopharyngeal angiofibroma. In: StatPearls—NCBI Bookshelf. https://www.ncbi.nlm.nih.gov/books/NBK545240/

Wang Y, Yang R, Zhao M et al (2020) Retrospective analysis of 98 cases of maxillary sinus squamous cell carcinoma and therapeutic exploration. World J Surg Oncol 18:90. https://doi.org/10.1186/s12957-020-01862-3

Yeh S-A (2010) Radiotherapy for head and neck cancer. Semin Plast Surg 24:127–136. https://doi.org/10.1055/s-0030-1255330

Reconstruction for Maxillary Sinus

15

Goran Latif Omer, Hawre Abdulsattar Hasan, Dastan Tahir Abdallah, Zhwan Sabah Hassan, Vyan Hiwa Mohammed Rouf, Sazgar Shahab Ali, Stefano Di Girolamo, Sahand Soran Ali, and Aland Salih Abdullah

Reconstruction and Cosmetic Surgery for Maxillary Sinus

Introduction

Maxillary sinus operations are usually conducted for the sake of treating sinus conditions that do not respond to medications or conditions that mandate surgical intervention. An example of the former is chronic sinusitis, and of the latter is the presence of polyps, congenital abnormalities, reconstruction after trauma or tumour resection, etc.

Regardless of the underlying aetiology necessitating the surgery, maxillary sinus reconstruction is a valuable procedure contributing to overall anatomic correction and functional enhancement, improving lifestyle of the patient.

Maxillary Sinus Reconstruction Following Fracture

Midfacial fractures account for 45.4% to 79.1% of all facial fractures and have a substantial effect on the appearance and functionality of patients (Akama 2005). The array consists of the digits 12, 3, 4, and 5. The AO CMF categorisation system

G. L. Omer (✉) · S. S. Ali · A. S. Abdullah
Department of Clinical Sciences, College of Medicine, University of Sulaimani, Sulaymaniyah, KRI, Iraq

H. A. Hasan · D. T. Abdallah · Z. S. Hassan · V. H. M. Rouf · S. S. Ali
Royal Hospital, Sulaymaniyah, KRI, Iraq

S. Di Girolamo
Department of Otorhinolaryngology, University of Rome Tor Vergata, Rome, Italy

© The Author(s), under exclusive license to Springer Nature Switzerland AG 2025
G. L. Omer, S. Di Girolamo (eds.), *Maxillary Sinus: A Comprehensive Guide*, https://doi.org/10.1007/978-3-031-83468-4_15

defines the midfacial region into distinct anatomical regions, such as zygoma, upper central midface, intermediate central midface, lower central midface, frontal, parietal, sphenoidal, and temporal (Whyne et al. 2020). The AO CMF categorisation system classifies the midfacial region into specific anatomical regions, including zygoma, upper central midface, intermediate central midface, lower central midface, frontal, parietal, sphenoidal, and temporal (Bächli et al. 2009). The symptoms of maxillary sinusitis include nasal congestion, nasal discharge, facial pain, and rhinocnesmus, among other manifestations (Li and Felländer-Tsai 2021). Acute maxillary sinusitis can have serious and sometimes life-threatening implications, while chronic disease can greatly affect a person's quality of life owing to frequent episodes and the discomfort they cause (Slavin et al. 2005). The goal of controlling facial fractures is to minimise the incidence of maxillary sinusitis. An assessment was carried out to evaluate the decrease of maxillary sinus wall fractures using Ellis's categorisation (Jiang et al. 2022).

Photos showing any asymmetry more than 2 mm were deemed to indicate an inadequate alignment of the fracture on the CT axial scan image. Our analysis found that not adequately reducing the maxillary sinus wall increased the likelihood of having postoperative maxillary sinus sickness. Prior research has indicated that the primary objectives in treating midfacial fractures are to rectify dental misalignment, enhance facial appearance, reinstate the height of the central region of the face, and mend the projection of the midface (Forrest and Antonyshyn 1998). The targeted reduction of the maxillary sinus wall has not been a well-defined therapeutic objective and is frequently disregarded. Nevertheless, our research highlights the significance of accurate reduction since an inaccurate reduction was linked to maxillary sinus sickness. Hence, it is imperative for surgeons to strive for precise alignment of maxillary sinus wall fractures during ORIF treatments (Rahpeyma and Khajehahmadi 2015).

Maxillary Sinus Floor Reconstruction

This article analyses the anatomical components that play a role in successful augmentation therapies, with a specific emphasis on sinus augmentation techniques and the anatomical factors that impact the stretching capacity of the Schneiderian membrane (Lundgren et al. 2004). Schneiderian membrane perforation occurs when the local stress exceeds its stretching capability, which is closely associated with structural anomalies of the maxillary sinus (Testori et al. 2019). The extensibility of the Schneiderian membrane impacts the selection of a surgical approach and the resulting clinical results. When assessing surgical techniques and clinical outcomes, physicians should consider not only the residual bone height but also the extensibility affected by the health state of the membrane, the morphologies of the maxillary sinus, and the presence of antral septate text iontained within the tags. After a tooth is lost, the alveolar ridge may become compromised because of the shrinkage and air-filled expansion of the maxillary sinus. This might, therefore, impede the success of dental repair (Wassef et al. 2012).

Maxillary sinus floor augmentation (MSFA) is a procedure that involves lifting the Schneiderian membrane to raise the height of the remaining bone in the back of the upper jaw (Velasco-Ortega et al. 2021). This increases the amount of bone available for placing dental implants in this area. The elevation of the membrane can be done through either a lateral or transcrestal approach (Lundgren et al. 2016). The lateral window sinus augmentation technique, initially developed by Tatum and later documented by Boyne and James, involves creating a bony opening in the lateral wall of the maxillary sinus (Wallace et al. 2012). However, this operation is associated with post-surgical problems, high expenses, and intricate steps. The transcrestal method, initially suggested by Tatum and then modified by Summers, is a minimally invasive technique. It involves making an incision without direct visualisation, resulting in a small wound, a brief operation duration, and a favourable patient outcome (Younes et al. 2017) provides evidence that MSFA, when implemented using both of the aforementioned methods, is both successful and safe. Advancements in surgical techniques and equipment have led to ongoing updates in the impact of anatomical parameters and the selection of surgical approaches. The MSFA procedure involves three main steps: raising a flap, entering the sinus cavity through a window, and elevating the Schneiderian membrane above the maxillary floor and beneath the Schneider membrane to increase the height of the alveolar bone and establish a restricted area (Díaz-Olivares et al. 2021). Upon examination of this enclosed area from the coronal perspective, it becomes evident that it is comprised of three distinct boundaries: the lateral wall of the maxillary sinus, the ridge at the top of the alveolar bone, and the expanded and elevated membrane of the maxillary sinus (Whyte and Boeddinghaus 2019). Studies have indicated that a stress of 7.3 N/mm^3 on average can result in the rupture of the sinus membrane (Lanzer 2015). The membrane can be stretched in one dimension up to 132.6% of its initial size and in two dimensions up to 124.7% (Pommer et al. 2009). Although MSFA procedures are generally predictable, the Schneiderian membrane can be perforated if the local tension exceeds its stretching capacity (Lyu et al. 2023).

Selection of Patients

Individuals with a medical history of sinusitis, allergies, or other sinus abnormalities may not be suitable candidates for maxillary sinus augmentation. These circumstances may lead to the formation of a dense membrane, which might make the process of lifting the membrane more challenging (Valentini 2023). If you have any preexisting sinus disorders or other related conditions, it is advisable to seek consultation with an ear, nose, and throat (ENT) specialist before proceeding with surgery (Cote et al. 2011). It is crucial to provide patients with comprehensive knowledge about the different consequences that can occur after sinus surgery (Senior et al. 1998). Smokers are at a heightened risk of experiencing several issues following sinus surgery as well as a significantly increased likelihood of implant failures. As a result, they are not considered ideal candidates for either treatment (Testori et al. 2019). Additional contraindications for sinus augmentation in dental implant procedures include unmanaged diabetes, chemotherapy, previous unsuccessful sinus surgeries, neoplasms, radiotherapy, or prior LeFort I surgery (Göçmen and Özkan 2017). It is crucial to carefully choose and educate patients about the surgery as well as ensure that the doctor doing the procedure has sufficient experience. This is necessary in order to reduce the likelihood of difficulties during and after the operation (Rothrock 2022).

Complications of Maxillary Sinus Augmentation

Perforation of the Schneiderian sinus membrane is the most prevalent surgical complication. This can happen in both the lateral window technique and the crestal approach (Díaz-Olivares et al. 2021). Failure to detect or adequately seal sinus perforations can lead to elevated occurrences of postoperative sinusitis, infection, and transplant failure (Testori et al. 2019). During the delicate process of lifting or after surgery, inflammatory fluid in the sinus might readily seep into the augmented site and hinder the healing of the graft (Katranji et al. 2008). This type of sinusitis is typically acute, and thankfully, infections rarely arise. Another commonly reported complication of sinus lifting surgery is profuse bleeding from the posterior superior alveolar artery, which can lead to the failure of the graft or even more severe consequences. Although uncommon, it is important to take into account the position and path of this artery following cone beam computed tomography (CBCT) prior to any surgical procedure. The complexity can be significantly decreased or removed by using the crestal surgical technique. Maxillary septa are bony structures that cross through the sinus. The anatomical barriers present make it difficult to elevate the sinus membrane without causing a tear. It is recommended to perform a CBCT examination of the sinus septa before conducting a lateral antrostomy. Techniques such as enlarging the bony opening or creating many lateral openings can resolve the problem of bony partitions.

Role of Prosthesis in Maxillary Reconstruction

Introduction

Reconstruction and aesthetic surgeries of the midface and maxillary region have become increasingly popular in recent years as advancements in medical technology have allowed for more precise and effective procedures. These surgeries can help patients improve their overall appearance and self-esteem as well as address functional issues that may be affecting their quality of life. With the help of skilled surgeons and innovative techniques, individuals can achieve natural-looking results that enhance their facial features and restore balance to their facial structure (Haleem et al. 2022).

Conventional cosmetic procedures may not always provide the desired outcome, as soft tissue grafting may not always be a suitable option for certain patients. Colour matching and proper anatomical reconstruction are major hurdles in that area. However, advancements in technology have led to the development of alternative methods, such as 3D printing, that can create custom implants tailored to each patient's unique facial structure. This personalised approach ensures a more precise and natural-looking result without the limitations of traditional techniques. By utilising cutting-edge technology, patients can now achieve the facial rejuvenation they desire with greater accuracy and satisfaction. This groundbreaking innovation is revolutionising the field of facial reconstruction and providing new possibilities for those seeking cosmetic enhancements (Bhatia et al. 2020; Butt et al. 2021; Herath and Jinendra 2024; Kalaj and Cohen 2020).

Epidemiology

The epidemiology of the maxillary defects is somehow hard to calculate because of the variety of conditions affecting the nasomaxillary complex. However, advancements in technology and medical knowledge are helping to improve our understanding and accurate tracking of these defects (Izzetti et al. 2021; Liu et al. 2020).

The Use of Prosthetics in Maxillary Reconstruction

Using prosthetics is a crucial aspect of restoring normal function and aesthetics for patients. By utilising prosthetics, surgeons can create custom-made structures that fit perfectly in the maxillary region, allowing for proper chewing, speaking, and breathing. Additionally, preserving the maxillary sinus during reconstruction helps maintain the integrity of the facial structure and prevents complications such as infection or sinusitis. Overall, the combination of prosthetics and preservation of the maxillary sinus is essential for successful maxillary reconstruction procedures (Kämmerer and Al-Nawas 2023; Schwarz et al. 2021; Rogers et al. 2022).

When considering maxillary reconstruction, it is important for surgeons to carefully assess the individual needs of each patient in order to achieve optimal results. This may involve considering factors such as bone density, soft tissue support, and overall facial symmetry. By tailoring the approach to each patient, surgeons can ensure that the final outcome not only restores function but also enhances the patient's appearance. Additionally, ongoing monitoring and follow-up care are essential to ensure the long-term success of the reconstruction and to address any potential issues that may arise. By combining expertise in prosthetics with a commitment to preserving the natural anatomy of the maxillary region, surgeons can provide patients with a comprehensive and effective solution for their reconstructive needs (Abdelwahab and Patel 2021; Aman et al. 2020; Petrides et al. 2021).

Types of Prosthetic Materials Used in Maxillofacial Reconstruction

The list includes silicone, acrylic, PEEK, MedPor, and titanium. Each material has its own unique properties and benefits, allowing surgeons to tailor the prosthesis to the specific needs and preferences of the patient. Silicone prosthetics, for example, are known for their flexibility and natural feel, making them ideal for facial reconstruction. Acrylic prosthetics, on the other hand, are more durable and can be easily customised to match the patient's skin tone and facial features. Titanium prosthetics are incredibly strong and lightweight, making them suitable for patients who require a more robust solution. Ultimately, the choice of material will depend on the individual patient's needs and the goals of the reconstruction surgery (Cristache and Totu 2020; Generalova et al. 2024; Khashaba et al. 2021; Larsen et al. 2015).

It is important for the prosthetist to work closely with the patient and their medical team to determine the best material for their specific situation. Factors such as skin sensitivity, lifestyle, and desired appearance all play a role in the decision-making process. By taking the time to carefully consider these factors, the prosthetist can ensure that the patient receives a prosthesis that not only meets their functional needs but also helps them feel confident and comfortable in their own skin. Additionally, ongoing communication and adjustments may be necessary to ensure that the prosthesis continues to fit properly and function effectively over time (Ghazali and Ariff 2023; Karasan et al. 2021; Montero 2021; Tribst et al. 2020).

However, in some cases, even with careful consideration and communication, a prosthesis may still fail to meet the patient's needs. For example, if a patient has a rare skin condition that makes it difficult for any material to be worn comfortably, no amount of adjustments or communication may fully resolve the issue. In such cases, alternative solutions or treatments may need to be explored in order to provide the patient with the best possible outcome. This could involve considering a different type of prosthesis, exploring surgical options, or seeking out specialised care from medical professionals who have experience with unique cases like this. It is important for healthcare providers to listen to the patient's concerns and work collaboratively to find a solution that works best for them. Ultimately, the goal is to ensure that the patient is able to live their life comfortably and confidently despite any challenges they may face with their prosthesis (Atallah et al. 2023; Meythaler 2001; Turner et al. 2021).

Techniques Used in Maxillary Sinus Reconstruction

The techniques used include bone grafting, sinus lift surgery, and implant placement. These procedures are often performed in stages to allow for proper healing and integration of the new bone. The prosthetist works closely with the oral surgeon to ensure that the prosthesis is compatible with the reconstruction process and can be securely attached to the newly formed bone. Regular follow-up appointments are essential to monitor the healing process and make any necessary adjustments to the prosthesis. In some cases, additional surgeries or treatments may be required to achieve the desired outcome. It is important for patients to communicate openly with their healthcare team and follow their recommendations to ensure the success of their maxillary sinus reconstruction. Patients undergoing maxillary sinus reconstruction should also be diligent in following postoperative care instructions, such as maintaining good oral hygiene and avoiding certain foods that could potentially disrupt the healing process. It is also important for patients to attend all scheduled follow-up appointments to track progress and address any concerns. By actively participating in their own care and staying informed about their treatment plan, patients can increase the likelihood of a successful outcome and an improved quality of life. It is crucial for patients to trust their healthcare team and feel comfortable asking questions or seeking clarification on any aspect of their treatment. Building a strong rapport with healthcare providers can help patients feel confident in their care and be more likely to adhere to their treatment plan. Patients should not hesitate to speak up about any discomfort or issues they may be experiencing, as early intervention can prevent complications. By taking an active role in their recovery, patients can empower themselves to make informed decisions and optimise their overall health and well-being. Remember, open communication and collaboration between patients and healthcare professionals are essential for achieving the best possible outcomes (Berrone et al. 2021; Dobrzański and Dobrzański 2020; Li and Felländer-Tsai 2021).

However, in some cases, even with a strong rapport with healthcare providers, patients may still feel hesitant to speak up about their discomfort or issues due to fear of being judged or dismissed. This lack of communication can lead to delayed or improper treatment, ultimately compromising the patient's recovery and overall health. It is important for patients to remember that their health is a priority, and they have the right to voice their concerns and ask questions. Healthcare professionals are there to help and support patients in their journey towards better health. By being proactive and assertive in communicating their needs, patients can ensure that they receive the quality care they deserve. Remember, your health is worth speaking up for, so don't be afraid to advocate for yourself in order to receive the best possible care (Farrell et al. 2021; Kayser et al. 2024; Larsen et al. 2022).

Production Methods for Maxillary and Facial Implants

These vary depending on the specific needs of the patient and the expertise of the surgeon. Some common techniques include computer-aided design and manufacturing (CAD/CAM) technology, which allows for precise customisation of the implant to fit the patient's unique anatomy. Other methods may involve 3D printing or traditional handcrafting techniques. The choice of production method will depend on factors such as the complexity of the reconstruction, the patient's overall health, and the surgeon's preferences. Ultimately, the goal is to create a durable and functional implant that will restore the patient's quality of life and improve their overall oral health (Ahmed et al. 2022; Copelli et al. 2024; Tanveer et al. 2021).

This level of customisation and precision in implant production has greatly improved outcomes for patients undergoing oral reconstruction. By utilising advanced technology and techniques, surgeons can ensure a better fit and the long-term success of the implant. Additionally, these advancements have allowed for quicker recovery times and reduced the risk of complications post-surgery. Overall, the field of oral reconstruction continues to evolve and improve, providing patients with better options for restoring their oral health and function (Guzzi and Tibbitt 2019; Kunrath 2020; Mobarak et al. 2023).

One of the key advancements in oral reconstruction is the use of 3D printing technology to create custom implants that perfectly match the patient's unique anatomy. This level of precision ensures a more comfortable fit and reduces the risk of complications. In addition, the use of advanced materials has also improved the durability and longevity of implants, allowing patients to enjoy the benefits of their new smile for years to come. With these advancements, oral reconstruction procedures have become more efficient and effective, ultimately improving the quality of life for patients (Ahmad et al. 2022; Nesic et al. 2020; Tian et al. 2021).

Furthermore, the integration of digital imaging and computer-aided design has revolutionised the planning process for oral reconstruction surgeries. This technology allows for detailed analysis of the patient's oral structure, enabling surgeons to accurately map out the placement of implants before the actual procedure. By utilising these tools, surgeons can ensure optimal positioning and alignment, leading to better functional and aesthetic outcomes for the patient. The combination of 3D printing, advanced materials, and digital technology has truly transformed the field of oral reconstruction, offering patients a higher level of care and satisfaction (Babu et al. 2024; Khan 2022; Nyirjesy et al. 2022).

Effects of Facial Implants on Maxillary Sinus Health

These effects have also been studied extensively, with research indicating that proper placement and design can minimise the risk of sinus complications post-surgery. In addition, advancements in imaging technology have allowed for more precise preoperative planning, reducing the likelihood of implant-related issues. As the field continues to evolve, the focus on patient safety and satisfaction remains paramount, driving further innovation and improvements in oral reconstruction techniques. Overall, the combination of improved implant design, careful placement techniques, and advanced imaging technology has significantly enhanced the success rate of facial implant procedures. This has not only reduced the risk of complications but has also increased patient comfort and confidence in the outcomes of their surgery. As researchers and practitioners continue to collaborate and innovate in the field of oral reconstruction, the future looks promising for further advancements that will benefit both patients and providers. With ongoing advancements in technology and techniques, the field of oral reconstruction is poised for even greater success in the years to come. Patients can look forward to safer and more effective procedures, while providers can offer cutting-edge solutions with confidence. The collaboration between researchers and practitioners will undoubtedly lead to continued progress and improved outcomes, ultimately enhancing the quality of care for those in need of facial implant procedures. As new innovations continue to emerge, the field of oral reconstruction will only continue to evolve, offering more personalised and efficient treatment options for patients. This collaboration between researchers and practitioners will drive further breakthroughs in the field, leading to enhanced patient satisfaction and improved long-term outcomes. With a focus on patient safety and comfort, the future of facial implant procedures is bright, promising a higher standard of care for those seeking oral reconstruction services. By staying at the forefront of technological advancements and constantly refining their techniques, oral reconstruction specialists will be able to provide patients with even better results and quicker recovery times. This dedication to innovation and patient-centred care ensures that individuals in need of facial implant procedures will receive the highest quality treatment possible. In the coming years, we can expect to see continued improvements in both the aesthetic and functional aspects of oral reconstruction, ultimately providing patients with a greater sense of confidence and satisfaction with their appearance (Comuzzi et al. 2023; Lafzi et al. 2021; Lyu et al. 2023; Mahajan et al. 2022; Rengo et al. 2021; Rocha et al. 2023).

Presentation of the Case

A 60-year-old patient with a history of squamous cell carcinoma on the tip of her nose was required to have immediate surgical intervention to remove the tumour and reconstruct the affected area. A total rhinectomy was performed with free surgical and pathological margins. The patient was able to fully recover and resume her normal activities, and she is now seeking reconstructive surgery to restore the appearance of her nose (Fig. 15.1).

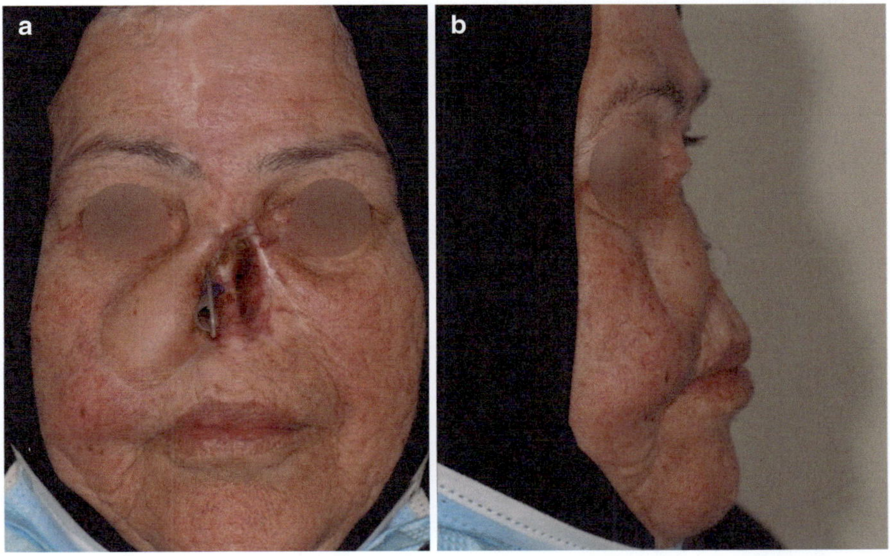

Fig. 15.1 Patient post-nasal resection; frontal (**a**) and lateral (**b**) perspectives

Approach

Following a comprehensive assessment, it was determined that the most suitable course of action for rehabilitation would be to use an implant-supported silicone nasal prosthesis with pre-made PEEK telescoping attachments. A presurgical planning computed tomogram (CT) was performed to evaluate the bone condition, identify any disease, and aid in the design of the subperiosteal implant. The subperiosteal implant was created with Mimics software developed by Materialise NV, located in Leuven, Belgium (Fig. 15.2). The design of the implant head was intended to replicate that of the ROOTT One-Piece Implant from ROOTT Global in Switzerland. The virtual model was carefully constructed to accurately match the patient's distinct nasal bone architecture. The ultimate design was subsequently fabricated using a laser additive metal 3D printing machine (Riton D-150, China) with titanium alloy (Ti Grade V) as the material. The selection of titanium as the material was based on its biocompatibility and strength, which guarantee long-term stability and support (Carretero et al. 2022).

The subperiosteal implant was surgically placed while the patient was under general anaesthesia. Precise cuts were performed to minimise noticeable scarring and ensure sufficient access to the nasal bone. The implant was placed with accuracy, and miniature screws were utilised to firmly fasten it to the underlying bone, guaranteeing stability (Fig. 15.3) (Rinaldi and Mommaerts 2023; Wazir 2023).

Postoperative treatment involved vigilant surveillance for any indications of infection or sequelae. The patient was given a prescription for prophylactic antibiotics and provided with instructions on how to properly care for the wound. Periodic follow-up appointments were arranged to evaluate the progress of healing and verify the durability of the implant (Javed et al. 2023).

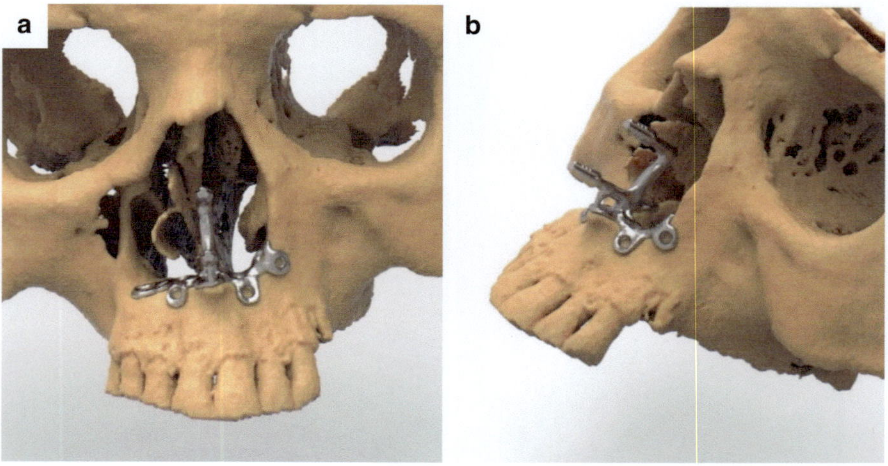

Fig. 15.2 The process of creating a subperiosteal implant. 3D-images are rendered in frontal (**a**) and oblique (**b**) views

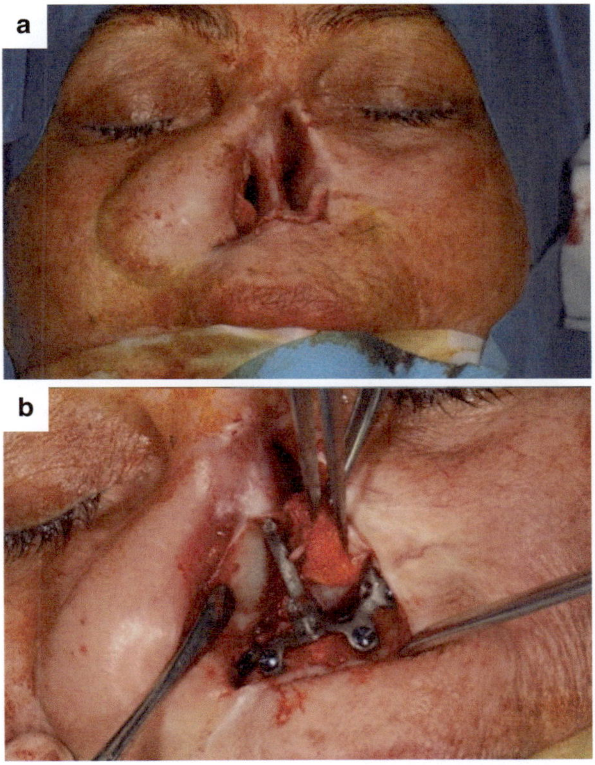

Fig. 15.3 The surgical procedure for positioning the subperiosteal implant. (**a**) shows a preoperative picture and (**b**) shows an intraoperative view of positioning the subperiosteal implant

Once the surgical area had fully healed, the patient underwent a facial scan utilising the Einscan SHINING 3D scanner from China. The prusament filament, produced by the Prusa 3D Printer 3.1 in the Czech Republic, was used to print a unique tray. To prevent the imprint material from sticking, petroleum jelly was put on the patient's eyebrows and eyelashes. To prevent the unwanted flow of material, wet gauze was inserted into the defect. Impression transfers (TRA, ROOTT Global, Switzerland) were then placed on the implant extension to limit movement. Hydrophilic vinyl polysiloxane putty body elastomeric impression material (Vonflex, VERICOM Co., Ltd., South Korea) was applied around the impression transfer to minimise distortion of the tissue bed. An impression of the defect and surrounding tissues was made using a hydrophilic vinyl polysiloxane light body elastomeric impression material (Vonflex, VERICOM Co., Ltd., South Korea) (Fig. 15.4). Following the impression, the root analogues (ROOTT Global-Switzerland) were inserted into the imprint transfers within the impression. Subsequently, the impression was filled with a type IV gypsum product (Kalabhai Karson, Mumbai, India) (Fig. 15.5). The patient's model was scanned using the CEREK Omnicam (Dentsply, Germany), and both STL files were overlaid to

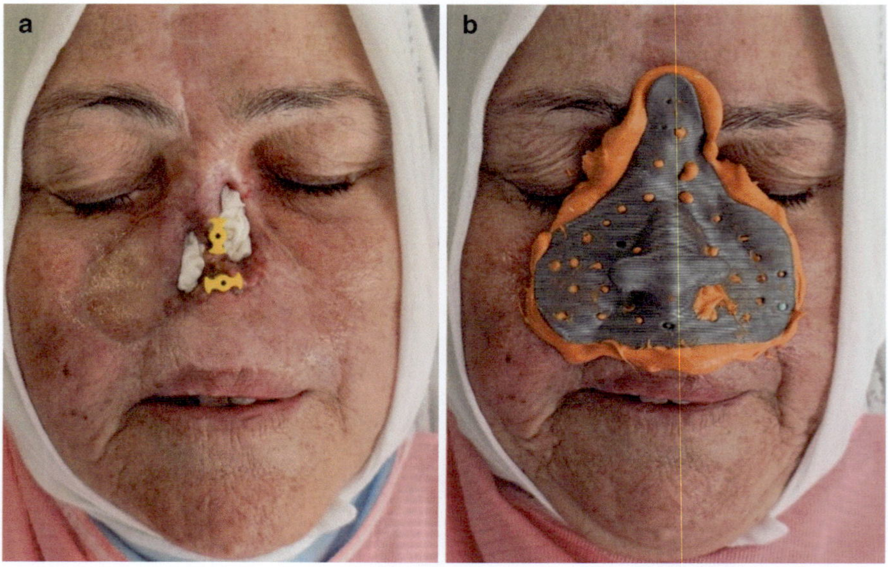

Fig. 15.4 In this figure, 2 pictures are seen, before (**a**) and after (**b**) positioning of the impression transfer

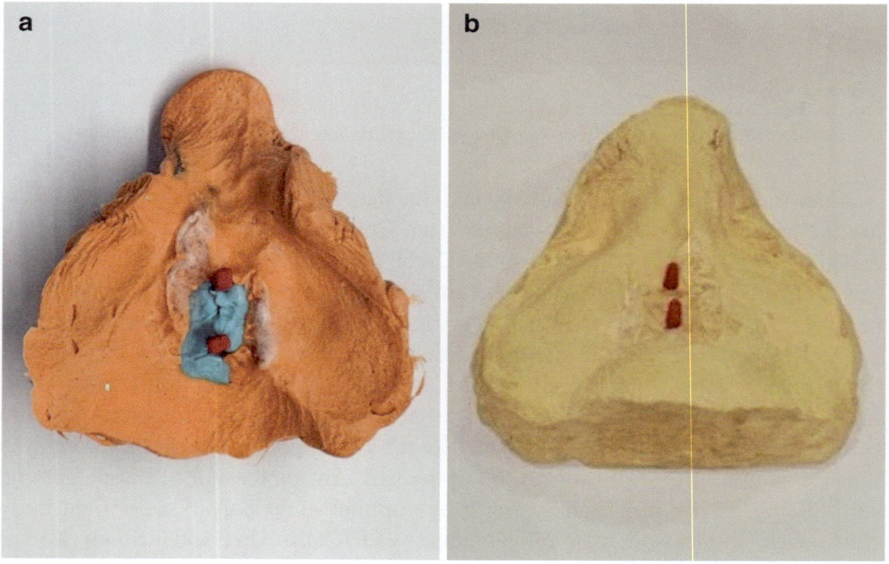

Fig. 15.5 The ultimate representation, featuring analogues (**a**) and the definitive model (**b**)

minimise the possibility of any alterations in dimensions (Albayrak et al. 2020; Al-Ibrahim et al. 2021; Jivănescu et al. 2021; Leven et al. 2022; Nagy et al. 2020; Schmidt et al. 2021).

The nose's virtual design was accomplished using Mimics software, developed by Materialise NV in Leuven, Belgium (Fig. 15.6). Upon receiving confirmation from the patient, the virtual nose was fabricated using Flexible 80A resin (Formlabs, USA) through the utilisation of an SLA 3D printer (Formlabs Form 2, USA) (Farook et al. 2020; Tanveer et al. 2021).

A prefabricated PEEK telescoping cap (PCE1, ROOTT Global-Switzerland) was utilised as a means of attachment for retention. It was then inserted into the acrylic resin to enhance its connection with the silicon material of the prosthesis (Fig. 15.7). Next, the fabricated nose was positioned onto the patient model and fastened using sculpting wax (Factor II, USA) (Fig. 15.8). Next, the pattern was encased with type III gypsum goods from Kalabhai Karson in Mumbai, India. Following the removal and cleaning of the final model, a coat of primer (A-330-G Platinum) was applied to the acrylic resin to improve the adhesion between the acrylic resin and the platinum silicon (Wang 2023).

The A-RTV 3040 medical-grade silicone, manufactured by Factor II in the USA, was mixed and placed in the mould after assessing the patient's skin tone. The process of layer-wise packing was utilised to create a prosthesis with multiple layers that possess inherent colouration. Following the completion of

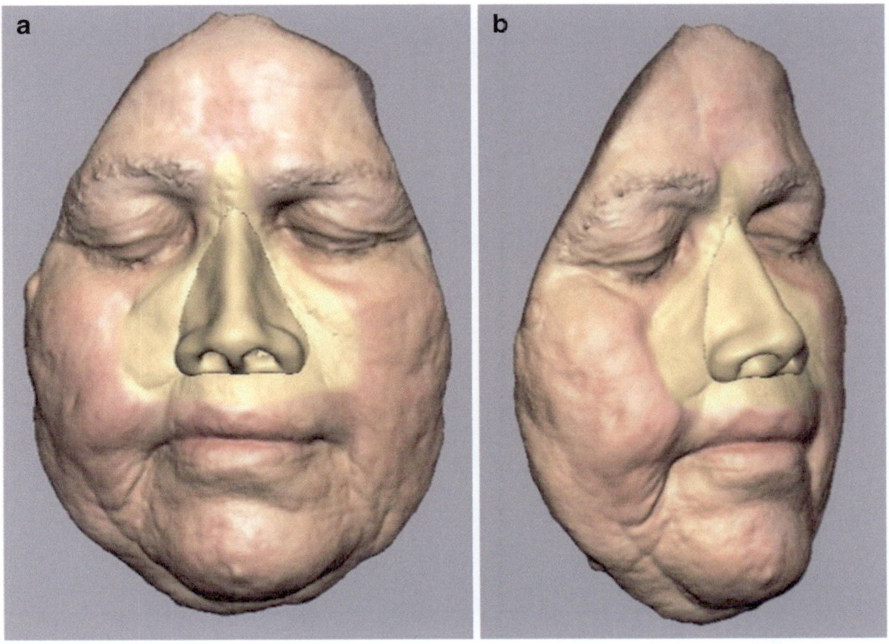

Fig. 15.6 The virtual representation of the nose in frontal (**a**) and oblique (**b**) views

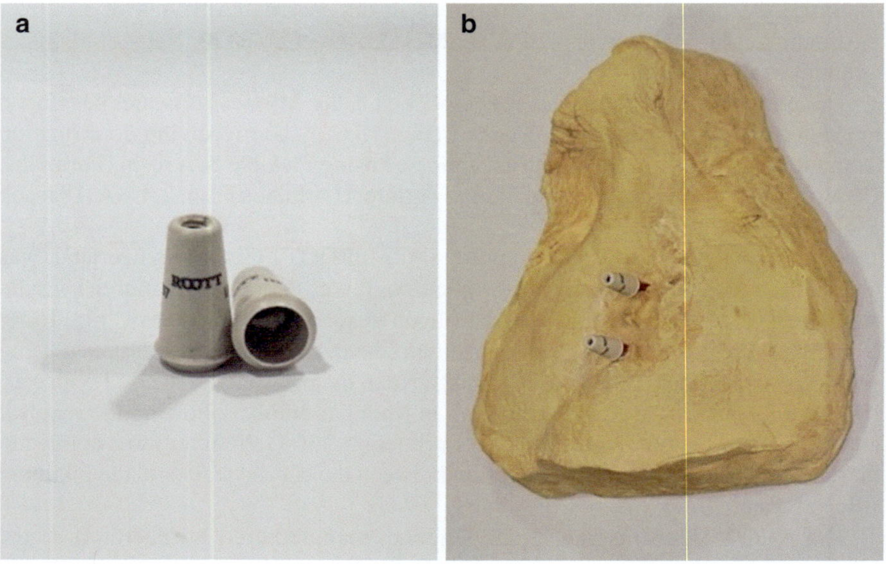

Fig. 15.7 Prefabricated PEEK telescopic attachments (**a**). The image shows the process of inspecting the attachment on the implant extension and inserting the attachment into the acrylic resin (**b**)

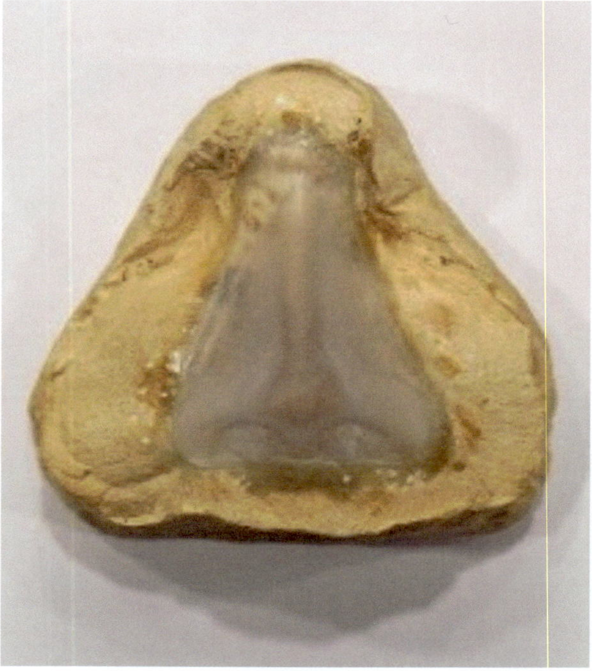

Fig. 15.8 Fastening the nose on the final prototype

packing, the mould was securely fastened under applied pressure at ambient temperature for a duration of 24 h. After the prosthesis was fully cured, it was removed from the flask, meticulously trimmed, and completed using scissors and silicone finishing burs. A small amount of flash was intentionally left on the edges of the nasal prosthesis to help the borders blend smoothly with the surrounding tissue (See Fig. 15.9).

An assessment was conducted on the patient's face to evaluate the prosthesis. The patient's skin tone was further matched using extrinsic colouration, namely the FE-199 Extrinsic Coloration Kit from Factor II, USA. The prosthesis was painted with a silicon dispersion (TS-564, Factor II, USA) according to the manufacturer's instructions for extrinsic colouration. Once the layer of TS-564 was dry to the touch, a very thin additional layer of acetoxy silicon adhesive (A-564, Factor II, USA) was applied. This layer was matted using slightly damp gauze. After dissolving 2 g of A-564 in 10 g of acetoxy matting dispersion (MD-564), the prosthesis was coated with a thin layer of the mixture to eliminate any glossy appearance resulting from the sealing operation.

The finalised nasal prosthesis was given to the patient, who expressed great satisfaction with the outcome of the therapy (Fig. 15.10). The patient received detailed information and demonstrations regarding the proper hygiene practices for the silicone, attachment, and metallic components of the nasal prosthesis. This involved providing the patient with guidance on a regular cleaning regimen. These endeavours would aid in maintaining the soft tissues free from reactions and minimising the likelihood of skin irritation or infection.

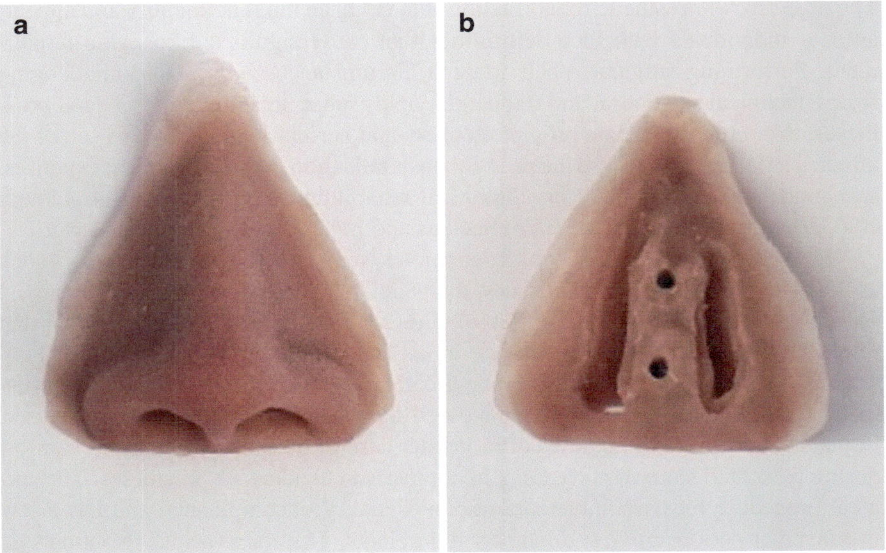

Fig. 15.9 The prosthesis, after being removed from the flask, front (**a**) and back (**b**) views

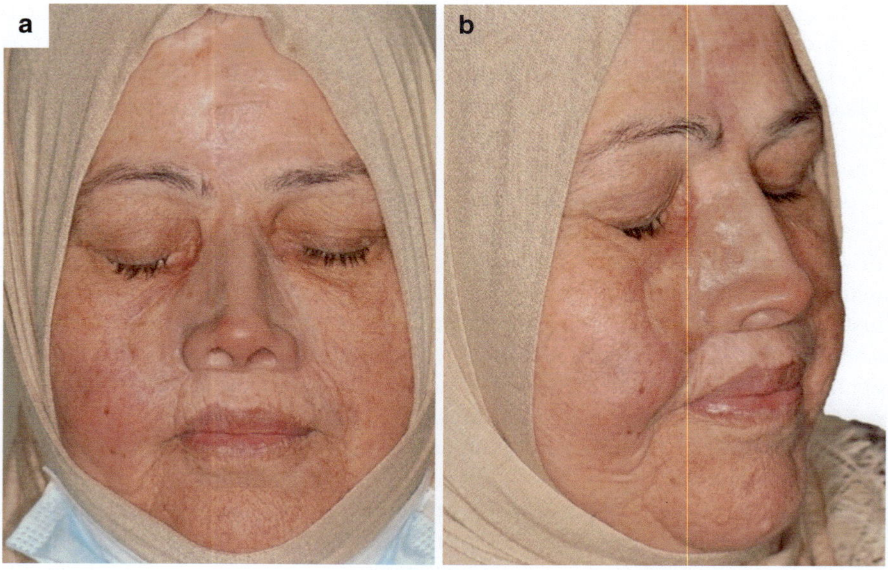

Fig. 15.10 The patient using a nasal prosthesis that is considered to be the final and conclusive version, in frontal (**a**) and oblique (**b**) views

Discussion

The objective of prosthetic rehabilitation is to enhance the functionality and appearance of individuals with face deformities that cause significant cosmetic impairment. Performing surgical repair in such circumstances is typically challenging from a technical standpoint and frequently yields suboptimal outcomes. Facial prostheses, in contrast, facilitate prompt recovery and permit regular examination of the affected area. They minimise the need for hospitalisation, reduce treatment expenses, and contribute to the timely psychological rehabilitation of patients (Barraclough et al. 2022; De Oliveira et al. 2024; Seelaus and Evans 2022).

The surgeon can determine which retention system to utilise based on factors such as the state of the surrounding tissues, the patient's expectations, and their financial status. While adhesive retention technologies continue to advance, it is evident that implant systems offer far superior retention. The range is from 16 to 18. Implant-retained facial prostheses have become a highly effective treatment choice in prosthetic rehabilitation and are often favoured by patients over adhesive prostheses. Implant-retained face prostheses offer greater ease of placement, enhanced comfort during wear, and simplified cleaning in comparison to adhesive prostheses. The surgical procedure for osseointegrated implants is very uncomplicated and has a low incidence of perioperative and long-term problems. There are various retention systems for implant superstructures that are now in use, including bar-clip retention, ball attachment, magnetic retention, locator abutment attachment, and the slant lock system (Fernandes et al. 2022; Rajani et al. 2020; Vazouras and Taylor 2021).

The implementation of extraoral endosseous implants for securing craniofacial prostheses was a significant advancement. The osseointegration system has been an established and authorised method for over 30 years for patients with craniofacial abnormalities. However, the presence of anatomic regions with inadequate bone volume poses a difficult condition for the insertion of a single screw implant. Therefore, the osteosynthesis technique was utilised to introduce plate-like titanium implants, resulting in additional progress in retention strategies. These systems can be equipped with several percutaneous abutments and are securely attached beneath the periosteum using various bone screws to distribute the stresses exerted on the plate. In 1991, Farmand collaborated with Leibinger GmbH to create the Epitec system, which is composed of a titanium grid with threaded holes. P. made other advancements. Federspil, PA. Federspil, and M. In 2000, Schneider and Medicon eG jointly introduced the epiplating technique. The 2.0 titanium miniplate system used in craniofacial trauma has been specifically designed to accommodate it. It is equipped with standardised plates for various anatomical locations, such as the orbital or nasal region.

While typical plate-like implants have proven to be a helpful method for prosthetic retention, it is important to acknowledge certain limitations. Customisation of standardised plates necessitates laborious and difficult intraoperative bending and adjustment to accommodate the unique anatomy of each patient. Repeated remodelling can lead to decreased metal quality, which can cause premature fatigue and failure. Considerable effort must be dedicated to achieving exact trimming as well as meticulously processing and beveling sharp edges. The effectiveness of positioning may be compromised due to the constraints of the plate's dimensions. Plate-like implants should be precisely positioned in the prosthetic device according to its shape without causing any obstruction. In addition, it is important for the prosthesis to have enough retention to prevent unintentional displacement. However, in anatomically challenging areas with incorrect anatomy, it is difficult to properly adjust and position the implant system while considering the aforementioned concerns. Accurately adapting the plates is a laborious operation that is challenging to accomplish manually, yet it is of paramount importance. Improper positioning of the implants can result in compromised production of the prosthesis, unsatisfactory aesthetic and functional results, or even complete failure of the prosthetic rehabilitation (Duong et al. 2022; Roy et al. 2020; Sailser et al. 2022).

The growing domain of computer-assisted technologies facilitates diverse medical applications. Prosthetic facial reconstruction has already made progress in utilising digital technologies, such as using CT scans to plan the placement of craniofacial implants and creating digital models for producing silicone prostheses. The text describes the utilisation of a pre-shaped Epitec system that applies stereolithographic techniques, together with the computer-assisted creation of a copy-milled bar for prosthetic reconstruction. This information may be found in references. However, the existing literature contains little data regarding patient-specific implants produced by computer-assisted design and manufacture for the purpose of retaining craniofacial prostheses. Customised titanium CAD/CAM implants have become a widely accepted method in reconstructive cranioplasty surgery and the treatment of orbital wall abnormalities. Additionally, they have also documented their efforts in repairing midface deformities (Alberga et al. 2022).

Prior to the treatment, patient-specific implants are carefully planned using a three-dimensional model, guaranteeing a predictable result. The virtual design allows for precise determination of the optimal place, size, and shape of the implant. When designing a retention system for prosthetic rehabilitation, it is important to prioritise achieving an optimal anatomical alignment of the implant's abutments. This will enable the subsequent insertion of the prosthesis in the best possible position, leading to enhanced cosmetic appearance and functional outcomes. Additionally, the design of the implant should allow for easy cleaning and maintenance by the patient. The concept of backward planning allows for the virtual evaluation and control of the implant's design by the anaplastology team, as well as its demonstration to the patient before the manufacturing process. The surgical operation is made easier by the implant's form-congruence to the recipient's anatomy, which allows for easy handling. There is no need for any further manual bending or adjustment, which reduces the stress on the tissue surrounding the implant and also shortens the surgical procedure. This leads to decreased surgical stress for the patient, allowing for a quicker recovery with enhanced clinical results. The use of computer-assisted navigation in the surgical process allows for the accurate transition of the implant's preplanned virtual anatomical position to its precise three-dimensional placement. It allows for the simultaneous alignment of the implant's position during surgery with the virtual surgical plan. In this particular example, the accurate positioning was determined due to the distinct three-dimensional alignment. However, it is advisable to use navigation-assisted control of position when there is a lack of conventional anatomic reference points. The drawbacks of prefabricated CAD/CAM-created implants undoubtedly involve challenges in coordinating the planning and design as well as the time and cost of manufacture (Nazar et al. 2021).

Various materials, including precious and non-precious metal alloys, zirconia, and PEEK, were utilised in the production of telescopic crowns. PEEK material was introduced as a key breakthrough in prosthetic and implant dentistry because of its exceptional mechanical and physical properties. PEEK has exhibited commendable flexibility, excellent mechanical wear resistance, and elevated tensile, fatigue, and flexural strengths. The study determined that the telescopic attachment, constructed from PEEK material, exhibits a consistent and reliable retention force of 38 units. Insufficient evidence exists regarding the wear characteristics of CAD-CAM polymer materials, particularly PEEK (Alfenas et al. 2023; Messias et al. 2021).

Final Remarks

Currently, the use of CAD/CAM implants is a feasible approach in medical practice, thanks to the widespread adoption of computer-assisted treatment planning and surgery. Patient-specific implants that are prefabricated via backward planning provide an excellent solution for securely attaching craniofacial prostheses in challenging anatomical conditions. In the future, we suggest using patient-specific implants for prosthetic reconstruction as the preferred treatment choice over traditional plate-like implants in typical instances. However, we deem them necessary in anatomically challenging and intricate cases since they facilitate a more reliable and efficient surgical process, followed by prosthetic rehabilitation in everyday practice (Ahmed et al. 2022; Sgarzani et al. 2022; Tanveer et al. 2021).

Several types of implants, such as screw-shaped, cylindrical, and plate-like titanium implants, have been used to secure facial prostheses. The surgical placement of screw-shaped Osseointegrated implants, usually performed in two stages with a recovery period of 3–4 months, has been extensively described. A one-stage technique has been recently described for the mastoid, although a two-stage approach is still advised for juvenile patients, orbit, midface applications, and irradiated patients. There have also been reports of one-stage procedures in the orbit. Both pre-cut and self-tapping threaded implants have demonstrated efficacy in both one-stage and two-stage procedures. By utilising CT scanning and implant installation simulation, the need for periosteal reflection may be eliminated. The placement of cylinder implants for face prostheses usually involves a two-stage process with a healing period of 3 months. However, it is not advisable to utilise cylindrical implants in the orbit due to the risk of microfracture of the orbital bone. The surgical placement of the plate-like implant system is distinct from that of the screw-shaped or cylindrical systems. Under specific circumstances and at certain anatomical sites, there may be a scarcity of bone for the implantation of screws or cylindrical implants. Typically, osseointegration systems are either screw-shaped or cylindrical, while the plate-like system is secured using mini-screws. The procedure for installing the plate-like system is analogous to the conventional installation of a bone plate. A 4-week healing interval has been employed prior to prosthetic fabrication. The plate-like device has been recommended for application in the mastoid, orbit, and nasal regions (Copelli et al. 2024; Nyirjesy et al. 2022; Tanveer et al. 2021).

Stem Cell Reconstruction

Stem Cell in Maxillary Reconstruction

Stem cell therapy has become a promising method for reconstructing the maxilla, providing prospective solutions to the difficulties presented by conventional bone grafting techniques. This emerging discipline integrates mesenchymal stem cells derived from several origins with sophisticated scaffolds and growth factors to rejuvenate bone structure in the maxillary area. However, in the initial phases of clinical implementation, stem cell-based approaches demonstrate significant potential for treating maxillary deformities caused by trauma, tumour removal, or congenital abnormalities.

Introduction to Stem Cell Therapy

Stem cell therapy has become a promising method in regenerative medicine, providing new opportunities for repairing and regenerating tissues in several medical areas, such as maxillofacial surgery. This novel method utilises the distinct characteristics of stem cells to facilitate the process of healing and rebuilding tissues in complex clinical situations.

Mesenchymal stem cells (MSCs) are a type of progenitor cell with the ability to differentiate into multiple cell types, such as osteoblasts, chondrocytes, and adipocytes (Egido-Moreno et al. 2021). Their capacity for self-renewal and differentiation into osteogenic cells makes them highly desirable for maxillary restoration. MSCs can be obtained from various sources such as bone marrow, adipose tissue, dental pulp, and umbilical cord. Each source has its own benefits and restrictions (Alfayez and Alghamdi 2022).

The utilisation of stem cell treatment in maxillary reconstruction seeks to overcome the constraints associated with conventional bone grafting methods, including complications at the donor site, restricted availability of grafts, and unpredictable rates of resorption (Vaswani et al. 2023). Researchers and physicians aim to enhance bone regeneration in the maxillofacial region by utilising stem cells, scaffolds, and growth factors in a manner that closely mimics the natural physiological processes.

Stem cell-based strategies for maxillary reconstruction typically involve the isolation and expansion of MSCs, their seeding onto biocompatible scaffolds, and the incorporation of growth factors to enhance osteogenic differentiation and bone formation (Nam et al. 2023). This approach has shown promise in various maxillofacial applications, including alveolar ridge augmentation, sinus lift procedures, and the repair of large bony defects resulting from trauma or tumour resection (Mangano 2015).

The promise of stem cell therapy in maxillary reconstruction has been further improved by recent developments in tissue engineering and biomaterial science have greatly raised the possibilities for stem cell treatment in maxillary reconstruction. For example, the development of 3D-printed scaffolds lets one create patient-specific constructions that precisely match the geometry of maxillary abnormalities (Chen et al. 2022). Furthermore, found to improve the osteogenic capacity of transplanted stem cells is the application of growth factors, including platelet-rich plasma (PRP) and bone morphogenetic proteins (BMPs) (Chen et al. 2022).

Although stem cell therapy for maxillary repair has shown encouraging outcomes in preclinical investigations and initial clinical trials, there are still some obstacles that need to be resolved before it can be widely implemented in clinical practice. These tasks involve enhancing cell supplies, refining scaffold designs, guaranteeing long-term safety, and surmounting regulatory obstacles (Ruan et al. 2023). However, the possibility of stem cell therapy to completely transform maxillary repair and enhance patient results remains a strong motivating factor for ongoing research and advancements in this area.

Stem Cell Sources

Various sources of mesenchymal stem cells (MSCs) have been investigated for maxillary reconstruction, each with unique advantages and considerations. The most commonly studied sources include:

1. Bone Marrow-Derived Mesenchymal Stem Cells (BM-MSCs)
   BM-MSCs are commonly utilised because of their demonstrated ability to generate bone tissue. Sauerbier et al. conducted a study that showed effective bone production in maxillary sinus augmentation by utilising BM-MSCs that were placed on β-tricalcium phosphate granules (Egido-Moreno et al. 2021). Nevertheless, the process of extracting bone marrow can be distressing and intrusive, perhaps resulting in complications at the donor site.
2. Adipose-Derived Mesenchymal Stem Cells:
   AD-MSCs have numerous benefits, such as being easily obtainable and plentiful, making them a good alternative to bone marrow stem cells for tissue engineering applications (Gentile et al. 2019).
3. Dental Pulp Stem Cells (DPSCs):
   DPSCs, derived from extracted teeth, have shown significant potential for maxillofacial bone regeneration. DPSCs could differentiate into osteoblasts and form bone tissue when transplanted in vivo (Vaswani et al. 2023). The use of DPSCs is particularly appealing in dentistry due to their neural crest origin and natural role in tooth development.
4. Periodontal Ligament Stem Cells (PDLSCs):
   PDLSCs have shown promise in periodontal regeneration and alveolar bone reconstruction. Successful regeneration of periodontal tissues, including alveolar bone, has been reported using PDLSCs in a porcine mode (Zhao et al. 2022).
5. Human Umbilical Cord-Derived Mesenchymal Stem Cells (hUCMSCs):
   hUCMSCs have gained attention due to their non-invasive collection and high proliferation capacity. The use of hUCMSCs seeded on a PCL-TCP scaffold for maxillary sinus augmentation has demonstrated enhanced bone formation compared to conventional techniques (Zhao et al. 2022).
6. Induced Pluripotent Stem Cells (iPSCs):
   While still in the early stages of research for maxillary reconstruction, iPSCs offer the potential for patient-specific treatments. The osteogenic differentiation of iPSCs and their potential for bone regeneration has been demonstrated in a rat calvarial defect model (Kato et al. 2022).

Each stem cell source has its own advantages and limitations. BM-MSCs and AD-MSCs are currently the most widely studied and clinically applied sources for maxillary reconstruction. However, dental-derived stem cells (DPSCs and PDLSCs) show particular promise due to their natural role in craniofacial development.

The choice of stem cell source may depend on factors such as accessibility, proliferation capacity, and osteogenic potential. For instance, AD-MSCs are easily accessible but may have lower osteogenic potential compared to BM-MSCs (Chen et al. 2022). Conversely, dental-derived stem cells have shown excellent osteogenic capabilities but are limited in quantity (Ruan et al. 2023).

Recent studies have looked into using different types of stem cells together to take advantage of their unique strengths, such as combining AD-MSCs and DPSCs, which has shown improved bone healing in a rat calvarial defect model (Lau et al. 2024).

Additionally, the advancement of cell-free methodologies that employ extracellular vesicles (EVs) derived from stem cells is increasing in popularity. These EVs contain bioactive molecules that can promote tissue regeneration without the necessity of cell transplantation. Bone regeneration in a rodent calvarial defect model has been demonstrated to be improved by EVs derived from BM-MSCs (Zhang et al. 2020).

As research in this field progresses, optimising the selection and application of stem cell sources will be crucial for improving the outcomes of maxillary reconstruction procedures. Future studies should focus on comparative analyses of different stem cell sources in standardised maxillary defect models to determine the most effective approaches for specific clinical scenarios.

Scaffolds and Growth Factors

Scaffolds and growth factors play crucial roles in stem cell-based maxillary reconstruction, providing structural support and biochemical cues to guide tissue regeneration. The selection of appropriate scaffolds and growth factors is essential for optimising the osteogenic potential of mesenchymal stem cells (MSCs) and achieving successful bone formation in the maxillary region.

Scaffolds serve as temporary extracellular matrices that support cell attachment, proliferation, and differentiation. Various biomaterials have been investigated for maxillary reconstruction, including:

1. Beta-tricalcium phosphate (β-TCP): This biocompatible and resorbable ceramic material has shown promising results in maxillary sinus augmentation procedures. A study by Sauerbier et al. demonstrated successful bone formation using β-TCP granules seeded with bone marrow-derived MSC (Egido-Moreno et al. 2021).
2. Poly(ε-caprolactone) (PCL): Polycaprolactone (PCL) is a biodegradable polymer that can be 3D-printed to create patient-specific scaffolds, which have been used successfully in maxillary reconstruction and bone regeneration, showing promising results in terms of volume conformity and bone density (Jeong et al. 2022).
3. Hydroxyapatite (HA): HA is a naturally occurring mineral component of bone that provides excellent osteoconductive properties. A study by Koppe et al. utilised HA scaffolds in combination with adipose-derived stem cells for maxillary sinus floor elevation (Shi et al. 2022).
4. Chitosan: This natural polymer derived from chitin has shown potential in bone tissue engineering due to its biocompatibility and antibacterial properties. A novel chitosan composite biomaterial with drug-eluting capacity has been developed for maxillary bone regeneration (Giordano-Kelhoffer et al. 2023).

Growth factors are essential signalling molecules that regulate cell behaviour and promote tissue regeneration. Several growth factors have been investigated for enhancing the osteogenic potential of MSCs in maxillary reconstruction:

1. Bone Morphogenetic Proteins (BMPs): BMPs, particularly BMP-2 and BMP-7, are potent osteoinductive factors. A study by Herford et al. demonstrated successful maxillary reconstruction using BMP-2 in combination with a collagen sponge carrier (Chenard et al. 2012).
2. Platelet-Rich Plasma (PRP): PRP contains various growth factors, including platelet-derived growth factor (PDGF) and transforming growth factor-beta (TGF-β). Marx et al. reported enhanced bone formation in maxillary sinus grafts using PRP in combination with autogenous bone (Rodriguez et al. 2014).
3. Vascular Endothelial Growth Factor (VEGF): VEGF promotes angiogenesis, which is crucial for successful bone regeneration. A study by Schliephake et al. showed improved bone formation in mandibular defects using VEGF-loaded scaffolds (Li et al. 2016).
4. Fibroblast Growth Factor-2 (FGF-2): FGF-2 stimulates osteoblast proliferation and differentiation. Kawaguchi et al. demonstrated enhanced bone regeneration in periodontal defects using FGF-2 (Nath and Raveendran 2014).

Combining the right scaffolds and growth factors can greatly improve the success of stem cell-based maxillary reconstruction. For instance, a study used a PCL-TCP scaffold with BMP-2 and human umbilical cord-derived MSCs for maxillary sinus augmentation, leading to better bone formation compared to traditional methods (Tollemar et al. 2016).

Furthermore, advanced scaffold fabrication techniques, such as 3D printing, allow for the creation of patient-specific constructs that can accurately match the geometry of maxillary defects. Park et al. demonstrated the feasibility of using 3D-printed PCL scaffolds loaded with BMP-2 for maxillary reconstruction in a canine model (Jeong et al. 2022).

Although there have been positive outcomes, there are still obstacles to overcome in order to improve the characteristics of the scaffold and the administration of growth factors for maxillary reconstruction. Future investigations should prioritise the development of smart scaffolds capable of delivering growth factors in a controlled manner, imitating the natural bone healing process. Additionally, investigating the synergistic effects of multiple growth factors and exploring novel biomaterials with improved mechanical and biological properties will be crucial for advancing stem cell-based maxillary reconstruction techniques.

Clinical Applications and Challenges

Stem cell therapy for maxillary reconstruction has shown promising results in both preclinical and early clinical studies. Several clinical applications have been explored, demonstrating the potential of this approach in addressing various maxillary defects.

One important use of stem cells is in maxillary sinus augmentation, where studies have shown that using bone marrow-derived mesenchymal stem cells (BM-MSCs) with different materials can significantly improve bone regeneration and implant success rates (Parnia et al. 2018).

Another important application is the reconstruction of alveolar cleft defects. Bajestan et al. reported a case of cleft alveolus reconstruction using a three-dimensional printed bioresorbable scaffold seeded with bone marrow cells. Six months post-transplantation, the newly regenerated bone volume was approximately 45% of the total defect volume, demonstrating the feasibility of this approach (Ahn et al. 2018).

Stem cell therapy has also been investigated for the treatment of medication-related osteonecrosis of the jaw (MRONJ). A clinical trial by Kaibuchi et al. used autologous BM-MSCs combined with platelet-rich plasma for MRONJ treatment, resulting in complete mucosal healing and significant improvement in bone regeneration in 7 out of 8 patients (Nifosì et al. 2021).

Despite these promising results, several challenges remain in the clinical application of stem cell therapy for maxillary reconstruction:

Standardisation remains a critical issue, as there is no consensus on protocols for stem cell isolation, expansion, and differentiation, leading to inconsistent outcomes across studies (Alfayez and Alghamdi 2022). Long-term safety data is limited, necessitating further research into potential adverse effects (Parnia et al. 2018). Regulatory hurdles complicate the clinical translation of stem cell-based therapies, and the high costs associated with these procedures may hinder widespread adoption (Bahari et al. 2023). Ensuring adequate vascularisation of large tissue-engineered constructs is particularly challenging for extensive maxillary defects (Nifosì et al. 2021). Additionally, while mesenchymal stem cells (MSCs) are generally considered immune privileged, the risk of immune rejection in allogeneic transplantation requires further investigation (Yoshida et al. 2020). Scaffold optimisation to balance mechanical properties with stem cell differentiation and tissue integration is an ongoing research focus (Nifosì et al. 2021).

Addressing these challenges will be crucial for advancing stem cell therapy in maxillary reconstruction from promising experimental approaches to widely adopted clinical treatments. Future research should focus on optimising cell sources, improving scaffold designs, and developing standardised protocols to enhance the efficacy and reproducibility of stem cell-based maxillary reconstruction techniques (Alfayez and Alghamdi 2022).

References

Abdelwahab M, Patel PN (2021) Conventional resection versus preservation of the nasal dorsum and ligaments. Facial Plast Surg Clin North Am 29:15–28. https://doi.org/10.1016/j.fsc.2020.08.005

Ahmad S, Hasan N, Fauziya N et al (2022) Review on 3D printing in dentistry: conventional to personalized dental care. J Biomater Sci Polym Ed 33:2292–2323. https://doi.org/10.1080/09205063.2022.2099666

Ahmed KS, Ibad H, Suchal ZA, Gosain AK (2022) Implementation of 3D printing and computer-aided design and manufacturing (CAD/CAM) in craniofacial reconstruction. J Craniofac Surg 33:1714–1719. https://doi.org/10.1097/scs.0000000000008561

Ahn G, Lee J-S, Yun W-S et al (2018) Cleft alveolus reconstruction using a three dimensional printed bioresorbable scaffold with human bone marrow cells. J Craniofac Surg 29:1880–1883. https://doi.org/10.1097/scs.0000000000004747

Akama MK (2005) Current pattern of road traffic accidents, maxillofacial and associated injuries in Nairobi. http://erepository.uonbi.ac.ke/handle/11295/24669

Albayrak B, Sukotjo C, Wee AG et al (2020) Three-dimensional accuracy of conventional versus digital complete arch implant impressions. J Prosthodont 30:163–170. https://doi.org/10.1111/jopr.13264

Alberga J, Eggels I, Visser A et al (2022) Outcome of implants placed to retain craniofacial prostheses—a retrospective cohort study with a follow-up of up to 30 years. Clin Implant Dent Relat Res 24:643–654. https://doi.org/10.1111/cid.13106

Alfayez E, Alghamdi F (2022) Clinical application of stem cell therapy in reconstructing maxillary cleft alveolar bone defects: a systematic review of randomized clinical trials. Curēus 14:e23111. https://doi.org/10.7759/cureus.23111

Alfenas E, Silva I, Oliveira D et al (2023) Intraoral and facial rehabilitation retained with zygomatic implants and magnets after complete resection of the maxilla, lip and nose: a clinical report. J Clin Exp Dent 15:e695–e699. https://doi.org/10.4317/jced.60659

Al-Ibrahim IK, Keeling AJ, Osnes C (2021) The effect of operator scanning speed on the trueness and precision of full-arch digital impressions captured in vitro using an intraoral scanner. www.journalofosseointegration.eu. https://doi.org/10.23805/JO.2021.13.S04.2

Aman HM, Alenezi A, Ducic Y, Reddy LV (2020) Secondary reconstruction of the zygomaticomaxillary complex. Semin Plast Surg 34:254–259. https://doi.org/10.1055/s-0040-1721761

Atallah H, Qureshi AZ, Msechu Z (2023) Satisfaction of individuals with partial-hand amputations after they were fitted with cosmetic silicone prostheses. Prosthetics Orthot Int 47:288–292. https://doi.org/10.1097/pxr.0000000000000196

Babu NN, Sameer NS, Sharma NS et al (2024) The impact of digital imaging and computer-assisted surgery in oral surgery: a narrative review. World J Adva Res Rev 21:2591–2598. https://doi.org/10.30574/wjarr.2024.21.3.0996

Bächli H, Leiggener C, Gawelin P et al (2009) Skull base and maxillofacial fractures: two centre study with correlation of clinical findings with a comprehensive craniofacial classification system. J Craniomaxillofac Surg 37:305–311. https://doi.org/10.1016/j.jcms.2009.01.008

Bahari M, Mokhtari H, Yeganeh F (2023) Stem cell therapy, the market, the opportunities and the threat. Int J Mol Cell Med 12:310–319. https://doi.org/10.22088/ijmcm.bums.12.3.310

Barraclough O, Patel J, Milne S et al (2022) Pathways for the rehabilitation of resection defects in the maxilla. Br Dent J 232:783–789. https://doi.org/10.1038/s41415-022-4342-3

Berrone M, Lajolo C, De Corso E et al (2021) Cooperation between ENT surgeon and dentist in head and neck oncology. Acta Otorhinolaryngol Ital 41:S124–S137. https://doi.org/10.14639/0392-100x-suppl.1-41-2021-13

Bhatia SK, Jagtap SS, Bedekar AA et al (2020) Recent developments in pretreatment technologies on lignocellulosic biomass: effect of key parameters, technological improvements, and challenges. Bioresour Technol 300:122724. https://doi.org/10.1016/j.biortech.2019.122724

Butt OM, Zulqarnain M, Butt TM (2021) Recent advancement in smart grid technology: future prospects in the electrical power network. Ain Shams Eng J 12:687–695. https://doi.org/10.1016/j.asej.2020.05.004

Carretero JLC, Del Castillo Pardo De Vera JL, García NM et al (2022) Virtual surgical planning and customized subperiosteal titanium maxillary implant (CSTMI) for three dimensional reconstruction and dental implants of maxillary defects after oncological resection: case series. J Clin Med 11:4594. https://doi.org/10.3390/jcm11154594

Chen R, Hao Z, Wang Y et al (2022) Mesenchymal stem cell–immune cell interaction and related modulations for bone tissue engineering. Stem Cells Int 2022:1–19. https://doi.org/10.1155/2022/7153584

Chenard KE, Teven CM, He T-C, Reid RR (2012) Bone morphogenetic proteins in craniofacial surgery: current techniques, clinical experiences, and the future of personalized stem cell therapy. J Biomed Biotechnol 2012:1–14. https://doi.org/10.1155/2012/601549

Comuzzi L, Tumedei M, Petrini M et al (2023) Clinical and radiological evaluation of a self-condensing bone implant in one-stage sinus augmentation: a 3-year follow-up retrospective study. Int J Environ Res Public Health 20:2583. https://doi.org/10.3390/ijerph20032583

Copelli C, Cacciatore F, Cocis S et al (2024) Bone reconstruction using CAD/CAM technology in head and neck surgical oncology. A narrative review of state of the art and aesthetic-functional outcomes. Acta Otorhinolaryngol Ital 44:S58–S66. https://doi.org/10.14639/0392-100x-suppl.1-44-2024-n2819

Cote MT, Segelnick SL, Rastogi A, Schoor R (2011) New York state ear, nose, and throat specialists' views on pre–sinus lift referral. J Periodontol 82:227–233. https://doi.org/10.1902/jop.2010.100344

Cristache CM, Totu EE (2020) 3D printing-processed polymers for dental applications. Springer, Cham, pp 141–164

De Oliveira Costa L, Soares SGM, Barreto BN et al (2024) Recommendations for post-rehabilitation care of maxillofacial prostheses. Braz J Oral Sci 23. https://doi.org/10.20396/bjos.v23i00.8669184

Díaz-Olivares LA, Brinkmann JC-B, Martínez-Rodríguez N et al (2021) Management of Schneiderian membrane perforations during maxillary sinus floor augmentation with lateral approach in relation to subsequent implant survival rates: a systematic review and meta-analysis. Int J Implant Dent 7:91. https://doi.org/10.1186/s40729-021-00346-7

Dobrzański LA, Dobrzański LB (2020) Dentistry 4.0 concept in the design and manufacturing of prosthetic dental restorations. Processes 8:525. https://doi.org/10.3390/pr8050525

Duong H, Roccuzzo A, Stähli A et al (2022) Oral health-related quality of life of patients rehabilitated with fixed and removable implant-supported dental prostheses. Periodontology 2000 88:201–237. https://doi.org/10.1111/prd.12419

Egido-Moreno S, Valls-Roca-Umbert J, Céspedes-Sánchez JM et al (2021) Clinical efficacy of mesenchymal stem cells in bone regeneration in oral implantology. Systematic review and meta-analysis. Int J Environ Res Public Health 18:894. https://doi.org/10.3390/ijerph18030894

Farook TH, Jamayet NB, Abdullah JY et al (2020) Designing 3D prosthetic templates for maxillofacial defect rehabilitation: a comparative analysis of different virtual workflows. Comput Biol Med 118:103646. https://doi.org/10.1016/j.compbiomed.2020.103646

Farrell SE, Bochatay N, Kim S (2021) Embracing or relinquishing sources of power in interprofessional communication: implications for patient-centered speaking up. J Interprof Care:1–8. https://doi.org/10.1080/13561820.2021.1975665

Fernandes AM, Dias PAC, Hoshino IAE, Anchieta RB (2022) Total rehabilitation with implant-supported and implant-retained prostheses in atrophic maxillae: aesthetic and functional resolution for totally edentulous patients. Res Soc Dev 11:e110111637232. https://doi.org/10.33448/rsd-v11i16.37232

Forrest CR, Antonyshyn OM (1998) Acute management of complex midface fractures. Oper Tech Plast Reconstr Surg 5:188–200. https://doi.org/10.1016/s1071-0949(98)80012-7

Generalova AN, Vikhrov AA, Prostyakova AI et al (2024) Polymers in 3D printing of external maxillofacial prostheses and in their retention systems. Int J Pharm 657:124181. https://doi.org/10.1016/j.ijpharm.2024.124181

Gentile P, Calabrese C, De Angelis B et al (2019) Impact of the different preparation methods to obtain human adipose-derived stromal vascular fraction cells (AD-SVFs) and human adipose-derived mesenchymal stem cells (AD-MSCs): enzymatic digestion versus mechanical centrifugation. Int J Mol Sci 20:5471. https://doi.org/10.3390/ijms20215471

Ghazali N, Ariff TFTM (2023) Fundamental properties and biocompatibility classification of extraoral prosthesis: a review. J Med Dev Technol 2:19–30. https://doi.org/10.11113/jmeditec.v1n1.27

Giordano-Kelhoffer B, Rodríguez-Gonzalez R, Perpiñan-Blasco M et al (2023) A novel chitosan composite biomaterial with drug eluting capacity for maxillary bone regeneration. Materials 16:685. https://doi.org/10.3390/ma16020685

Göçmen G, Özkan Y (2017) Maxillary sinus augmentation for dental implants. InTech eBooks, London

Guzzi EA, Tibbitt MW (2019) Additive manufacturing of precision biomaterials. Adv Mater 32. https://doi.org/10.1002/adma.201901994

Haleem A, Javaid M, Singh RP, Suman R (2022) Medical 4.0 technologies for healthcare: features, capabilities, and applications. Internet Things Cyber Phys Syst 2:12–30. https://doi.org/10.1016/j.iotcps.2022.04.001

Herath HMWAI, Jinendra BMS (2024) Advancing efficiency and consistency in agarwood inoculum production through agarwood-induce inoculum mixing machine. J Agrotechnol Rural Sci 3:1–9. https://doi.org/10.4038/atrsj.v3i2.50

Izzetti R, Nisi M, Aringhieri G et al (2021) Basic knowledge and new advances in panoramic radiography imaging techniques: a narrative review on what dentists and radiologists should know. Appl Sci 11:7858. https://doi.org/10.3390/app11177858

Javed H, Olanrewaju OA, Owusu FA et al (2023) Challenges and solutions in postoperative complications: a narrative review in general surgery. Curēus. 15:e50942. https://doi.org/10.7759/cureus.50942

Jeong W-S, Kim Y-C, Min J-C et al (2022) Clinical application of 3D-printed patient-specific polycaprolactone/beta tricalcium phosphate scaffold for complex zygomatico-maxillary defects. Polymers 14:740. https://doi.org/10.3390/polym14040740

Jiang L, Wu M, Li H et al (2022) Risk factors for maxillary sinus pathology after surgery for midfacial fracture: a multivariate analysis. J Clin Med 11:6299. https://doi.org/10.3390/jcm11216299

Jivănescu A, Bara A, Faur A-B, Rotar RN (2021) Is there a significant difference in accuracy of four intraoral scanners for short-span fixed dental prosthesis? A comparative in vitro study. Appl Sci 11:8280. https://doi.org/10.3390/app11188280

Kalaj M, Cohen SM (2020) Postsynthetic modification: an enabling technology for the advancement of metal–organic frameworks. ACS Cent Sci 6:1046–1057. https://doi.org/10.1021/acscentsci.0c00690

Kämmerer PW, Al-Nawas B (2023) Bone reconstruction of extensive maxillomandibular defects in adults. Periodontology 2000 93:340–357. https://doi.org/10.1111/prd.12499

Karasan D, Fehmer V, Ligoutsikou M et al (2021) The influence of patient-related factors and material selection on the clinical outcomes of fixed and removable complete implant prostheses: an overview on systematic reviews. Int J Prosthodont 34:s46–s62. https://doi.org/10.11607/ijp.7070

Kato H, Watanabe K, Saito A et al (2022) Bone regeneration of induced pluripotent stem cells derived from peripheral blood cells in collagen sponge scaffolds. J Appl Oral Sci 30:e20210491. https://doi.org/10.1590/1678-7757-2021-0491

Katranji A, Fotek P, Wang H-L (2008) Sinus augmentation complications: etiology and treatment. Implant Dent 17:339–349. https://doi.org/10.1097/id.0b013e3181815660

Kayser JD, Ersbøll AK, Kolbe M et al (2024) Medical students' speak up barriers: a randomized controlled trial with written vignettes. J Patient Saf 20:323. https://doi.org/10.1097/pts.0000000000001227

Khan MK (2022) Modern digital pediatric dentistry with the advent of intraoral sensors, computer-aided design/computer-aided manufacturing, and three-dimensional printing technologies: a comprehensive review. J Dent Res Rev 9:195. https://doi.org/10.4103/jdrr.jdrr_83_22

Khashaba MM, Shaheen HA, Ibrahim WH, AlDainy DG (2021) Accuracy of patient-specific temporal implants using PEKK. J Craniofac Surg 49:943–949. https://doi.org/10.1016/j.jcms.2021.05.001

Kunrath MF (2020) Customized dental implants: manufacturing processes, topography, osseointegration and future perspectives of 3D fabricated implants. Bioprinting 20:e00107. https://doi.org/10.1016/j.bprint.2020.e00107

Lafzi A, Atarbashi-Moghadam F, Amid R, Sijanivandi S (2021) Different techniques in transalveolar maxillary sinus elevation: a literature review. J Adv Periodontol Implant Dent 13:35–42. https://doi.org/10.34172/japid.2021.004

Lanzer P (2015) PanVascular medicine. Springer, Cham

Larsen M, Mishra R, Miller M, Dean D (2015) Craniofacial and dental tissue. Elsevier, Amsterdam, pp 191–213

Larsen BH, Lundeby T, Gerwing J et al (2022) "Eh—what type of cells are these—flourishing in the liver?" Cancer patients' disclosure of existential concerns in routine hospital consultations. Patient Educ Couns 105:2019–2026. https://doi.org/10.1016/j.pec.2021.11.010
Lau CS, Park SY, Ethiraj LP et al (2024) Role of adipose-derived mesenchymal stem cells in bone regeneration. Int J Mol Sci 25:6805. https://doi.org/10.3390/ijms25126805
Leven R, Schmidt A, Binder R et al (2022) Accuracy of digital impression taking with intraoral scanners and fabrication of CAD/CAM posts and cores in a fully digital workflow. Materials 15:4199. https://doi.org/10.3390/ma15124199
Li Y, Felländer-Tsai L (2021) The bone anchored prostheses for amputees—historical development, current status, and future aspects. Biomaterials 273:120836. https://doi.org/10.1016/j.biomaterials.2021.120836
Li B, Wang H, Qiu G et al (2016) Synergistic effects of vascular endothelial growth factor on bone morphogenetic proteins induced bone formation in vivo: influencing factors and future research directions. Biomed Res Int 2016:1–11. https://doi.org/10.1155/2016/2869572
Liu Y, Wang Y, He X et al (2020) An exploration of multidisciplinary team care with digital technology for complicated cranio-maxillofacial bone defects and fractures. J Craniofac Surg 31:1914–1919. https://doi.org/10.1097/scs.0000000000006674
Lundgren S, Andersson S, Gualini F, Sennerby L (2004) Bone reformation with sinus membrane elevation: a new surgical technique for maxillary sinus floor augmentation. Clin Implant Dent Relat Res 6:165–173. https://doi.org/10.1111/j.1708-8208.2004.tb00217.x
Lundgren S, Cricchio G, Hallman M et al (2016) Sinus floor elevation procedures to enable implant placement and integration: techniques, biological aspects and clinical outcomes. Periodontology 2000 73:103–120. https://doi.org/10.1111/prd.12165
Lyu M, Xu D, Zhang X, Yuan Q (2023) Maxillary sinus floor augmentation: a review of current evidence on anatomical factors and a decision tree. Int J Oral Sci 15:41. https://doi.org/10.1038/s41368-023-00248-x
Mahajan K, Das M, Kumar GA (2022) Post surgical immediate prosthetic reconstruction in patients with rhinocerebral mucormycosis: case series. J Family Med Prim Care 11:379. https://doi.org/10.4103/jfmpc.jfmpc_1192_21
Mangano FG (2015) Mesenchymal stem cells in maxillary sinus augmentation: a systematic review with meta-analysis. World J Stem Cells 7:976. https://doi.org/10.4252/wjsc.v7.i6.976
Messias A, Nicolau P, Guerra F (2021) Different interventions for rehabilitation of the edentulous maxilla with implant-supported prostheses: an overview of systematic reviews. Int J Prosthodont 34:s63–s84. https://doi.org/10.11607/ijp.7162
Meythaler J (2001) Physical medicine and rehabilitation clinics of North America: preface. 12
Mobarak MH, Islam MA, Hossain N et al (2023) Recent advances of additive manufacturing in implant fabrication—a review. Appl Surf Sci Adv 18:100462. https://doi.org/10.1016/j.apsadv.2023.100462
Montero J (2021) A review of the major prosthetic factors influencing the prognosis of implant prosthodontics. J Clin Med 10:816. https://doi.org/10.3390/jcm10040816
Nagy Z, Simon B, Mennito A et al (2020) Comparing the trueness of seven intraoral scanners and a physical impression on dentate human maxilla by a novel method. BMC Oral Health 20:97. https://doi.org/10.1186/s12903-020-01090-x
Nam J-H, Almansoori AA, Kwon O-J et al (2023) Sinus augmentation with poly(ε)caprolactone-β tricalcium phosphate scaffolds, mesenchymal stem cells and platelet rich plasma for one-stage dental implantation in minipigs. J Periodont Implant Sci 53:218. https://doi.org/10.5051/jpis.2300660033
Nath Sameera G, Raveendran R (2014) An insight into the possibilities of fibroblast growth factor in periodontal regeneration. J Indian Soc Periodontol 18:289. https://doi.org/10.4103/0972-124x.134560
Nazar SA, Nair VV, Harsha Kumar K, Ravichandran R (2021) Retention in maxillofacial prosthetics: a review. Int J Appl Dent Sci 7:568–573. https://doi.org/10.22271/oral.2021.v7.i2i.1265

Nesic D, Schaefer BM, Sun Y et al (2020) 3D printing approach in dentistry: the future for personalized oral soft tissue regeneration. J Clin Med 9:2238. https://doi.org/10.3390/jcm9072238
Nifosì G, Nifosì L, Nifosì AF (2021) Mesenchymal stem cells in the treatment of osteonecrosis of the jaw. J Korean Assoc Oral Maxillofac Surg 47:65–75. https://doi.org/10.5125/jkaoms.2021.47.2.65
Nyirjesy SC, Heller M, Von Windheim N et al (2022) The role of computer aided design/computer assisted manufacturing (CAD/CAM) and 3- dimensional printing in head and neck oncologic surgery: a review and future directions. Oral Oncol 132:105976. https://doi.org/10.1016/j.oraloncology.2022.105976
Parnia F, Yazdani J, Dizaj SM (2018) Applications of mesenchymal stem cells in sinus lift augmentation as a dental implant technology. Stem Cells Int 2018:1–7. https://doi.org/10.1155/2018/3080139
Petrides GA, Hicks G, Dunn M et al (2021) Dentoalveolar outcomes in maxillary reconstruction: a retrospective review of 85 maxillectomy reconstructions. ANZ J Surg 91:1472–1479. https://doi.org/10.1111/ans.17001
Pommer B, Unger E, Sütö D et al (2009) Mechanical properties of the Schneiderian membrane in vitro. Clin Oral Implants Res 20:633–637. https://doi.org/10.1111/j.1600-0501.2008.01686.x
Rahpeyma A, Khajehahmadi S (2015) Open sinus lift surgery and the importance of preoperative cone-beam computed tomography scan: a review. PubMed Central (PMC). https://www.ncbi.nlm.nih.gov/pmc/articles/PMC4589707/
Rajani A, Mistry G, Sardar C, Kini A (2020) Rekindle maxillofacial prosthesis with extra oral implants as retention system. Int J Appl Dent Sci 6(3):1–6. http://www.oraljournal.com/archives/2020/6/3/A/6-2-100
Rengo C, Fiorino A, Cucchi A et al (2021) Patient-reported outcomes and complication rates after lateral maxillary sinus floor elevation: a prospective study. Clin Oral Investig 25:4431–4444. https://doi.org/10.1007/s00784-020-03755-x
Rinaldi M, Mommaerts MY (2023) Additively manufactured subperiosteal jaw implant (AMSJI). Springer, Cham, pp 277–315
Rocha RS, Vianna CP, Trojan LC et al (2023) Comparison of sinusitis rate after sinus lift procedure and zygomatic implant surgery: a meta-analysis. Oral Maxillofac Surg 28:63–77. https://doi.org/10.1007/s10006-023-01159-1
Rodriguez IA, Kalaf EA, Bowlin GL, Sell SA (2014) Platelet-rich plasma in bone regeneration: engineering the delivery for improved clinical efficacy. Biomed Res Int 2014:1–15. https://doi.org/10.1155/2014/392398
Rogers SN, Adatia A, Hackett S et al (2022) Changing trends in the microvascular reconstruction and oral rehabilitation following maxillary cancer. Eur Arch Otorrinolaringol 279:4113–4126. https://doi.org/10.1007/s00405-022-07277-y
Rothrock JC (2022) Alexander's care of the patient in surgery. Elsevier
Roy S, Maji S, Paul R et al (2020) A comparison of cost and cost-effectiveness analysis of two- implant-retained overdentures versus other removable prosthodontic treatment options for edentulous mandible: a systematic review. J Indian Prosthodont Soc 20:162. https://doi.org/10.4103/jips.jips_393_19
Ruan C, Zhu Y, Xiong J (2023) Stem cell therapy in oral medicine: status and clinical application prospects. J Med Health Sci 5(3):1–10. https://www.stemmpress.com/jmhs/jmhs20234/531.html
Sailser I, Karasan D, Todorovic A et al (2022) Prosthetic failures in dental implant therapy. Periodontology 2000 88:130–144. https://doi.org/10.1111/prd.12416
Schmidt A, Benedickt C, Schlenz M et al (2021) Accuracy of four different intraoral scanners according to different preparation geometries. Int J Prosthodont 34:756–762. https://doi.org/10.11607/ijp.6233
Schwarz F, Schär A, Nelson K et al (2021) Recommendations for implant-supported full-arch rehabilitations in edentulous patients: the oral reconstruction foundation consensus report. Int J Prosthodont 34:s8–s20. https://doi.org/10.11607/ijp.consensusreport
Seelaus R, Evans PL (2022) Anaplastology and facial prosthetics. Elsevier, Amsterdam, pp 318–338

Senior BA, Kennedy DW, Tanabodee J et al (1998) Long-term results of functional endoscopic sinus surgery. Laryngoscope 108:151–157

Sgarzani R, Meccariello G, Iannella G et al (2022) Computer-aided design and manufacturing technology applied to total nasal reconstruction. Eur J Plast Surg 46:433–440. https://doi.org/10.1007/s00238-022-02014-4

Shi J, Dai W, Gupta A et al (2022) Frontiers of hydroxyapatite composites in bionic bone tissue engineering. Materials 15:8475. https://doi.org/10.3390/ma15238475

Slavin RG, Spector SL, Bernstein IL et al (2005) The diagnosis and management of sinusitis: a practice parameter update. J Allergy Clin Immunol 116:S13–S47. https://doi.org/10.1016/j.jaci.2005.09.048

Tanveer W, Ridwan-Pramana A, Molinero-Mourelle P et al (2021) Systematic review of clinical applications of CAD/CAM technology for craniofacial implants placement and manufacturing of nasal prostheses. Int J Environ Res Public Health 18:3756. https://doi.org/10.3390/ijerph18073756

Testori T, Weinstein T, Taschieri S, Wallace SS (2019) Risk factors in lateral window sinus elevation surgery. Periodontology 2000 81:91–123. https://doi.org/10.1111/prd.12286

Tian Y, Chen C, Xu X et al (2021) A review of 3D printing in dentistry: technologies, affecting factors, and applications. Scanning 2021:1–19. https://doi.org/10.1155/2021/9950131

Tollemar V, Collier ZJ, Mohammed MK et al (2016) Stem cells, growth factors and scaffolds in craniofacial regenerative medicine. Genes Dis 3:56–71. https://doi.org/10.1016/j.gendis.2015.09.004

Tribst JPM, De Oliveira Dal Piva AM, Borges ALS et al (2020) Does the prosthesis weight matter? 3D finite element analysis of a fixed implant-supported prosthesis at different weights and implant numbers. J Adv Prosthodont 12:67. https://doi.org/10.4047/jap.2020.12.2.67

Turner S, Belsi A, McGregor AH (2021) Issues faced by people with amputation(s) during lower limb prosthetic rehabilitation: a thematic analysis. Prosthetics Orthot Int 46:61–67. https://doi.org/10.1097/pxr.0000000000000070

Valentini P (2023) How to prevent and manage postoperative complications in maxillary sinus augmentation using the lateral approach: a review. Int J Oral Maxillofac Implants 38:1005–1013. https://doi.org/10.11607/jomi.10145

Vaswani BK, Mundada BP, Bhola N et al (2023) Stem-cell therapy: filling gaps in oro-maxillofacial region. Curēus. 15:e47171. https://doi.org/10.7759/cureus.47171

Vazouras K, Taylor T (2021) Full-arch removable vs fixed implant restorations: a literature review of factors to consider regarding treatment choice and decision-making in elderly patients. Int J Prosthodont 34:s93–s101. https://doi.org/10.11607/ijp.7016

Velasco-Ortega E, Sierra-Baztan A, Jiménez-Guerra A et al (2021) Long-term clinical study of implants placed in maxillary sinus floor augmentation using beta-tricalcium phosphate. Int J Environ Res Public Health 18:9975. https://doi.org/10.3390/ijerph18199975

Wallace SS, Tarnow DP, Froum SJ et al (2012) Maxillary sinus elevation by lateral window approach: evolution of technology and technique. J Evid Based Dent Pract 12:161–171. https://doi.org/10.1016/s1532-3382(12)70030-1

Wang J (2023) Novel 3D bioprinting of biomaterials: application of statistical modeling & machine learning. https://repositories.lib.utexas.edu/items/3b758e59-9257-427e-864b-6cbe59a26d18

Wassef SN, Batra PS, Barnett S (2012) Skull base inverted papilloma: a comprehensive review. ISRN Surg 2012:1–34. https://doi.org/10.5402/2012/175903

Wazir HU (2023) Development of precision 3D-printed medical implants. https://opus.lib.uts.edu.au/handle/10453/172746

Whyne C, Fialkov J, Engineering B (2020) Improving workflow and accuracy in craniofacial reconstruction with computer-assisted surgical planning. In: TSpace Repository. https://tspace.library.utoronto.ca/handle/1807/103460

Whyte A, Boeddinghaus R (2019) The maxillary sinus: physiology, development and imaging anatomy. Dentomaxillofac Radiol 48:20190205. https://doi.org/10.1259/dmfr.20190205

Yoshida S, Miyagawa S, Toyofuku T et al (2020) Syngeneic mesenchymal stem cells reduce immune rejection after induced pluripotent stem cell-derived allogeneic cardiomyocyte transplantation. Sci Rep 10. https://doi.org/10.1038/s41598-020-58126-z

Younes R, Nader N, Khoury G (2017) Sinus grafting techniques. Springer, Cham

Zhang B, Tian X, Hao J et al (2020) Mesenchymal stem cell-derived extracellular vesicles in tissue regeneration. Cell Transplant 29:096368972090850. https://doi.org/10.1177/0963689720908500

Zhao Z, Liu J, Weir MD et al (2022) Periodontal ligament stem cell-based bioactive constructs for bone tissue engineering. Front Bioeng Biotechnol 10. https://doi.org/10.3389/fbioe.2022.1071472

Cleft Palate

16

Goran Latif Omer, Hawre Abdulsattar Hasan,
Dastan Tahir Abdallah, Zhwan Sabah Hassan,
Vyan Hiwa Mohammed Rouf, Sazgar Shahab Ali,
Aran Aso Ahmed, Brian Sommerlad, Stefano Di Girolamo,
Sahand Soran Ali, and Aland Salih Abdullah

Introduction

A cleft palate is a defect in the development of the hard palate. This defect is responsible for communication between the oral cavity with the nasal cavities (Phalke and Goldman 2023). With a prevalence of 0.5–1.6 in 1000 newborns, cleft lip and/or palate is regarded as the most common congenital anomaly of the head and neck worldwide (Panamonta et al. 2015). Clefts have a wide spectrum of severity ranging from small incomplete cleft of the lip to complete bilateral cleft of the lip and palate. Cleft conditions affect the functional and aesthetic aspects of the life of a person. Functionally, clefs face feeding and speech difficulties, while aesthetically, their atypical appearance has a profound psychological impact because of a lack of community acceptance and social stigma to poor achievements in life (Hunt et al. 2005). Clefts disproportionately affect low-resource countries where many barriers prevent individuals from reaching appropriate management (Munabi and Alonso 2021).

G. L. Omer (✉) · S. S. Ali · A. S. Abdullah
Department of Clinical Sciences, College of Medicine, University of Sulaimani, Sulaymaniyah, KRI, Iraq

H. A. Hasan · D. T. Abdallah · Z. S. Hassan · V. H. M. Rouf · S. S. Ali · A. A. Ahmed
Royal Hospital, Sulaymaniyah, KRI, Iraq

B. Sommerlad
Great Ormond Street Hospital, London, UK

S. Di Girolamo
Department of Otorhinolaryngology, University of Rome Tor Vergata, Rome, Italy

© The Author(s), under exclusive license to Springer Nature Switzerland AG 2025
G. L. Omer, S. Di Girolamo (eds.), *Maxillary Sinus: A Comprehensive Guide*,
https://doi.org/10.1007/978-3-031-83468-4_16

Embryology

The face develops from a fusion of five prominences surrounding the primitive mouth or stomodeum: one frontonasal, two maxillary, and two mandibular prominences (Kirschner and LaRossa 2000). The normal palate develops by the fusion of medial nasal/palatine prominence and nasal septum (derived from frontonasal prominence) and lateral palatine shelves (derived from maxillary prominences). The primary palate includes medial palatine prominence and nasal septum, while the secondary palate includes lateral palatine shelves. The incisive foramen is the landmark between these two embryonic units (Eberlin et al. 2014). The primary palate fuses in the fifth to sixth week of gestation from behind forwards, whereas the secondary palate fuses from incisive foramen backwards in the seventh to eighth week of gestation. Arrest of these processes at any point is responsible for different types of clefts of the lip and palate (Guyuron 2009).

Epidemiology

Cleft lip and palate are the most common congenital anomalies of the face and comprise about 13% of all reported congenital malformations (Batra et al. 2003). The commonest diagnosis is cleft lip and palate (46%), followed by isolated cleft palate (33%) and isolated cleft lip (21%). Approximately, 35% of clefts are associated with other congenital anomalies, more commonly cleft palate. Unilateral clefts are nine times as common as bilateral clefts. A cleft lip is more common in males, while an isolated cleft palate has female predominance (Swanson 2021). The highest reported prevalence is among Asian and Amerindian populations 1/500, intermediate prevalence is in European-derived populations 1/1000, and African-derived populations have the lowest prevalence 1/2500 (Dixon et al. 2011). 30% of clefts have associated syndrome, suggesting a genetic cause of the cleft (Figueiredo et al. 2015).

Aetiology

Failure of fusion of palatal shelves may be due to:

- Dysplasia: tongue or rarely hamartomas or other space-occupying lesions may prevent the joining of palatal shelves.
- Hypoplasia: because of their small size, they fail to join at a critical time.
- Breakdown: related to tenuous union in some situations.

The aetiology of cleft palate is multifactorial, which includes:

- Genetic: cleft lip and palate is 40 times more common in first-degree relatives (offspring or sibling).
- Teratogens: maternal smoking, alcohol intake, and some antiepileptic drugs increase the incidence of clefts.

- Syndromes: Pierre Robin Sequence (PRS), velocardiofacial syndrome (22q11.2 deletion syndrome), Van Der Woude syndrome, Apert and Crouzon syndromes.

Pierre-Robin Sequence

Babies with this sequence have cleft palate (usually U-shaped) associated with the triad of micrognathia, a retrodisplaced tongue, and airway problems during the neonatal period. This sequence also includes Sticklers syndrome, which is an autosomal dominant condition where there is associated myopia, joint disorders, craniofacial microsomia, and Treacher-Collins syndrome.

Velocardiofacial Syndrome

This syndrome may be associated with overt cleft palate, classical SMCP or varying degrees of less classical SCMP, or in some cases, merely velopharyngeal incompetence with no obvious abnormality of the palate. The microdeletion associated with this syndrome (22q11.2 deletion syndrome) is identified by the fluorescent in situ hybridisation test.

Van Der Woude Syndrome

This syndrome (autosomal dominant) is usually diagnosed with associated lower lip pits. There may occasionally be either cleft lip with or without cleft palate or isolated CP.

Apert and Crouzon syndromes: These syndromes are associated with an unusually high-arched palate (Guyuron 2009).

Anatomy

Vascular Supply of Palate

The main blood supply of the palate is the greater palatine artery, which is a branch of the maxillary artery. It emerges from the greater palatine foramen adjacent to the second maxillary molar tooth. It is accompanied by nerves and venous channels, which drain into the pterygoid plexus (Drake et al. 2023).

Muscles of Soft Palate (Velum)

The musculature of cleft palate is disordered. The levator veli palati muscle in the normal palate is located in the middle 40% of the soft palate, while in the cleft palate, it inserts to the cleft margin in the anterior half of the velum (not to the back of the hard palate as commonly stated).

The palatoglossus and palatopharyngeus muscles are attached somewhat anteriorly, and fibres occupy anterior two-thirds to three-quarters of the soft palate in comparison with normal anatomy in which fibres rarely reach the back of the hard palate. The presence of musculus uvulae muscle in the cleft is controversial and rarely seen. The tensor veli palati muscle is not actually a palatal muscle where in the cleft, its tendon partially attaches to the pterygoid hamulus and back of the hard palate; compared to the normal palate, the tensor tendon hooks around the hamulus and then fans out to form palatal aponeurosis in the anterior third of the velum (Boorman and Sommerlad 1985).

Classification

The cleft palate is classified surgically as unilateral, bilateral, or submucous. Submucous cleft results from epithelial fusion of the soft palate without the programmed mesenchymal fusion explained in the embryology section. The width of the cleft is noted as it informs the difficulty of closure.

Although the most commonly used classification during the initial assessment of patients is the descriptive classification of cleft deformities, other systems of classification are often used for record-keeping and outcome research. Kernahan and Stark's "stripped Y" diagrammatic classification system and its modifications are used in many cleft centres.

Kriens introduced a palindromic acronym for the organisation of cleft deformities. The acronym LAHSHAL indicates the bilateral anatomy of lip (L), alveolus (A), hard (H), and soft (S) palates, from right to left by convention. Lowercase letters denote incomplete clefts of the structure; a period indicates no cleft (Thorne et al. 2013).

Veau Classification (1931)

This is widely used in many cleft units. The proposed groups are as follows:

- Group I: Cleft of the soft palate only.
- Group II: Cleft of the hard and soft palates up to the incisive foramen.
- Group III: Complete unilateral cleft of the soft, hard palate, lip, and alveolar ridge.
- Group IV: Complete bilateral cleft of the soft, hard palate, lip, and alveolar ridge (McGregor 1959).

Antenatal Detection and Management

Prognosis depends on the type of cleft, which makes antenatal detection of the cleft and its type critical. Parent counselling about foetal prognosis, treatment plan, and the risk of recurrence is mandatory. Multidisciplinary team management is needed from the prenatal period till adulthood (Bach-Ségura 2012; Jones 2002).

Ultrasonography

Its diagnostic accuracy in the antenatal period is highly operator and technique-dependent. Type of the cleft, amniotic fluid volume, fetal position, and maternal body habitus affect the antenatal diagnosis. In 20 weeks of gestation detection rate of two-dimensional ultrasound ranges from 16% to 93% (Maarse et al. 2010; Shaikh et al. 2001). The detection rate of cleft lip and palate is about 93%, isolated cleft lip 67%, isolated cleft palate 22%, and 65% for facial clefts (Cash et al. 2001).

Three-dimensional ultrasonic examination enhances accuracy and is used as an adjunct to two-dimensional ultrasound for confirmation of the defect (Ghi et al. 2009).

Magnetic Resonance Imaging

MRI helps in the more precise detection of the cleft together with the diagnosis and evaluation of the associated anomalies (Bekiesińska-Figatowska 2014; Mailáth-Pokorny et al. 2010).

Treatment

Multidisciplinary Cleft Care

Cleft patients need care from multiple specialities to optimise the outcome. The national standard is in a centre with a multidisciplinary cleft team dedicated to treating clefts from birth to adulthood. Typical members of the cleft team include a plastic surgeon, paediatrician, geneticist, audiologist, otolaryngologist, dentist, orthodontist, nutritionist/dietitian, psychologist, nurse, speech pathologist, and social worker. The success of primary surgeries will increase with good team care, especially in the first few months of life, by preparing the infant and family medically, physically, and psychologically (Thorne et al. 2013).

Psychological Support

Parents of a child with cleft are often devastated and depressed. Ensuring psychological support and creating a supportive parent–child relationship is vital for the child's development (Grollemund et al. 2010; Hunfeld et al. 1999).

Genetic Counselling

Seventeen percent of children with cleft lip and palate have a positive family history (Kot 2007). If one parent is affected with cleft lip and palate, the risk of a child being affected is 3.2% and 6.8% if the parent is affected with cleft palate. If a sibling is affected with cleft lip and palate, the risk of the next child being affected is 4.4% and 2.5% in case of cleft palate. If one parent and one sibling are affected, the risk becomes as high as 15%, and 9% if two children are affected (Bixler et al. 1971; Curtis 1961; Ross 1972).

Feeding and Nutrition

Infants with cleft palate have difficulty feeding due to reduced ability to suck. Breastfeeding can only be achieved with effort and modification of technique. In developed countries, cleft palate infants are mainly bottle-fed, though many mothers use expressed milk. Modified teat and a soft bottle needed to deliver a stream of milk.

Airway

Infants born with PRS have retrodisplaced tongue, which may obstruct both the nasal and the oral airway and produce significant airway problems (Guyuron 2009). The majority can be treated with positioning and anti-reflux medication. More severe cases may need nasopharyngeal airway protection, gavage feeding and apnoea monitoring. A few of them may need surgical intervention like tongue-lip adhesion, mandibular distraction or tracheostomy. Often, their palatoplasty is delayed several months compared with other cleft palate closures (Thorne et al. 2013).

Hearing

Hearing assessment is crucial. If the infant suffers from persistent hearing loss or glued ear, ventilation tubes (grommets) may need to be inserted at the time of palate repair. There is some evidence of Eustachian function improvement after repair of palate musculature which in turn enhances hearing (Guyuron 2009).

Presurgical Orthopaedics

Its role is controversial. Those of the palate may be active or passive. Two prospective randomised controlled trials have failed to show benefits for feeding and speech (Masarei et al. 2007; Niranjane et al. 2014).

Timing of Repair

There is considerable support in the literature that palate repair (specially velum) should be done before the age of 12 months (Dorf and Curtin 1982); there is evidence from a randomised controlled trial that speech is better if the palate is repaired at 6 months rather than 12 months as the children with cleft repaired at 6 months did not develop compensatory articulation, whereas in those repaired at 12 months, there was an incidence of compensatory articulation (Ysunza et al. 1998). The best environment will provide for early acquisition of consonant and speech development if repair is performed before babbling commences and also feeding improves (Friede and Enemark 2001).

Techniques for Closure of the Palate

Techniques for closure of the palate include:

- Von Langenbeck Repair.
- Veau-Wardill-Kilner push back.
- Two-flap (Bardach).
- Furlow's double-opposing Z-plasty.
- No palatal incisions (Sommerlad).

Von Langenbeck Repair

Many surgeons use lateral releasing incisions to reduce tension in the repair. The incision begins behind the alveolus, passes forward around the posterior border of the alveolus and backwards (if required) into the soft palate. The incision is carried down to the bone of the hard palate, lateral to the neurovascular bundle at the junction of the gingival and oral mucoperiosteal mucosa. Then flaps mobilise medially and sutured together (von Langenbeck 1862; Langenbeck 1861).

Veau and Wardill-Kilner Pushback Technique

These techniques believed that V to Y pushback of the oral mucoperiosteum would result in palatal lengthening and, therefore, improve speech:

- Has not been shown to produce effective lengthening.
- Result in maxillary arch collapse.
- Impairment of anteroposterior maxillary growth.

- Difficult fistulae at the junction of the flaps.
- Commonly used in low-resource countries, which resulted in disadvantaged patients (JAMA 1932; Kilner 1958; Losee and Kirschner 2015; Wardill 1937).

Two-Flap Repair

It involves the raising of two long posteriorly-based flaps on a greater palatine neurovascular bundle extending to the alveolar margin with the belief that raising the flaps facilitates exposure of soft palate musculature (Salyer et al. 1991).

Furlow's Double-Opposing Z-Plasty

It is popular in many centres worldwide. It may be combined with lateral releasing incisions. Its goal is to lengthen the soft palate through Z-plasty and retrodisplacement of the musculature.

- Possible advantages are:
  - Easy to perform.
  - Lengthening.
  - Better vascularisation of muscles.
- Disadvantages are:
  - Lateral tightening.
  - Less effective lengthening.
  - Reconstruction of muscles is less anatomic.
  - Not suitable for wide clefts.
  - Repair is not symmetric (Furlow 1986).

Sommerlad's Repair

This technique has now used in our centre (Sommerlad's centre for cleft lip and palate in Slemani Burn, Plastic and Reconstructive Surgery Hospital) since 2012 when Sir Dr. B.C. Sommerlad visited our hospital for the first time, and from that time, annual workshops were held in our center supervised by him.

The operative steps are as follows:

- Insertion of a modified mouth gag, which allows good exposure, especially with an operating microscope and avoids compression of the endotracheal tube.
- Insertion of throat pack (gauze).
- Local anaesthetic infiltration (with epinephrine).
- An incision along the margin of the cleft at the junction of the oral and nasal mucosa and elevation of the oral flaps in a subperiosteal plane.
- Elevation of the oral mucoperiosteal flaps extends to the posterior edge of the hard palate. Dimples are frequently seen on the oral side of the palate, which represents the side of attachment of oral mucous glands, care must be taken to elevate them intact.
- In wide clefts, a dental scaler is passed behind the greater palatine neurovascular bundle to free it.

- To achieve mobilisation of the oral layer, if necessary, the oral component of the tensor is incised, which lies behind the greater palatine vessels.
- The dissection continued into the soft palate in a plane between oral mucosa and underlying musculature (palatoglossus and palatopharyngeus muscles) which was performed by a combination of knife and blunt dissection.
- If necessary, the nasal mucosa is mobilised from the nasal surface of the palatal shelves in the subperiosteal plane.
- Insertion of the stay suture in the oral mucosa.
- The nasal mucosa/muscle layer is sutured using absorbable sutures (5-0 Monocryl) inserted close to the edge of the nasal mucosa.
- An incision is made on each side of the midline, starting 3–5 mm from the midline posteriorly and then passing closer to the midline anteriorly. This knife dissection was carried out down to the nasal mucosa, which was identified because of its almost blue colour. A plane developed between the nasal mucosa and the palatal muscles, then the nasal surface of the levator veli palati muscle is recognised,
- The Palatopharyngeus medially and the nasal component of the tensor palati tendon are divided from the back of the hard palate, and the beginning of the retrodisplacement of the musculature is performed.
- The tensor tendon is divided from the just medial to the hamulus.
- The combined levator palate and palatopharyngeus muscle are further retrodisplaced with a combination of sharp and blunt dissection.
- To avoid hematoma, a stab incision is made in the nasal mucosa.
- Using non-absorbable 4-0 or 5-0 nylon sutures, the muscle united usually in the posterior half of the velum.
- Closure of the oral layer begins with inserting the first suture in front of the retrodisplaced muscle sling picking up the nasal mucous glands using a twisted loop mattress suture. The aim of this suture is to unite oral and nasal layers, keeping the muscle sling in a posterior position to close the dead space and further reduce the chances of hematoma. 4-0 Monocryl suture on a modified 5/8 curved needle is used.
- In very wide clefts (usually >10 mm in width at the back of the hard palate), lateral releasing incisions are sometimes necessary (10% of cases) (Sommerlad 2003).
- After removal of the throat pack and aspiration of the pharynx suction test is performed by putting a sucker in one nostril, occluding the nose around it and testing the passive length and mobility of the velum, it has a grading system as follows: no closure, closure only after gentle, spontaneous closure, closure that remains after removing the sucker from the nose. This predicts the outcome in both primary repair and palate re-repairs (Sommerlad et al. 2002).
- Submucous cleft palate repair using a similar technique with some differences:
  - Oral flaps elevated subperiosteally but do not have to reach as far forwards.
  - Greater palatine vessel mobilisation and division of the oral component of the tensor palate tendon is not needed.
  - The nasal layer is kept intact.
  - The thin nasal layer in the midline should be protected during dissection lateral to the midline (Sommerlad et al. 2004).

Postoperative Care

Analgesia

Adequate analgesia should be given.

Feeding

As soon as the infant is awake, feeding is started using the same method that was used before the operation.

Antibiotics

Peri- and postoperative prophylaxis against the B-hemolytic streptococcus (Guyuron 2009).

Arm Restraints

Following a randomised controlled trial its use is abandoned (Jigjinni et al. 1993).

Complications

Early Complication

- Airway obstruction.
- Bleeding.

Later Complications

- Dehiscence.
- Fistula formation (Guyuron 2009).

References

(1932) Division palatine, anatomie, chirurgie, phonétique. JAMA 99:1017. https://doi.org/10.1001/jama.1932.02740640059036

Bach-Ségura P (2012) Facial clefts diagnosed before birth: routine ultrasound screening at the multi-disciplinary center for prenatal diagnosis (PCPD). J Dentofac Anom Orthodont 15:402. https://doi.org/10.1051/odfen/2012302

Batra P, Duggal R, Parkash H (2003) Genetics of cleft lip and palate revisited. J Clin Pediatr Dent 27:311–320. https://doi.org/10.17796/jcpd.27.4.k7j3628944237392

Bekiesińska-Figatowska M (2014) The role of magnetic resonance imaging in the prenatal diagnosis of cleft lip and palate. Dev Period Med 18:27–32

Bixler D, Fogh-Andersen P, Conneally PM (1971) Incidence of cleft lip and palate in the offspring of cleft parents. Clin Genet 2:155–159. https://doi.org/10.1111/j.1399-0004.1971.tb00271.x

Boorman JG, Sommerlad BC (1985) Levator palati and palatal dimples: their anatomy, relationship and clinical significance. Br J Plast Surg 38(3):326–332. https://doi.org/10.1016/0007-1226(85)90236-X

Cash C, Set P, Coleman N (2001) The accuracy of antenatal ultrasound in the detection of facial clefts in a low-risk screening population. Ultrasound Obstet Gynecol 18:432–436. https://doi.org/10.1046/j.0960-7692.2001.00508.x

Curtis EJ (1961) Congenital cleft lip and palate. Am J Dis Child 102:853. https://doi.org/10.1001/archpedi.1961.02080010855007

Dixon MJ, Marazita ML, Beaty TH, Murray JC (2011) Cleft lip and palate: understanding genetic and environmental influences. Nat Rev Genet 12:167–178. https://doi.org/10.1038/nrg2933

Dorf DS, Curtin JW (1982) Early cleft palate repair and speech outcome. Plast Reconstr Surg 70:74–79. https://doi.org/10.1097/00006534-198207000-00015

Drake RL, Vogl AW, Mitchell AWM (2023) Gray's anatomy for students. 5th ed. Philadelphia: Elsevier. ISBN: 978-0-323-93423-7

Eberlin KR, Vyas RM, Patel KB, Hamdan US (2014) Anatomy and embryology of cleft lip and palate. In: Rogers DJ, Hartnick CJ, Hamdan US (eds) Video atlas of cleft lip and palate surgery. Plural Publishing Inc., San Diego, pp 3–7

Figueiredo JC, Ly S, Magee KS et al (2015) Parental risk factors for oral clefts among Central Africans, Southeast Asians, and Central Americans. Birth Defects Res 103:863–879. https://doi.org/10.1002/bdra.23417

Friede H, Enemark H (2001) Long-term evidence for favorable midfacial growth after delayed hard palate repair in UCLP patients. Cleft Palate Craniofac J 38:323–329. https://doi.org/10.1597/1545-1569_2001_038_0323_lteffm_2.0.co_2

Furlow LT (1986) Cleft palate repair by double opposing Z-plasty. Plast Reconstr Surg 78:724–736. https://doi.org/10.1097/00006534-198678060-00002

Ghi T, Arcangeli T, Radico D et al (2009) Three-dimensional sonographic imaging of fetal bilateral cleft lip and palate in the first trimester. Ultrasound Obstet Gynecol 34:119–120. https://doi.org/10.1002/uog.6430

Grollemund B, Galliani E, Soupre V et al (2010) L'impact des fentes labiopalatines sur les relations parents-enfant. Arch Pediatr 17:1380–1385. https://doi.org/10.1016/j.arcped.2010.06.026

Guyuron B (2009) Plastic surgery. Saunders, Philadelphia, PA

Hunfeld JA, Tempels A, Passchier J et al (1999) Brief report: parental burden and grief one year after the birth of a child with a congenital anomaly. J Pediatr Psychol 24:515–520. https://doi.org/10.1093/jpepsy/24.6.515

Hunt O, Burden D, Hepper P, Johnston C (2005) The psychosocial effects of cleft lip and palate: a systematic review. Eur J Orthod 27:274–285. https://doi.org/10.1093/ejo/cji004

Jigjinni V, Kangesu T, Sommerlad BC (1993) Do babies require arm splints after cleft palate repair? Br J Plast Surg 46:681–685. https://doi.org/10.1016/0007-1226(93)90200-u

Jones MC (2002) Prenatal diagnosis of cleft lip and palate: detection rates, accuracy of ultrasonography, associated anomalies, and strategies for counseling. Cleft Palate Craniofac J 39:169–173. https://doi.org/10.1597/1545-1569_2002_039_0169_pdocla_2.0.co_2

Kilner TP (1958) The management of the patient with cleft lip and/or palate. Am J Surg 95:204–210. https://doi.org/10.1016/0002-9610(58)90503-8

Kirschner RE, LaRossa D (2000) Cleft lip and palate. Otolaryngol Clin N Am 33:1191–1215. https://doi.org/10.1016/s0030-6665(05)70277-2

Kot M (2007) Analysis of family incidence of cleft lip and/or palate. Med Sci Monit 13:CR231–CR234

Langenbeck B (1861) Weitere Erfahrungen im Gebiete der Uranoplastic mittels Ablusung des mucosperriostealen Gumenuberzuges. Arch Klin Chir 5:170. AbeBooks

Losee JE, Kirschner RE (2015) Comprehensive cleft care, vol 2, 2nd edn. Thieme, Stuttgart

Maarse W, Bergé SJ, Pistorius L et al (2010) Diagnostic accuracy of transabdominal ultrasound in detecting prenatal cleft lip and palate: a systematic review. Ultrasound Obstet Gynecol 35:495–502. https://doi.org/10.1002/uog.7472

Mailáth-Pokorny M, Worda C, Krampl-Bettelheim E et al (2010) What does magnetic resonance imaging add to the prenatal ultrasound diagnosis of facial clefts? Ultrasound Obstet Gynecol 36:445–451. https://doi.org/10.1002/uog.7743

Masarei AG, Wade A, Mars M et al (2007) A randomized control trial investigating the effect of presurgical orthopedics on feeding in infants with cleft lip and/or palate. Cleft Palate Craniofac J 44:182–193. https://doi.org/10.1597/05-184.1

McGregor IA (1959) The treatment of cleft lip and palate. Scott Med J 4:276–299. https://doi.org/10.1177/003693305900400602

Munabi NCO, Alonso N (2021) Burden of cleft disease and opportunity for impact. Springer, Cham, pp 9–16

Niranjane PP, Kamble RH, Diagavane SP et al (2014) Current status of presurgical infant orthopaedic treatment for cleft lip and palate patients: a critical review. Indian J Plast Surg 47:293–302. https://doi.org/10.4103/0970-0358.146573

Panamonta V, Pradubwong S, Panamonta M, Chowchuen B (2015) Global birth prevalence of orofacial clefts: a systematic review. J Med Assoc Thai 98(Suppl 7):S11–S21

Phalke N, Goldman JJ (2023) Cleft palate. In: StatPearls—NCBI Bookshelf. https://www.ncbi.nlm.nih.gov/books/NBK563128/#:~:text=Cleft%20palate%20is%20a%20developmental

Ross RB (1972) Cleft lip and palate [by] R. B. Ross [and] M. C. Johnston. With contributions by W. K. Lindsay [and]... Catalogue | National Library of Australia. https://catalogue.nla.gov.au/catalog/1014964

Salyer KE, Bardach J, Salyer K (1991) Surgical techniques in cleft lip and palate. Mosby Year Book, Saint Louis

Shaikh D, Mercer NS, Sohan K et al (2001) Prenatal diagnosis of cleft lip and palate. Br J Plast Surg 54:288–289. https://doi.org/10.1054/bjps.2001.3575

Sommerlad BC (2003) A technique for cleft palate repair. Plast Reconstr Surg 112:1542–1548. https://doi.org/10.1097/01.prs.0000085599.84458.d2

Sommerlad BC, Mehendale FV, Birch MJ et al (2002) Palate re-repair revisited. Cleft Palate Craniofac J 39:295–307. https://doi.org/10.1597/1545-1569_2002_039_0295_prrr_2.0.co_2

Sommerlad BC, Fenn C, Harland K et al (2004) Submucous cleft palate: a grading system and review of 40 consecutive submucous cleft palate repairs. Cleft Palate Craniofac J 41:114–123. https://doi.org/10.1597/02-102

Swanson JW (2021) Global cleft care in low-resource settings. Springer, Cham

Thorne CH, Chung KC, Gosain AK et al (2013) Grabb and Smith's plastic surgery. 7th ed. In: Northwestern Scholars. https://www.scholars.northwestern.edu/en/publications/grabb-and-smiths-plastic-surgery-seventh-edition

von Langenbeck B (1862) Die Uranoplastik mittels Ablösung des mucoperiostalen Gaumenüberzuges. Arch Klin Chir 2:205.

Wardill WEM (1937) The technique of operation for cleft palate. Br J Surg 25:117–130. https://doi.org/10.1002/bjs.1800259715

Ysunza A, Pamplona C, Mendoza M et al (1998) Speech outcome and maxillary growth in patients with unilateral complete cleft lip/palate operated on at 6 versus 12 months of age. Plast Reconstr Surg 102:675–679. https://doi.org/10.1097/00006534-199809030-00009

MIX
Papier aus verantwortungsvollen Quellen
Paper from responsible sources
FSC® C105338

If you have any concerns about our products,
you can contact us on
ProductSafety@springernature.com

In case Publisher is established outside the EU,
the EU authorized representative is:
Springer Nature Customer Service Center GmbH
Europaplatz 3, 69115 Heidelberg, Germany

Printed by Libri Plureos GmbH
in Hamburg, Germany